Shoulder

Spine

ORTHOPAEDIC SURGICAL APPROACHES

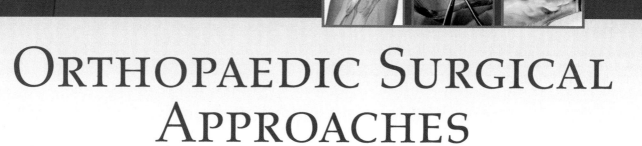

ORTHOPAEDIC SURGICAL APPROACHES

MARK D. MILLER, MD
Professor
Department of Orthopaedic Surgery
Head, Division of Sports Medicine
University of Virginia School
of Medicine
Charlottesville, Virginia

A. BOBBY CHHABRA, MD
Associate Professor
Division Head, Hand,
and Upper Extremity Surgery
Co-Director,
University of Virginia Hand Center
University of Virginia School
of Medicine
Charlottesville, Virginia

SHEPARD HURWITZ, MD
Executive Director
American Board
of Orthopaedic Surgery
Professor of Orthopaedic Surgery
University of North Carolina
Chapel Hill, North Carolina

WILLIAM M. MIHALKO, MD, PHD
Associate Professor
Department of Orthopaedic Surgery
University of Virginia School of Medicine
Department of Mechanical and Aerospace
Engineering
Charlottesville, Virginia

FRANCIS H. SHEN, MD
Assistant Professor
Division of Spine Surgery
Co-Director, Spine Fellowship
Department of Orthopaedic Surgery
University of Virginia School of Medicine
Charlottesville, Virginia

Associate Editor:

JENNIFER HART, MPAS, PA-C
Department of Orthopaedic Surgery
Division of Sports Medicine
University of Virginia
Charlottesville, Virginia

Illustrators:

ANITA IMPAGLIAZZO, MA, CMI
Medical Illustration & Graphics
Charlottesville, Virginia

TIFFANY S. DaVANZO, MA, CMI
BURT FALGUI, MS
TrialSight Medical Media LLC
Glen Allen, Virginia

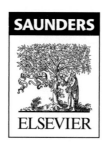

SAUNDERS

ELSEVIER

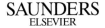

1600 John F. Kennedy Blvd.
Ste 1800
Philadelphia, PA 19103-2899

Notice

Knowledge and best practice in this field are constantly changing. As new research and experience broaden our knowledge, changes in practice, treatment, and drug therapy may become necessary or appropriate. Readers are advised to check the most current information provided (i) on procedures featured or (ii) by the manufacturer of each product to be administered, to verify the recommended dose or formula, the method and duration of administration, and contraindications. It is the responsibility of the practitioner, relying on their own experience and knowledge of the patient, to make diagnoses, to determine dosages and the best treatment for each individual patient, and to take all appropriate safety precautions. To the fullest extent of the law, neither the Publisher nor the Authors assume any liability for any injury and/or damage to persons or property arising out of or related to any use of the material contained in this book.

The Publisher

Library of Congress Cataloging-in-Publication Data (in PHL)
Orthopaedic surgical approaches / Mark D. Miller ... [et al.] ; editorial
assistant, Jennifer Hart ; illustrators, Anita Impagliazzo, Tiffany S. DaVanzo. – 1st ed.
      p. ; cm.
   ISBN 978-1-4160-3446-9
   1. Orthopedic surgery–Atlases. I. Miller, Mark D.
   [DNLM: 1. Orthopedic Procedures–Atlases. 2. Musculoskeletal Diseases–surgery–Atlases.
   3. Musculoskeletal System–surgery–Atlases. WE 17 O773 2008]
   RD733.2.O78 2008
   617.4'7–dc22

                                                            2007032522

Publishing Director: Kimberly Murphy
Developmental Editor: Lucia Gunzel
Publishing Services Manager: Linda Van Pelt
Project Manager: Francisco Morales
Design Direction: Steven Stave

Printed in Canada

Last digit is the print number: 9 8 7 6 5 4 3 2 1

We dedicate this book to all surgeons who just need a little help "getting there." We encourage you to continue to pursue "life-long learning," to know what to do once you get there!

To my Lord, who has given me the talents; I hope and pray that I have used them wisely.
To my family, whom I love and cherish more than any project I have undertaken.
And to my students—fellows, residents, medical students, undergraduates, volunteers:
Let the passion that burns in me catch fire in your ambitions and goals!

—M.M.

To my wife, for her unconditional love, support, and patience.
To my children, for their smiles, laughter, and daily hugs.
To my parents, for their guidance and understanding.
To all of the residents, fellows, and medical students I have had the privilege of working with: Thanks for challenging me every day and making me a better physician and person.

—B.C.

Endless gratitude to the three women who make it all worthwhile—Gretta, Zoe, and Leah.

—S.H.

To my mother and father, who gave me the opportunities in life to achieve all I can be.
To my wife and children, who give me my purpose in life from day to day.
To my past mentors, Ken and Leo, for their support, education, and knowledge, which have created my passion for my career.
And to all of my past residents and fellows, who have made me strive and teach them to obtain excellence for my patients on a daily basis.

—W.M.

To my loving daughter, Mia, the light of my life; and to my family, especially my parents, who are an endless source of inspiration.

—F.S.

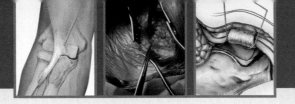

Consultants

Video Support

Derek W. Weichel, MD
University of Virginia
Charlottesville, Virginia

Pelvis, Hip, and Thigh

Thomas E. Brown, MD
University of Virginia
Charlottesville, Virginia

Quanjun Cui, MD
University of Virginia
Charlottesville, Virginia

Khaled J. Saleh, MD, MSc
University of Virginia
Charlottesville, Virginia

Shawn Brubaker, DO
University of Virginia
Charlottesville, Virginia

Abhijit Manaswi, MD
University of Virginia
Charlottesville, Virginia

William Hozack, MD
Rothman Institute
Philadelphia, Pennsylvania

Mark J. Anders, MD
State University of New York at Buffalo
Buffalo, New York

Kenneth A. Krackow, MD
State University of New York at Buffalo
Buffalo, New York

Shoulder, Arm, Knee, and Lower Leg

David R. Diduch, MD
University of Virginia
Charlottesville, Virginia

Marc R. Safran, MD
Stanford University
San Francisco, California

Elbow, Wrist, and Hand

Sara D. Rynders, MPAS, PA-C
Division of Hand and Upper Extremity Surgery
University of Virginia Health System
Charlottesville, Virginia

Spine

Ian Marks, PA-C
University of Virginia
Charlottesville, Virginia

Dino Samartzis, DSc, PhD(C), MSc, MA(C), Dip EBHC
Graduate Division, Harvard University
Cambridge, Massachusetts
Department of Epidemiology, Radiation Effects Research
   Foundation
Hiroshima, Japan

Foot and Ankle

Abhijit Manaswi, MD
University of Virginia
Charlottesville, Virginia

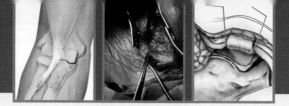

International Advisory Board

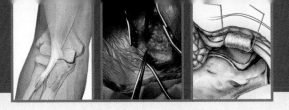

Contributors

Mark D. Miller, MD
Professor
Department of Orthopaedic Surgery
Head,
Division of Sports Medicine
University of Virginia School of Medicine
Charlottesville, Virginia

A. Bobby Chhabra, MD
Associate Professor
Division Head, Hand and Upper Extremity Surgery
Co-Director,
University of Virginia Hand Center
University of Virginia School of Medicine
Charlottesville, Virginia

Shepard Hurwitz, MD
Executive Director
American Board of Orthopaedic Surgery
Professor of Orthopaedic Surgery
University of North Carolina
Chapel Hill, North Carolina

William M. Mihalko, MD, PhD
Associate Professor
Department of Orthopaedic Surgery
University of Virginia School of Medicine
Department of Mechanical and Aerospace Engineering
Charlottesville, Virginia

Francis H. Shen, MD
Assistant Professor
Division of Spine Surgery
Co-Director, Spine Fellowship
Department of Orthopaedic Surgery
University of Virginia School of Medicine
Charlottesville, Virginia

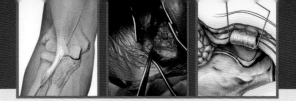

Preface

It is said that a picture is worth a thousand words. In that case, with the publication of *Orthopaedic Surgical Approaches,* we have millions of words for you! Although many textbooks and atlases on surgical exposure in orthopaedic surgery are available, we found those texts to be deficient in several areas. The main problem is that the illustrations, while typically beautiful, often do not tell the real story of what it's like to be there at surgery. For this book, therefore, we decided to marry illustrations—also beautifully done—with real-life surgical photos. These images are presented side by side throughout the text, giving simultaneous views of both the ideal and the real. We attempted to keep the scope of the book as comprehensive as possible, including all commonly used approaches while omitting approaches that were of purely historical interest. Because so much of what the orthopaedic surgeon does is aided by arthroscopic images, considerable useful material on this aspect of orthopaedic surgical practice also has been included in the relevant chapters. A DVD providing cadaveric demonstrations of all approaches is included with the text-based illustrations.

As with all such endeavors, a virtual army of support was necessary for completion of this project. From its inception, the publisher, Elsevier, made the project a priority, lending much-appreciated impetus to our efforts in both the preparation and book production phases. Our illustrators, Anita Impagliazzo, Tiffany DaVanzo, and Burt Falgui worked assiduously, with an inspired eye for detail, to produce beautiful and accurately depicted images that highlight our most important teaching points. We extend special thanks to Jennifer Hart, who has become an expert in book production, and to all of our colleagues who provided support during the preparation of this text.

"If you would thoroughly know anything, teach it to others."
—TRYON EDWARDS (1809–1894)

Mark D. Miller, MD
A. Bobby Chhabra, MD
Shepard Hurwitz, MD
William M. Mihalko, MD, PhD
Francis H. Shen, MD

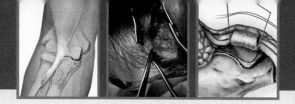

Contents

CHAPTER 6

Hip and Pelvis   331

CHAPTER 7

Knee and Lower Leg   423

CHAPTER 8

Foot and Ankle   491

Index   591

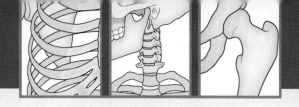

INTRODUCTION: APPROACH TO THE SURGICAL PATIENT

—

MARK D. MILLER

A. BOBBY CHHABRA

SHEPARD R. HURWITZ

FRANCIS H. SHEN

WILLIAM MIHALKO

- This book uses a bulleted text format and original color illustrations paired side-by-side with operative photographs to present orthopaedic anatomy and surgical approaches clearly

Regional Anatomy

▧ *Regional Anatomy* for each section is presented in the following order

Osteology (Bones)

▧ There are 206 bones in the human skeleton (FIGURE 1-1)

   ● 80 in the axial skeleton
   ● 126 in the appendicular skeleton

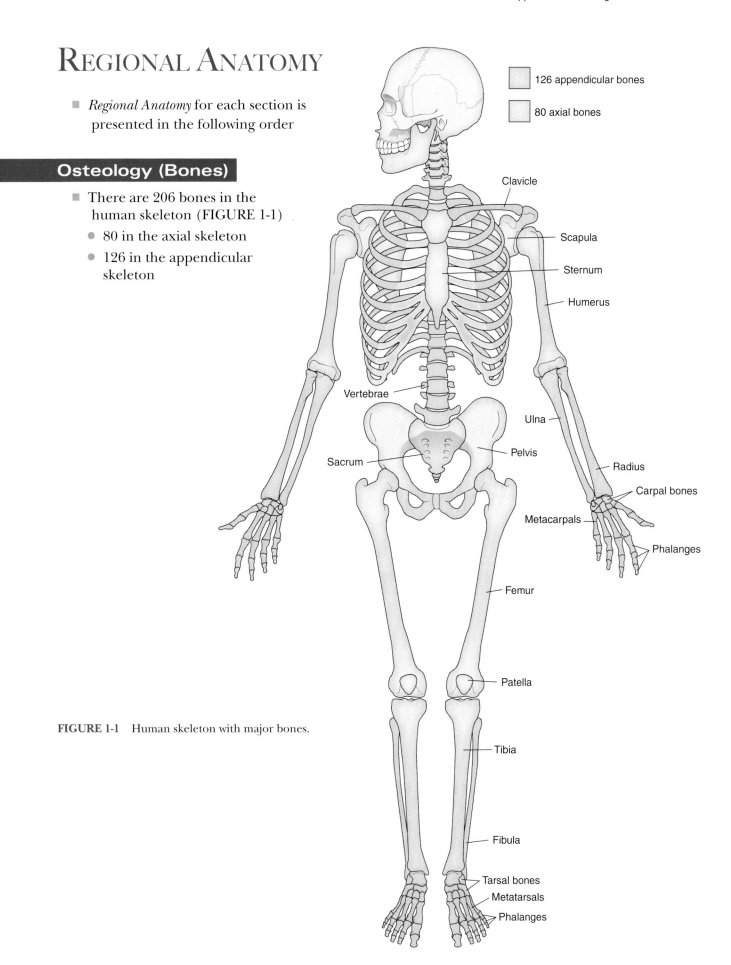

126 appendicular bones

80 axial bones

Clavicle

Scapula

Sternum

Humerus

Vertebrae

Ulna

Sacrum

Pelvis

Radius

Carpal bones

Metacarpals

Phalanges

Femur

Patella

Tibia

Fibula

Tarsal bones

Metatarsals

Phalanges

FIGURE 1-1   Human skeleton with major bones.

Arthrology (Joints)

- Diarthrodial joints with hyaline cartilage, synovial membranes, capsules, and ligaments are emphasized
  - Uniaxial joints allow motion in one plane and include ginglymus (hinge) and trochoid (pivot) types of articulations
  - Biaxial joints allow movement in two planes and include condyloid, ellipsoid, and saddle joints
  - Polyaxial joints allow movement in any direction and include spheroidal (ball-and-socket) joints
  - Gliding or plane joints allow sliding of surfaces
- Amphiarthrodial joints have limited motion, hyaline cartilage, and intervening discs

Myology (Muscles)

- Function to move the joint that they cross
- Have an origin and insertion
- Surgical approaches usually involve intervals between muscles with different innervations

Nerves

- Typically are branches from plexus
- Commonly supply groups of muscles
- May be motor or sensory or both

Vessels (with an emphasis on the arteries)

- Emphasis is on avoiding these structures

CROSS-SECTIONAL ANATOMY

- *Cross-Sectional Anatomy* emphasizes key structures and their relationships with each other at critical levels

TOPOGRAPHICAL LANDMARKS

- *Topographical Landmarks* are illustrated to assist in planning surgical incisions

HAZARDS

- *Hazards*—a detailed description of structures at risk and how to protect them—are included for each anatomical region

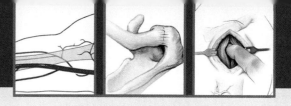

CHAPTER

2

SHOULDER AND ARM

—

MARK D. MILLER, MD

REGIONAL ANATOMY

Osteology

● Scapula (Figure SA-1)

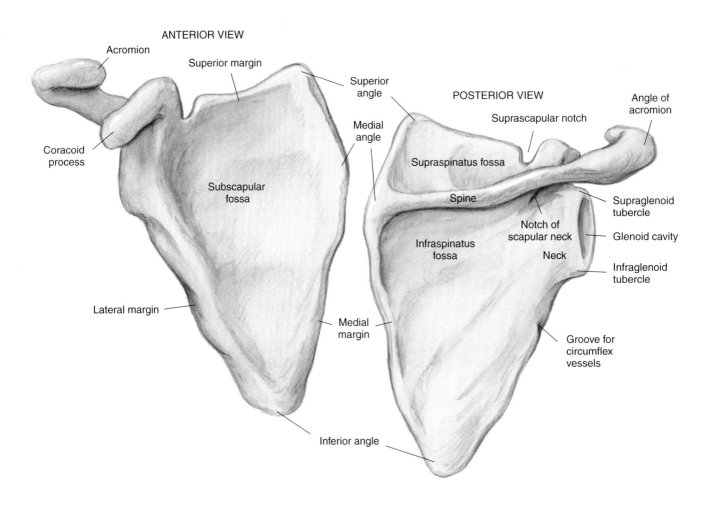

FIGURE SA-1   Scapula. Note the acromion, coracoid, spine, and supraspinatus fossa.

- Broad flat bone that serves as an attachment for 17 muscles and 4 ligaments
- Glenoid (socket) is retroverted 5 degrees
- Scapular spine is the superior aspect of the scapula
- Coracoid is the anterior projection that serves as the origin for several muscles and ligaments
- Acromion protects the superior aspect of the glenohumeral joint and is the origin of much of the deltoid and trapezius muscles; it articulates with the clavicle

● Clavicle (Figure SA-2)

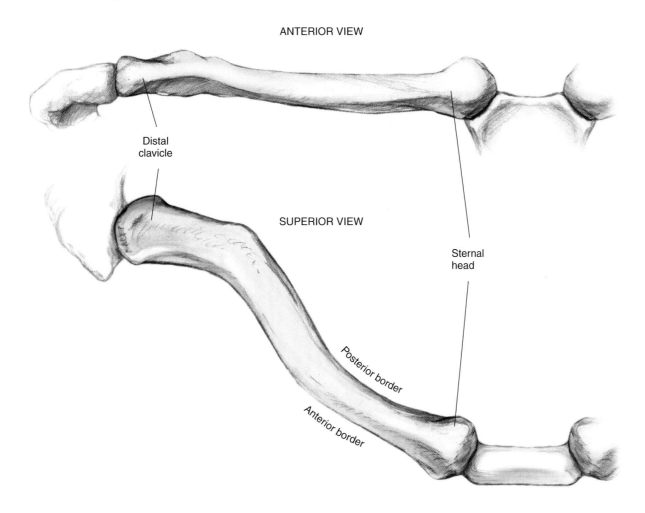

ANTERIOR VIEW

Distal
clavicle

SUPERIOR VIEW

Sternal
head

Posterior border

Anterior border

FIGURE SA-2   Clavicle. Note its curved "S" shape.

- ▓ S-shaped, rounded bone that serves as a fulcrum for lateral movement of the arm
- ▓ First bone in the body to ossify and the last to fuse

● Humerus (Figure SA-3)

- Largest diaphyseal bone in the upper extremity
- Hemispherical head is retroverted approximately 30 degrees
- Anatomical neck is directly below the head
- Surgical neck is approximately 2 cm distal to the anatomical neck
- Greater tuberosity is the attachment for most of the rotator cuff muscles
- Lesser tuberosity is the attachment for the subscapularis muscle

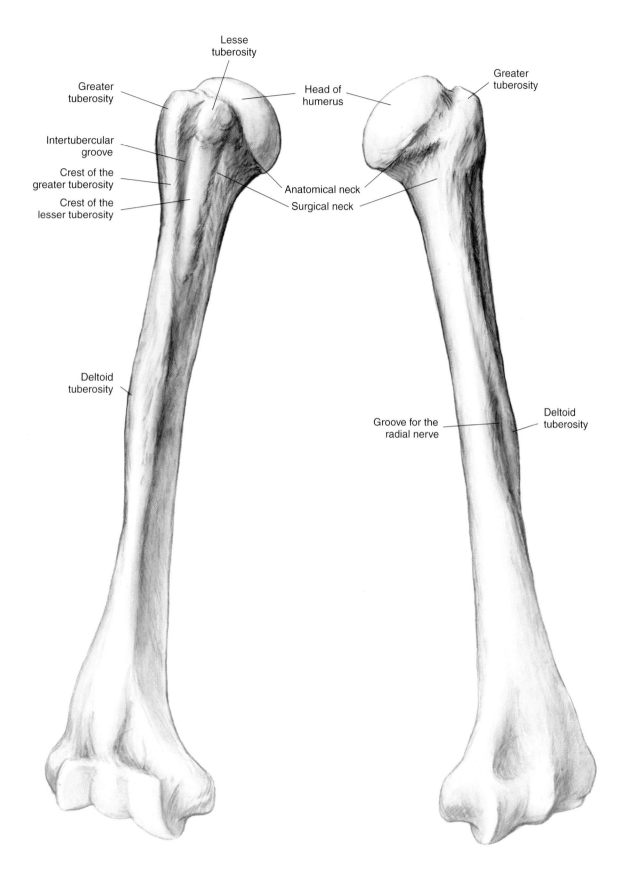

Lesse
tuberosity

Greater
tuberosity

Head of
humerus

Greater
tuberosity

Intertubercular
groove

Crest of the
greater tuberosity

Crest of the
lesser tuberosity

Anatomical neck

Surgical neck

Deltoid
tuberosity

Groove for the
radial nerve

Deltoid
tuberosity

FIGURE SA-3   Humerus. Note tuberosities and head.

Arthrology

- Glenohumeral joint (Figure SA-4)
  - Spheroidal (ball-and-socket) joint designed for motion over stability
  - Static restraints are as follows
    - Articular congruity
    - Labrum—deepens socket and provides a barrier against excessive translation
    - Negative intra-articular pressure
    - Capsule
    - Ligaments
      - Glenohumeral ligaments (superior, middle, inferior)
        - Resists anterior translation
      - Coracohumeral ligament
        - Resists inferior translation
      - Coracoclavicular ligament
        - Resists superior translation
  - Dynamic restraints
    - Rotator cuff muscles
    - Biceps tendon
    - Coupled scapulothoracic motion

- Acromioclavicular (AC) joint (Figure SA-5)
  - Plane (gliding) joint that stabilizes the clavicle to the acromion
  - Ligaments
    - Capsule
      - Resists anteroposterior translation
    - Coracoclavicular ligaments (trapezoid and conoid)
      - Resists superior translation

- Sternoclavicular joint
  - Plane (gliding) joint that stabilizes the clavicle to the sternum
  - Ligaments
    - Capsule
    - Sternoclavicular ligaments
    - Costoclavicular ligament

- Scapulothoracic joint
  - Located at ribs 2-7, allows coupled motion with glenohumeral abduction in a 2:1 ratio

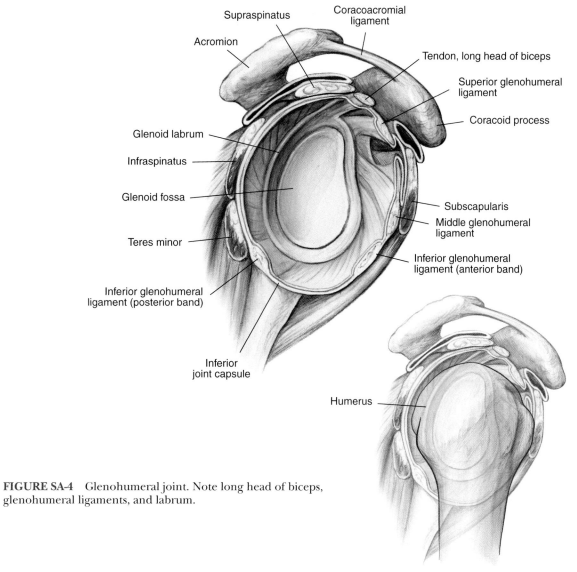

Supraspinatus
Coracoacromial ligament
Acromion
Tendon, long head of biceps
Superior glenohumeral ligament
Coracoid process
Glenoid labrum
Infraspinatus
Glenoid fossa
Subscapularis
Middle glenohumeral ligament
Teres minor
Inferior glenohumeral ligament (anterior band)
Inferior glenohumeral ligament (posterior band)
Inferior joint capsule
Humerus

FIGURE SA-4 Glenohumeral joint. Note long head of biceps, glenohumeral ligaments, and labrum.

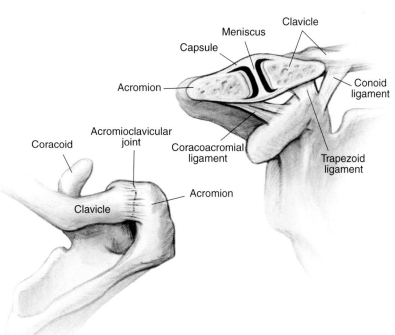

Clavicle
Meniscus
Capsule
Acromion
Conoid ligament
Coracoid
Acromioclavicular joint
Coracoacromial ligament
Trapezoid ligament
Acromion
Clavicle

FIGURE SA-5 AC joint. Note the coracoclavicular ligaments (conoid and trapezoid) and joint capsule.

Muscles

- **Shoulder muscle groups (Figure SA-6 and Table SA-1)**
  - Connect upper limb to axial skeleton
    - Trapezius, latissimus, rhomboid major and minor, levator scapulae
  - Connect upper limb to thoracic wall
    - Pectoralis major and minor, subclavius, serratus anterior
  - Act on glenohumeral joint
    - Deltoid, teres major and minor, supraspinatus, infraspinatus, subscapularis

- **Arm muscles (Figure SA-6D and Table SA-2)**
  - Three anterior muscles—coracobrachialis, biceps, brachialis
  - One posterior muscle (triceps)

TABLE SA–1   Muscles of the Shoulder

Muscle	Origin	Insertion	Action	Innervation
Trapezius	Spinous process C7-T12	Clavicle, scapula (acromion, spinous process)	Rotate scapula	Cranial nerve XI
Lateral dorsi	Spinous process T6-S5, ilium	Humerus (ITG)	Extend, adduct, IR humerus	Thoracodorsal
Rhomboideus major	Spinous process T2-T5	Scapula (medial border)	Adduct scapula	Dorsal scapular
Rhomboideus minor	Spinous process C7-T1	Scapula (medial spine)	Adduct scapula	Dorsal scapular
Levator scapulae	Transverse process C1-C4	Scapula (superior medial)	Elevate, rotate scapula	C3, C4
Pectoralis major	Sternum, ribs, clavicle	Humerus (lateral ITG)	Adduct, IR arm	Mid and lower PN
Pectoralis minor	Ribs 3-5	Scapula (coracoid)	Protract scapula	MPN
Subclavius	Rib 1	Inferior clavicle	Depress clavicle	Upper trunk
Serratus anterior	Ribs 1-9	Scapula (ventral medial)	Prevent winging	Long thoracic
Deltoid	Lateral clavicle, scapula	Humerus (deltoid tuberosity)	Abduct arm (2)	Axillary
Teres major	Inferior scapula	Humerus (medial ITG)	Adduct, IR, extend	Lower subscapular
Subscapularis	Ventral scapula	Humerus (lesser tuberosity)	IR arm, anterior stability	Upper and lower subscapular
Supraspinatus	Superior scapula	Humerus (GT)	Abduct (1), ER arm stability	Suprascapular
Infraspinatus	Dorsal scapula	Humerus (GT)	Stability, ER arm	Suprascapular
Teres minor	Scapula (dorsolateral)	Humerus (GT)	Stability, ER arm	Axillary

GT, greater tuberosity; ITG, intertubercular groove.

TABLE SA–2   Muscles of the Arm

Muscle	Origin	Insertion	Action	Innervation
Coracobrachialis	Coracoid	Mid humerus medial	Flexion, adduction	Musculocutaneous
Biceps	Coracoid (SH) Supraglenoid (LH)	Radial tuberosity	Supination, flexion	Musculocutaneous
Brachialis	Anterior humerus	Ulnar tuberosity (anterior)	Flexes forearm	Musculocutaneous, radial
Triceps	Infraglenoid (LH) Posterior humerus (LH) Posterior humerus (MH)	Olecranon	Extends forearm	Radial

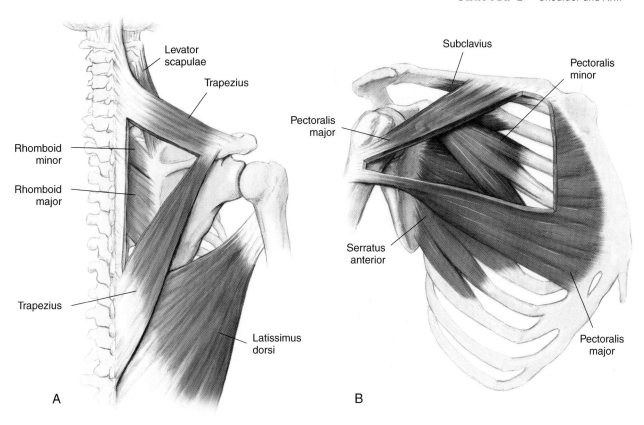

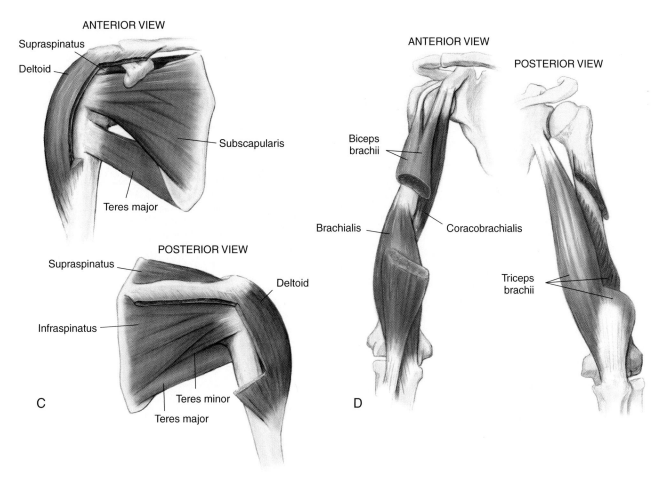

FIGURE SA-6   Muscles of the shoulder and arm.

Nerves

● Brachial plexus (Figure SA-7)

  ▓ From ventral rami of C5-T1
  ▓ Organized into five components
    ● Roots
    ● Trunks
    ● Divisions
    ● Cords
    ● Branches
  ▓ Preclavicular branches
    ● Dorsal scapular nerve
    ● Long thoracic nerve
    ● Suprascapular nerve
    ● Nerve to subclavius

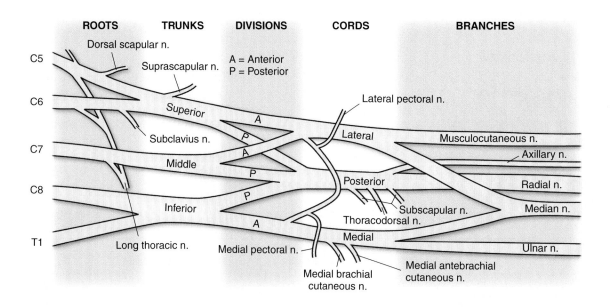

FIGURE SA-7 Brachial plexus. Note arrangement of roots, trunks, divisions, cords, and branches.

● Major arm branches (Figure SA-8)

- ▨ Musculocutaneous nerve (lateral cord)
  - ● Runs from medial to central anteriorly
  - ● Supplies biceps (short head), coracobrachialis, and part of the brachialis
- ▨ Radial nerve (posterior cord)
  - ● Spirals behind the humerus from medial to lateral
  - ● Supplies triceps (all three heads) in the arm
- ▨ Median nerve (medial and lateral cords)
  - ● Runs just medial to the brachial artery in the medial arm
  - ● No major branches in the arm
- ▨ Ulnar nerve (medial cord)
  - ● Runs just lateral to the brachial artery in the medial arm
  - ● No major branches in the arm

FIGURE SA-8   Major nerves in the arm.

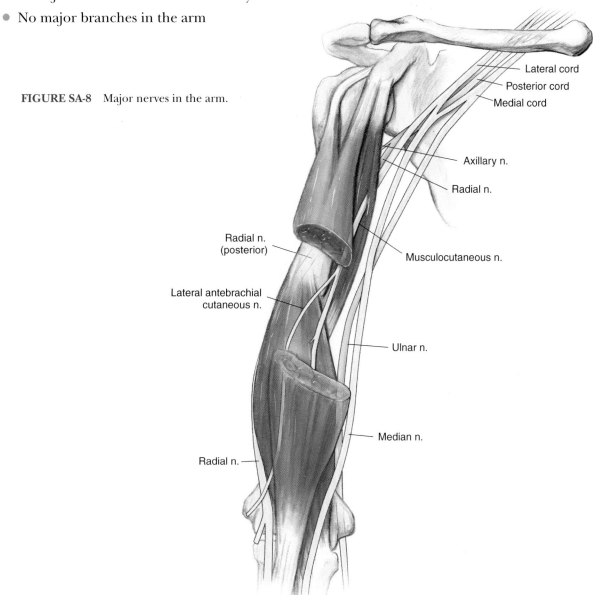

Vascularity (Figure SA-9)

- Subclavian artery
  - Becomes axillary artery at outer border of the first rib

- Axillary artery
  - Three divisions based on relationship to pectoralis minor [(1) proximal, (2) deep, (3) distal] [Table SA-3]
    - (1) Proximal: supreme thoracic
    - (2) Deep: thoracoacromial and lateral thoracic (deltoid, acromial, pectoralis, clavicular)
    - (3) Distal: subscapular, anterior and posterior humeral circumflex

- Brachial artery
  - Named at the lower border of the teres major
  - Lies medial in the arm and crosses centrally at the elbow
  - Major branches
    - Anterior humeral circumflex
    - Posterior humeral circumflex
    - Profunda brachii (deep brachial)

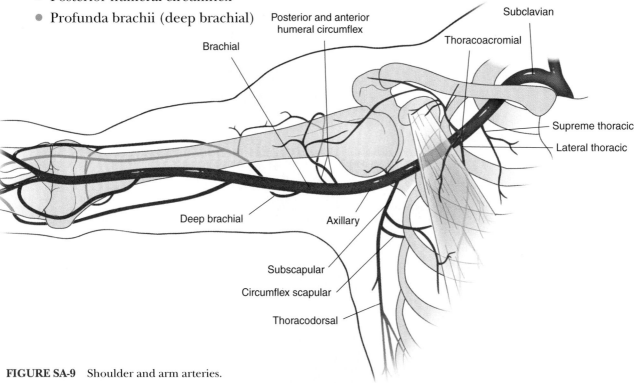

FIGURE SA-9   Shoulder and arm arteries.

TABLE SA–3   Axillary Artery Branches

Part	Branch	Course
1	Supreme thoracic	Medial to serratus anterior and pectorals
2	Thoracoacromial	Four branches (deltoid, acromial, pectoralis, clavicular)
	Lateral thoracic	Descends to serratus anterior
3	Subscapular	Two branches (thoracodorsal and circumflex scapular [triangular space])
	Anterior humeral circumflex	Blood supply to humeral head–arcuate artery lateral to bicipital groove
	Posterior humeral circumflex	Branch in quadrangular space accompanying axillary nerve

CROSS-SECTIONAL ANATOMY (Figure SA-10)

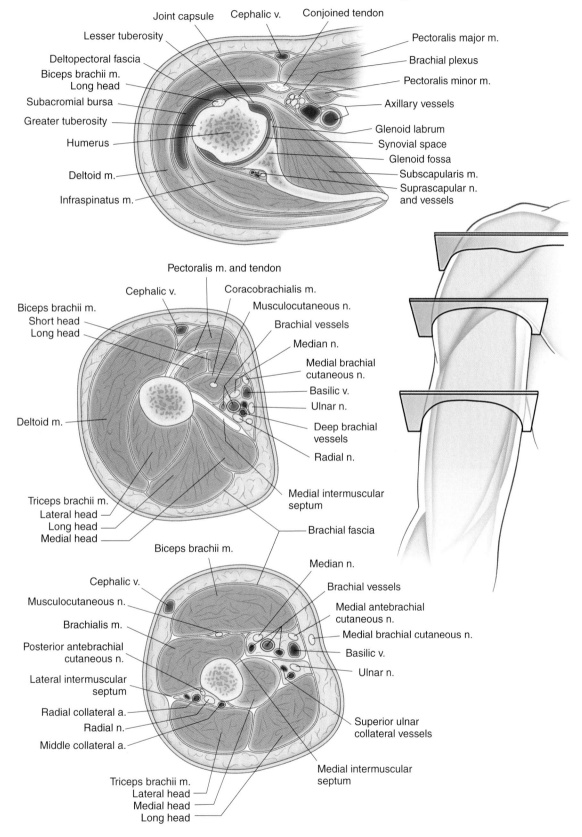

FIGURE SA-10 Cross-sectional anatomy of the shoulder and arm.

LANDMARKS (Figure SA-11)

- Coracoid process
- Acromion
- Clavicle
- Scapular spine
- Supraspinatus fossa

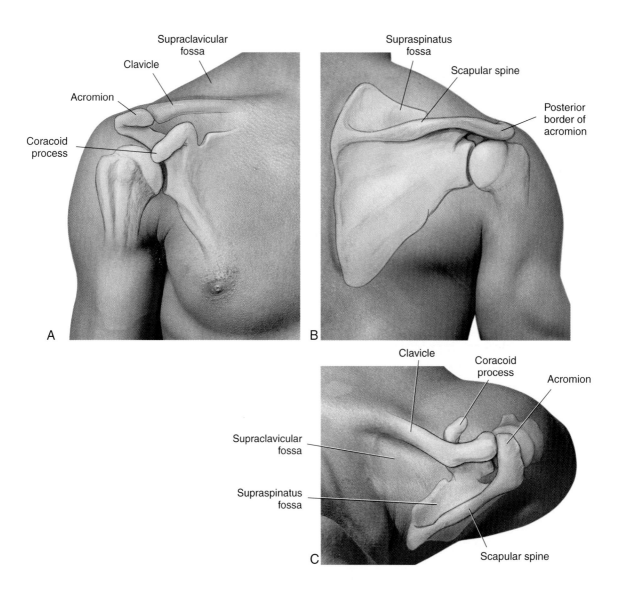

FIGURE SA-11   Landmarks. **A,** Anterior. **B,** Posterior. **C,** Superior.

HAZARDS

Shoulder (Figure SA-12)

NERVES

- **Axillary nerve**
  - Branch of posterior cord that supplies the deltoid and teres minor muscles
  - At risk
    - Inferiorly as it transverses just below the glenohumeral joint
      - Adduct and externally rotate the arm, and stay directly on the neck of the glenoid with dissection
      - Avoid retractor placement below the subscapularis and capsule
      - Palpate the nerve with blunt dissection, and use electrocautery without muscle relaxation
    - Laterally with any incision or dissection 5 cm or more distal to the lateral acromion
      - Place a marking suture at that location, and do not dissect below it
    - Posteriorly, in quadrangular space
      - Do not dissect below the teres minor

- **Musculocutaneous nerve**
  - Branch of the lateral cord that supplies the coracobrachialis, short head of the biceps, and a portion of the brachialis, and terminates as the lateral antebrachial cutaneous nerve
  - At risk
    - Approximately 5 cm below the coracoid
      - Be careful with medial retraction

- **Suprascapular nerve**
  - Preclavicular branch of the upper trunk that supplies the supraspinatus and infraspinatus
  - At risk
    - Excessive medial retraction or dissection, or both, can injure this nerve and affect one or both of the muscles it innervates

VASCULARITY

- **Subclavian artery and vein**
  - Runs inferior to clavicle
    - Dissect subperiosteally when exposing the undersurface of the clavicle

- **Acromial branch of the thoracoacromial artery**
  - Runs in the medial aspect of the coracoacromial ligament
    - Coagulate or tie this vessel off with superior dissection

● **Arcuate artery**

  ▪ Ascending branch of the anterior humeral circumflex artery that is the main blood supply to the humeral head

    ● Avoid excessive dissection or cautery lateral to the bicipital groove

● **Cephalic vein**

  ▪ Defines the interval between the deltoid and the pectoralis major (deltopectoral approach)

    ● Carefully dissect the vein, and tie off or coagulate larger branches

    ● The vein is usually more easily reflected from the medial side and is retracted with the deltoid

Arm

● **Radial nerve and profunda brachii artery**

  ▪ Vulnerable as they spiral around posterior humerus

    ● Palpate and protect radial nerve and profunda brachii artery

● **Medial structures (brachial artery, median and ulnar nerves)**

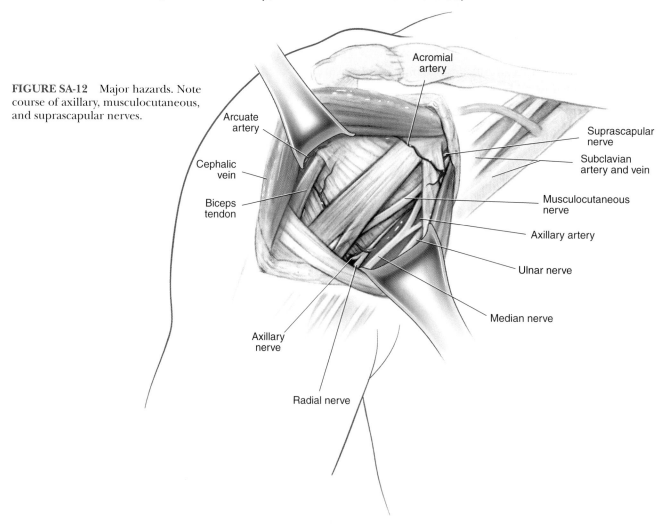

FIGURE SA-12   Major hazards. Note course of axillary, musculocutaneous, and suprascapular nerves.

ANTERIOR (DELTOPECTORAL) APPROACH TO THE SHOULDER

Indications: Open capsulorrhaphy, shoulder arthroplasty, proximal humerus fractures

POSITIONING

- Beach-chair position (Figure SA-13)
    - Head is secured in a Mayfield headrest or commercially available beach-chair attachment
    - Upper torso is elevated 45 to 60 degrees
        - Can cause transient hypotension
    - Opposite arm, legs, and other prominences are padded and secured
    - Operative shoulder and arm are positioned off the side of the operative table for full access
        - Bump placed under ipsilateral scapula may improve access
    - Rotating and airplaning the bed away from the operative side can be helpful
    - Commercially available arm holders or positioners may be helpful

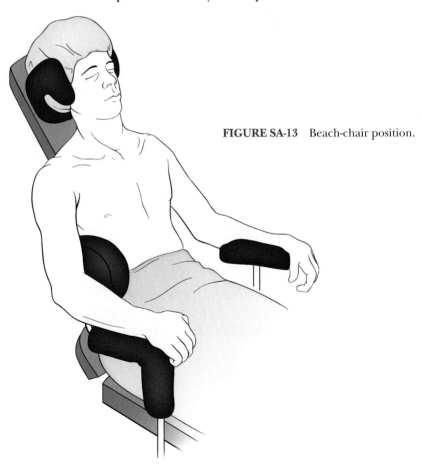

FIGURE SA-13 Beach-chair position.

INCISION

- ● Extended deltopectoral incision (Figure SA-14)
  - ▪ Typically used for arthroplasty and fracture care
  - ▪ A 10-15 cm oblique incision is made from just lateral to the coracoid down to deltoid insertion

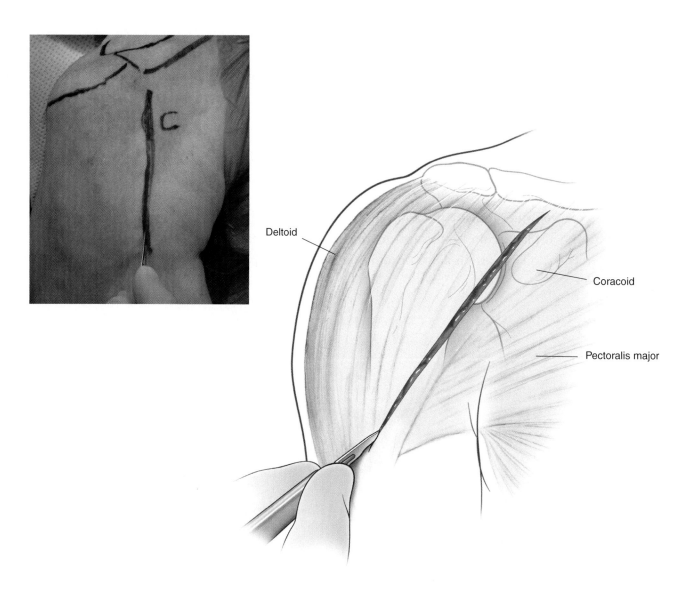

FIGURE SA-14   Extended deltopectoral incision.

● Limited anterior incision (Figure SA-15)

■ Typically used for capsulorrhaphy

■ A 5 cm vertical incision is made in the inferior axillary crease

● Can be extended superiorly for better exposure

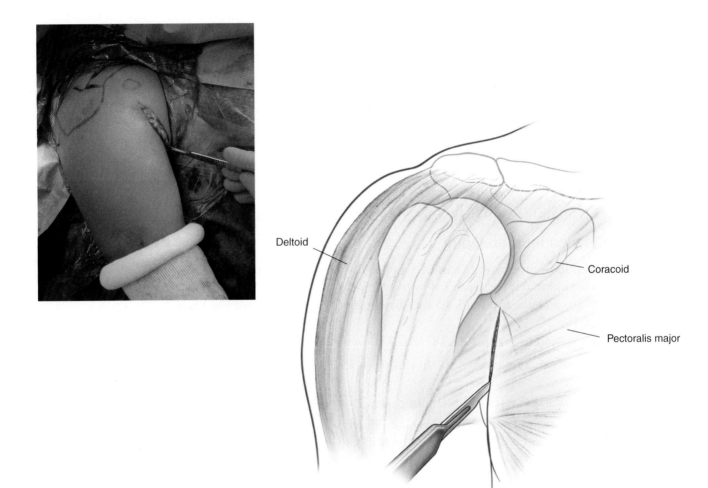

FIGURE SA-15   Limited anterior incision.

SUPERFICIAL DISSECTION

- Identify and dissect the deltopectoral interval (Figure SA-16)
    - The cephalic vein is the key landmark
        - Identification may be easier distally
            - Muscle fiber orientation (deltoid more vertical, pectoralis more horizontal), a groove, and perivascular fat may be helpful
        - Typically, the vein is more easily dissected free from the pectoralis major, and it is retraced with the deltoid
        - Small tributaries should be coagulated

- Retract the deltoid laterally and pectoralis major medially (Figure SA-17)
    - Commercially available self-retaining retractors are useful
        - Dissect the clavicopectoral fascia to expose the deeper structures

DEEP DISSECTION

- Identify subscapularis muscle and conjoint tendon (Figure SA-18)
- Expose the glenohumeral joint
    - The subscapularis and capsule can be taken down together by making a vertical incision approximately 1 cm medial to the bicipital groove, placing traction sutures in the capsule and tendon, and dissecting along the neck of the humerus (Figure SA-19)
        - Most often used for arthroplasty
        - The capsule can be dissected further inferiorly, directly off the neck of the humerus
            - The axillary nerve should be identified and protected with inferior dissection
    - The subscapularis and capsule can be taken down separately by making a vertical incision approximately 1 cm medial to the bicipital groove and carefully "teasing" the subscapularis off the underlying capsule (Figure SA-20)
        - Traction sutures are placed in the subscapularis, and a small elevator is used to assist in the dissection
            - The leash of humeral circumflex vessels at the inferior border of the subscapularis should be identified and either protected or coagulated and tied off for this approach and the previous approach
        - A capsulotomy can be made in a variety of fashions depending on the intended procedure (e.g., a T-capsular shift is made with a longitudinal incision over the humerus or glenoid, and a horizontal incision in the middle of the capsule)
    - The subscapularis can be split in a horizontal direction (Figure SA-21)
        - This gives limited access to the capsule and glenohumeral joint, but can be used for a modified capsulorrhaphy

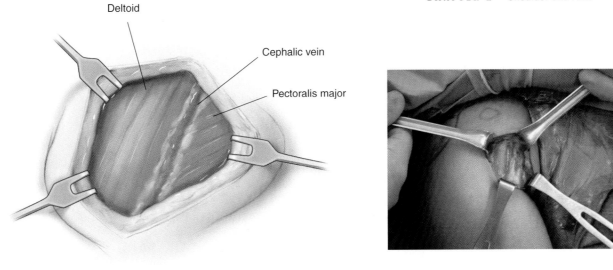

FIGURE SA-16   Identification of the deltopectoral interval

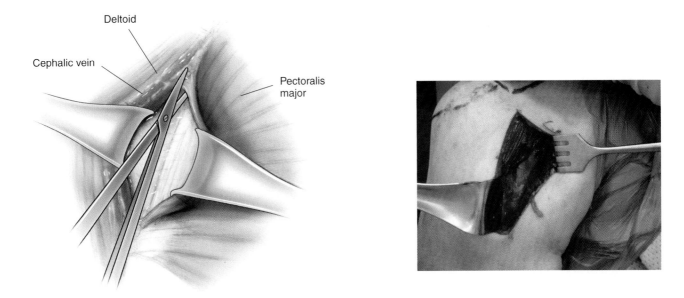

FIGURE SA-17   Retraction of the deltoid (laterally) and pectoralis (medially).

FIGURE SA-18   Exposure of the subscapularis.

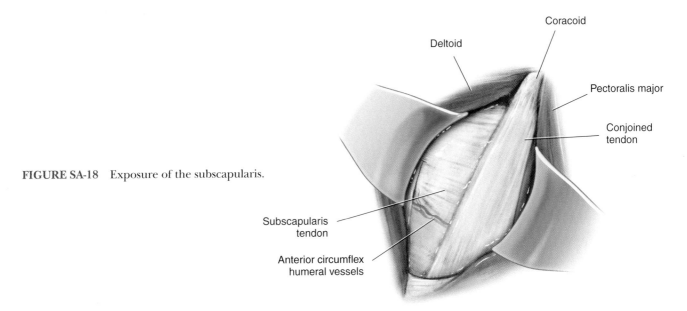

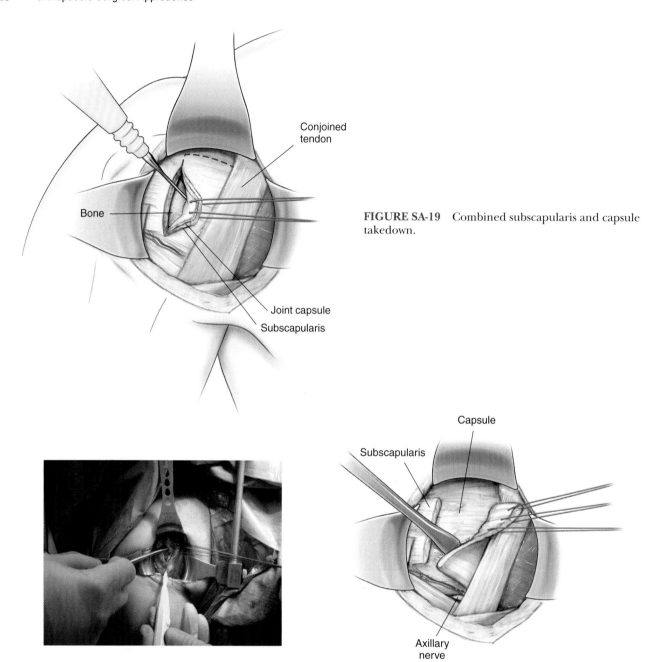

FIGURE SA-19   Combined subscapularis and capsule takedown.

Conjoined tendon

Bone

Joint capsule

Subscapularis

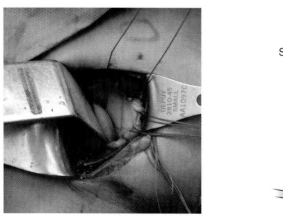

FIGURE SA-20   Capsular exposure by carefully reflecting the subscapularis from the underlying capsule.

Capsule

Subscapularis

Axillary nerve

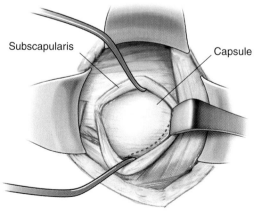

Subscapularis

Capsule

FIGURE SA-21   Limited capsular exposure through a subscapularis split.

- Expose the glenoid
  - Special forked and ring retractors can be used to expose the glenoid
  - Capsular releases can be performed (dissecting the glenoid articular surface circumferentially) and may be required for total shoulder arthroplasty

CLOSURE

- Depending on the procedure, the capsule and subscapularis are closed separately or together
  - Special care should be taken to reattach the subscapularis to the proximal humerus because this can lead to a major iatrogenic problem if it detaches

- The deltopectoral interval usually is not closed, but simply allowed to fall back into position
  - The cephalic vein should be preserved and protected
    - Small lacerations to the vein should be repaired

POSTERIOR APPROACH TO THE SHOULDER

Indications: Posterior capsulorrhaphy, posterior glenoid fractures

POSITIONING

- Lateral decubitus position (Figure SA-22)
  - Can follow arthroscopy in this position
  - Beanbag is typically used with operative side up
  - Nonoperative side must be well protected
    - Axillary roll
    - Pad elbow, fibular head, and ankles
    - Secure the head
  - Position and drape the operative arm free

- Beach-chair position
  - More difficult, but with planing of the operative table, can be done

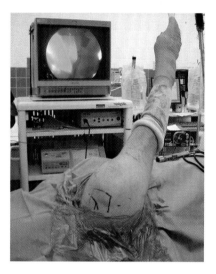

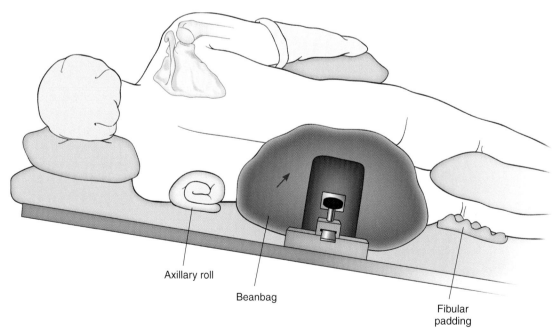

Axillary roll

Beanbag

Fibular padding

FIGURE SA-22 Lateral decubitus position.

INCISION (FIGURE SA-23)

- A 6-8 cm vertical incision is made directly over the glenohumeral joint and extended into the axilla

  - Incision is typically 2 cm medial to the posterolateral edge of the acromion and can incorporate a posterior arthroscopic portal

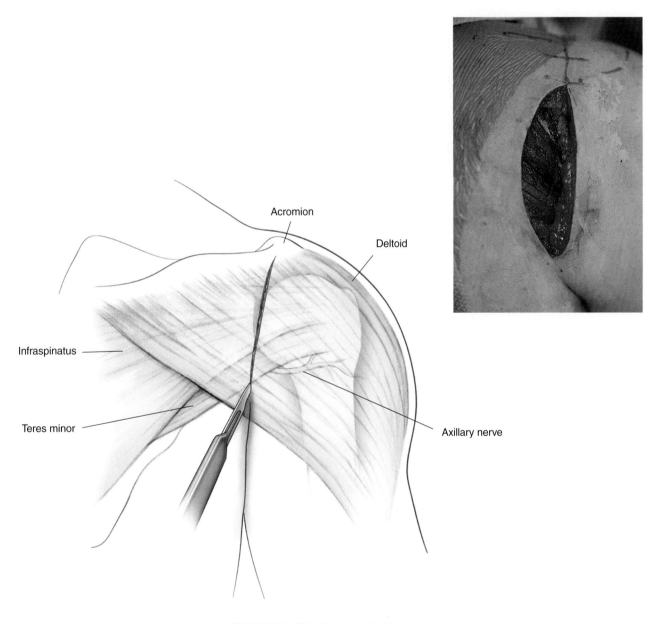

FIGURE SA-23 Posterior incision.

SUPERFICIAL DISSECTION

- The deltoid is typically split in line with its fibers (Figure SA-24)

- Occasionally, the deltoid can be retracted anteriorly

- Detachment of the deltoid off the spine of the acromion has fallen out of favor

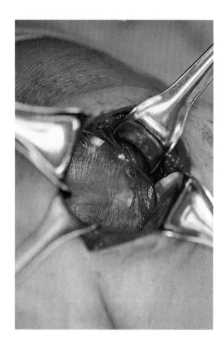

FIGURE SA-24   Deltoid split.

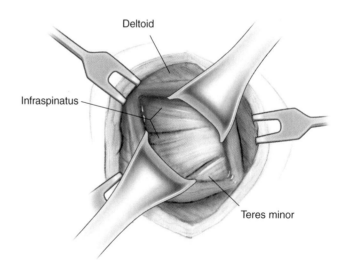

DEEP DISSECTION

■ Typically, the interval between the infraspinatus and teres minor is developed by blunt dissection, and the posterior capsule is exposed by retraction of these muscles (Figure SA-25)

■ Alternatives include taking down the infraspinatus from its humeral insertion or splitting the two heads of the infraspinatus and using this interval

■ Do not dissect below the teres minor muscle because of risk to the axillary nerve and posterior humeral circumflex artery

  ● There may be fat at the inferior border of the teres minor to help identify that you have gone too low

FIGURE SA-25   Infraspinatus–teres minor interval.

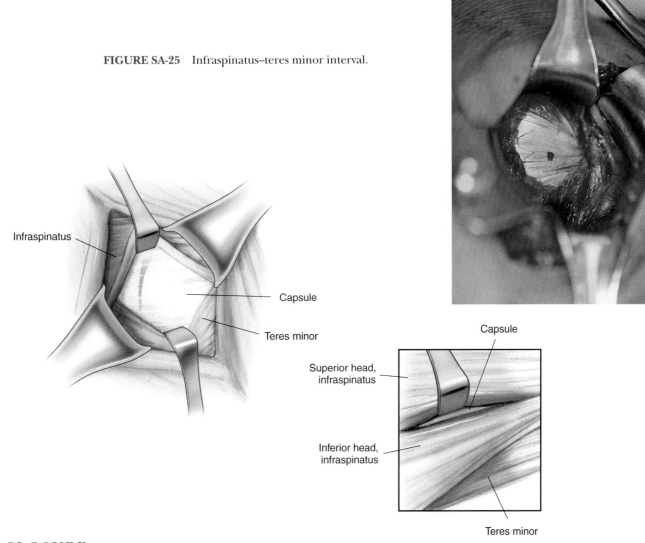

CLOSURE

■ If the infraspinatus or deltoid were detached, they must be reapproximated to bone

■ Otherwise, only the subcutaneous tissues and skin require closure

SUPEROLATERAL APPROACH TO THE SHOULDER

Indications: Rotator cuff repair, acromion fractures

POSITIONING

● Beach-chair position (see previous descriptions)

INCISION (FIGURE SA-26)

▪ A 5 cm saber-type incision is made in Langer's lines

▪ If a distal clavicle resection also is planned, the incision can be based more medially

SUPERFICIAL DISSECTION

▪ The deltoid muscle is attached to the acromion, and it can be split or subperiosteally dissected off the anterolateral acromion depending on the exposure needed (Figure SA-27)

   ● The deltoid can be split at the anterolateral border of the acromion (raphe) and extended 5 cm distally for exposure for rotator cuff repair

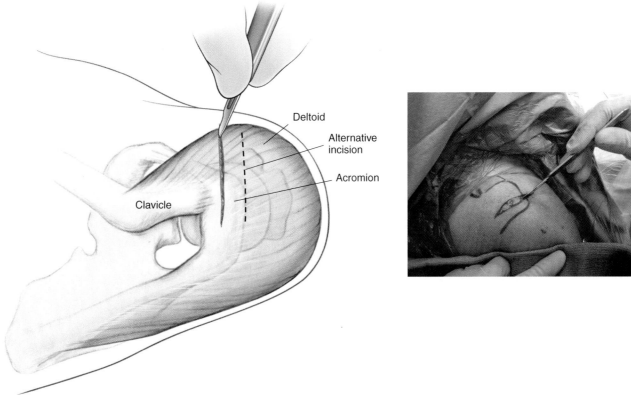

FIGURE SA-26   Skin incision for open rotator cuff repair.

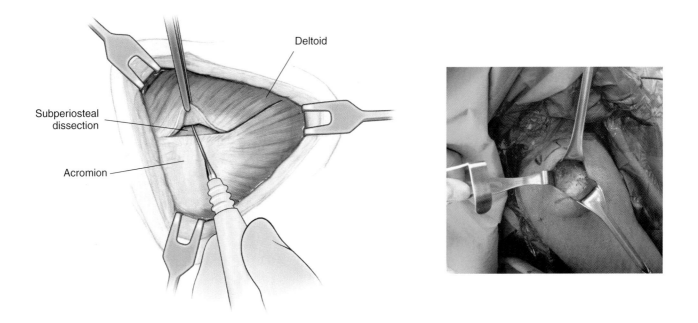

FIGURE SA-27   Deltoid reflection.

DEEP DISSECTION

■ The coracoacromial ligament can be incised, protected, or tagged, depending on the surgical plan

■ The supraspinatus tendon and overlying bursa are exposed and explored by rotating the arm (Figure SA-28)

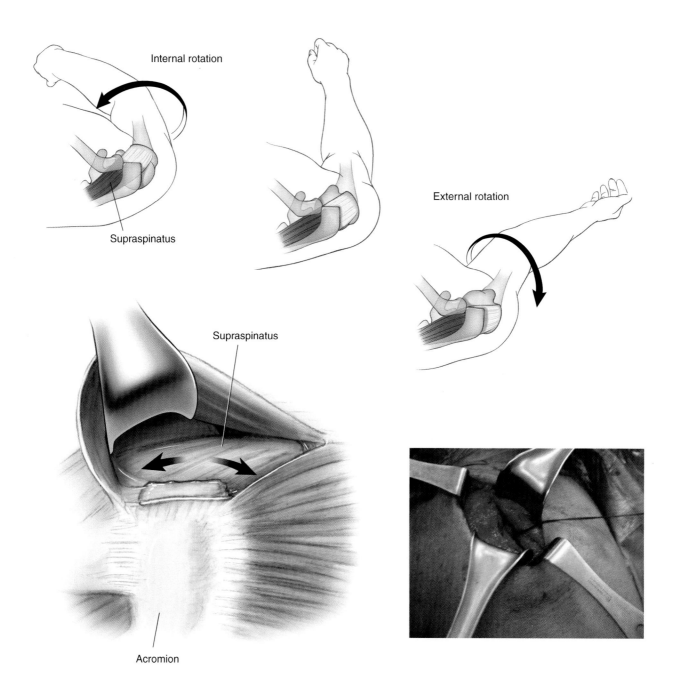

FIGURE SA-28   Exposure of the supraspinatus tendon. Rotation of the arm can facilitate inspection of the cuff.

CLOSURE

- If the deltoid was detached, it is crucial that it be reattached through drill holes into the acromion (Figure SA-29)

- The skin and subcutaneous tissues are closed in the standard fashion

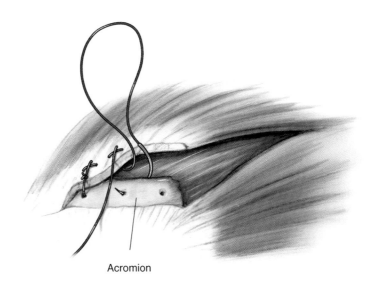

Acromion

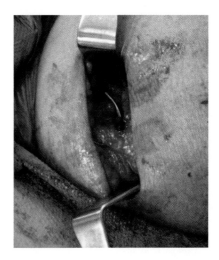

FIGURE SA-29   Closure of the deltoid back to bone through drill holes.

LATERAL (DELTOID SPLITTING [MINI-OPEN]) APPROACH TO THE SHOULDER

- Indications: Rotator cuff repair, shoulder arthroplasty

POSITIONING

- Beach-chair position (see previous descriptions)

INCISION (FIGURE SA-30)

- A longitudinal incision up to 5 cm is made from the midportion of the lateral acromion distally

  - An arthroscopic lateral portal can be extended for this approach

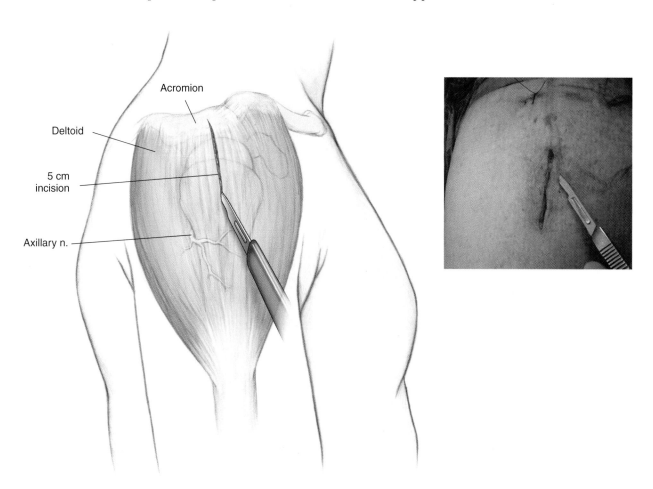

FIGURE SA-30   Deltoid splitting (mini-open) approach.

SUPERFICIAL DISSECTION

■ The deltoid muscle is split in line with its fibers being careful not to extend this 5 cm distal to the acromion (Figure SA-31)

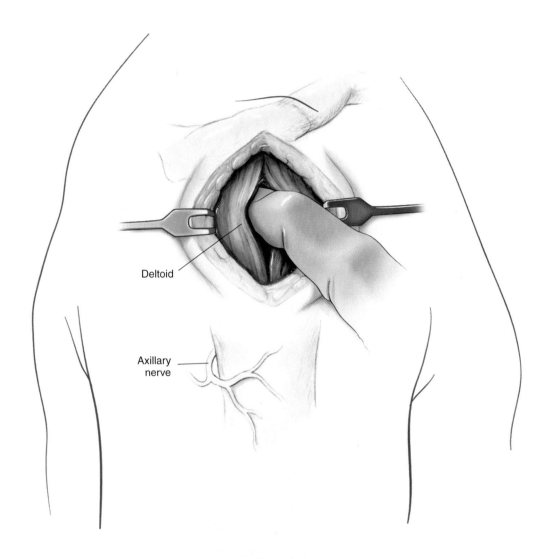

Deltoid

Axillary
nerve

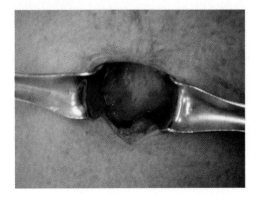

FIGURE SA-31 Deltoid split. This should not be extended more than 5 cm distal to the lateral acromion.

DEEP DISSECTION

- The subdeltoid bursa and supraspinatus insertion on the greater tuberosity can be exposed (Figure SA-32)

- If the supraspinatus is torn and retracted, it may be necessary to place sutures in the tendon arthroscopically before making this approach

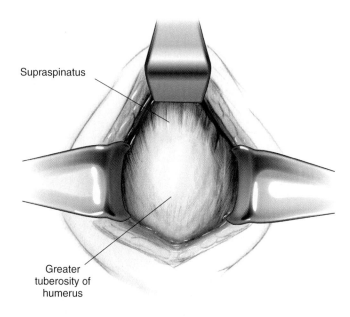

Supraspinatus

Greater tuberosity of humerus

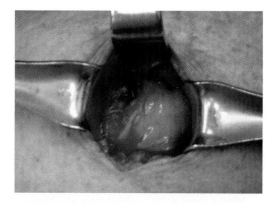

FIGURE SA-32   Exposure of the bursa and supraspinatus tendon.

CLOSURE

- If the deltoid was disrupted during this approach, it is crucial that it be repaired or reattached

- The skin and subcutaneous tissues are closed in the standard fashion

Approach to the AC Joint

Indications: AC pathology (arthrosis, instability)

POSITIONING

- Beach-chair position (see previous descriptions)

INCISION

- A 2-3 cm saber-type incision is made in Langer's lines directly over the AC joint (Figure SA-33)
  - If an anterior portal is used, it often can be extended superiorly for this approach
  - For AC reconstruction procedures, the incision is placed more medially and can be extended more distally to allow access to the coracoid (Figure SA-34)

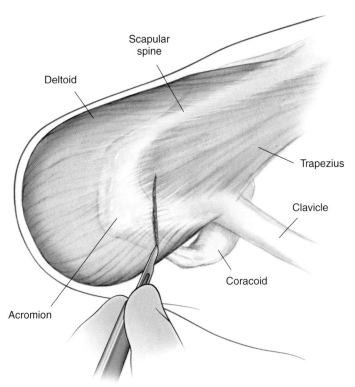

FIGURE SA-33   Skin incision for exposure of the AC joint.

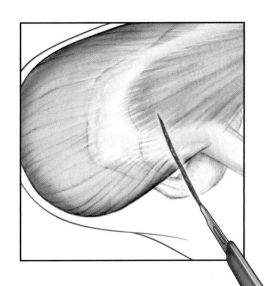

FIGURE SA-34   Extended incision for AC reconstruction.

SUPERFICIAL DISSECTION

■ Subperiosteally dissect the deltoid and trapezius attachments off of the distal clavicle (Figure SA-35)

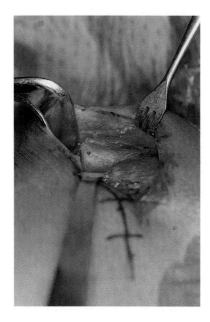

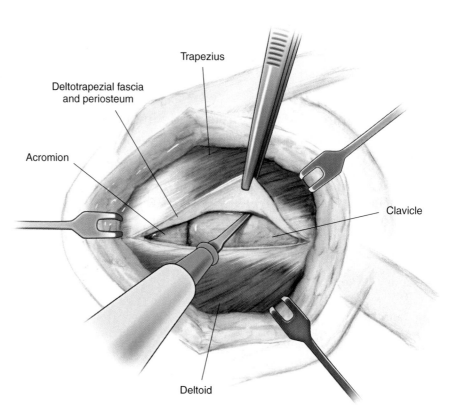

FIGURE SA-35   Distal clavicle exposure.

DEEP DISSECTION

■ Expose or resect the distal clavicle, or both, depending on the operative plan

■ If an AC reconstruction (modified Weaver-Dunn) operation is planned, do the following

  • Dissect the coracoacromial ligament from the undersurface of the acromion, and place a Bunnell-type suture in it

  • Bluntly dissect around the coracoid, and place a passing suture under it (Figure SA-36)

  • Proceed based on the surgical plan

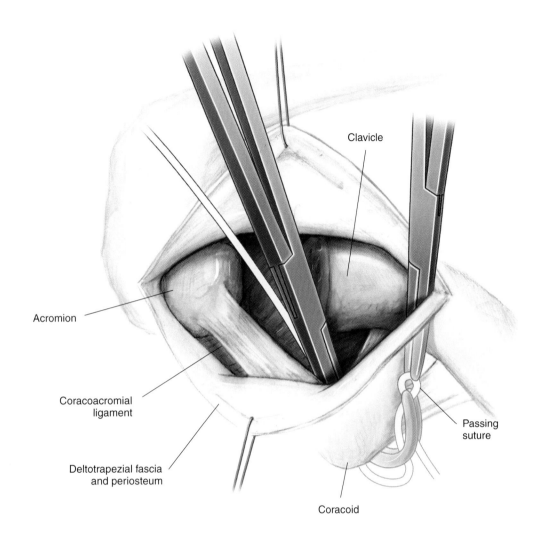

FIGURE SA-36 Coracoid exposure.

CLOSURE

- Reattach the deltotrapezial fascia over the distal clavicle or over the interval where the clavicle was resected

- The skin and subcutaneous tissues are closed in the standard fashion

SUPERIOR APPROACH TO THE SUPRASPINATUS FOSSA

Indications: Suprascapular nerve entrapment

POSITIONING

● Beach-chair position (see previous descriptions)

INCISION

▪ A 6 cm longitudinal incision is made just anterior (superior) and parallel to the spine of the scapula (Figure SA-37)

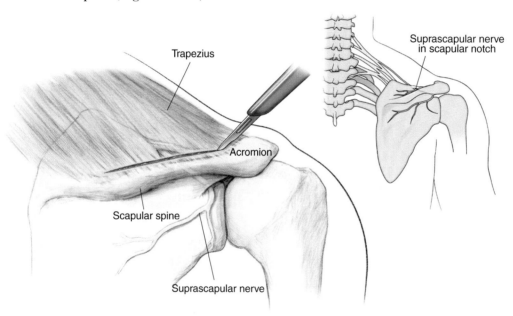

FIGURE SA-37   Incision for supraspinatus fossa approach.

SUPERFICIAL DISSECTION

▪ The trapezius muscle is identified and is reflected anteriorly, off the spine of the scapula (Figure SA-38)

DEEP DISSECTION

● Expose the supraspinatus muscle deep to the trapezius

▪ There is usually a layer of fat below the trapezius, and the fiber orientation is different (trapezius fibers are oblique, and supraspinatus fibers go directly from medial to lateral)

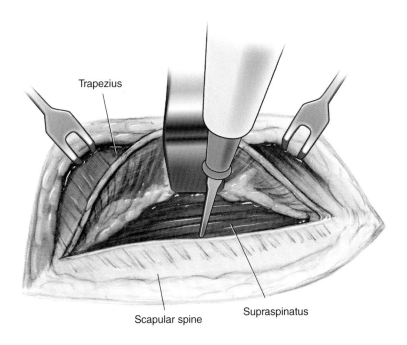
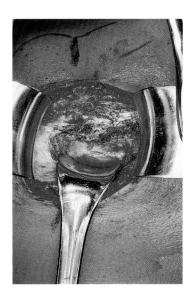

Trapezius

Scapular spine   Supraspinatus

FIGURE SA-38   Reflection of the trapezius muscle.

- Retract the supraspinatus anteriorly
- Expose the suprascapular notch (Figure SA-39)
- Palpate the coracoid base, and then palpate approximately 1 cm medially to locate the notch
- The suprascapular ligament is dissected
  - It may be covered with fat
  - The suprascapular artery must be identified and protected

CLOSURE

- The trapezius muscle must be reattached to the scapular spine through drill holes in bone

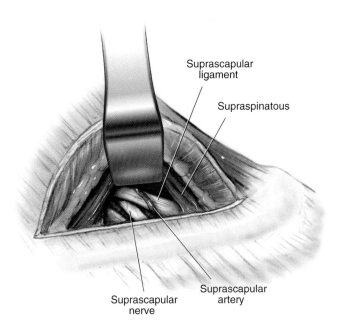
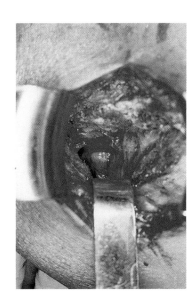

Suprascapular ligament

Suprascapinatous

Suprascapular nerve   Suprascapular artery

FIGURE SA-39   Exposure of the suprascapular notch. The artery travels above the ligament, and the nerve travels below it.

APPROACH TO THE CLAVICLE

Indications: Clavicular fractures

POSITIONING

● Beach-chair position (see previous descriptions)

INCISION

▪ A 5-8 cm longitudinal incision is made just superior and parallel to the clavicle (Figure SA-40)

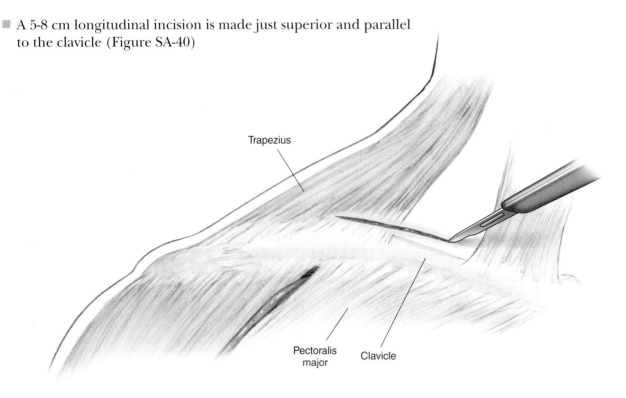

Trapezius

Pectoralis
major

Clavicle

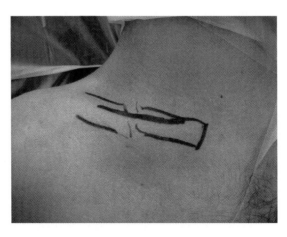

FIGURE SA-40 Standard incision for clavicle exposure.

- A smaller oblique incision can be made in Langer's line if only limited exposure is required (Figure SA-41)
  - ▪ Can be used for intramedullary fixation of the clavicle
  - ▪ Can limit injury to the suprascapular cutaneous nerves

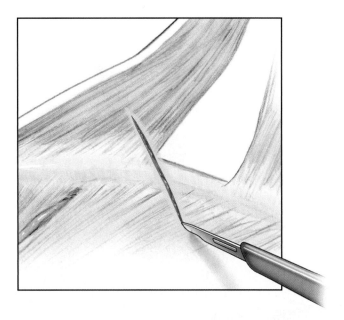

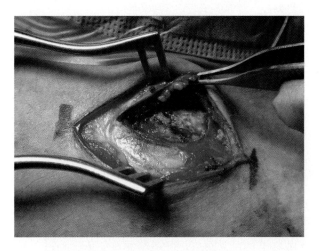

FIGURE SA-41   Modified incision for limited clavicle exposure (intramedullary fixation).

SUPERFICIAL OR DEEP DISSECTION

- The deltotrapezial fascia is subperiosteally stripped off the clavicle (Figure SA-42)
  - Dissection is continued the amount necessary for reduction and fixation

CLOSURE

- The deltotrapezial fascia is closed over the clavicle
- Skin and subcutaneous tissue are closed

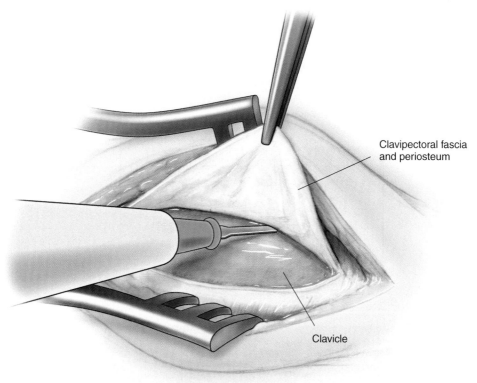

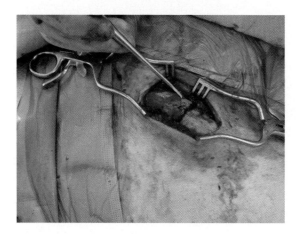

FIGURE SA-42 Clavicle exposure by subperiosteal dissection.

ANTERIOR APPROACH TO THE HUMERUS

Indications: Humerus fractures

POSITIONING

● **Supine with arm board**

- ▪ Opposite arm, legs, and bony prominences are padded and protected
- ▪ Bump may be helpful
- ▪ A sterile tourniquet may be useful

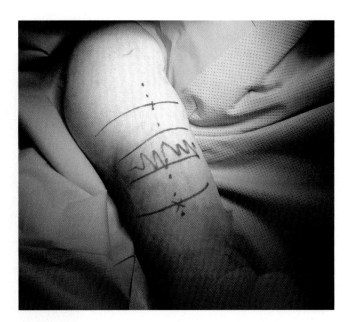

INCISION

- ▪ An 8-12 cm incision is made along the lateral border of the biceps
- ▪ A deltopectoral incision can be extended distally for this incision (Figure SA-43)

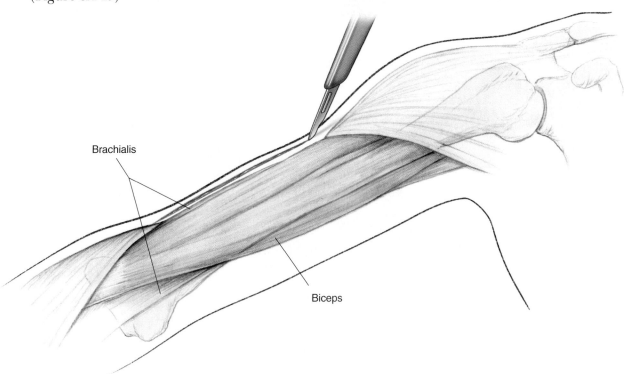

Brachialis

Biceps

FIGURE SA-43 Skin incision for anterolateral approach to the humerus. A deltopectoral incision can be extended for this approach.

SUPERFICIAL DISSECTION

- Develop the interval between the biceps and the brachialis (Figure SA-44)
- Alternatively, split the brachialis (which has two nerves)

DEEP DISSECTION

- Expose the humerus by developing this interval and subperiosteal dissection of the bone

CLOSURE

- Standard closure of the subcutaneous tissues and skin is accomplished

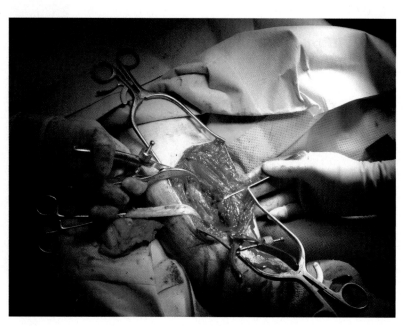

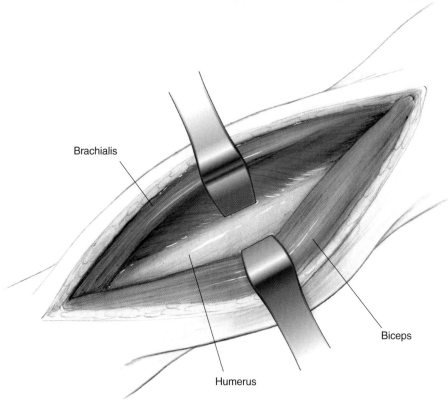

FIGURE SA-44   The biceps-brachialis interval is developed. Alternatively, the brachialis can be split.

POSTERIOR APPROACH TO THE HUMERUS

- Indications: Humerus fractures and radial nerve exploration

POSITIONING

- Lateral or Prone
  - Padding of prominent structures is important

INCISION (FIGURE SA-45)

  - A 10-15 cm midline longitudinal incision is made directly posteriorly

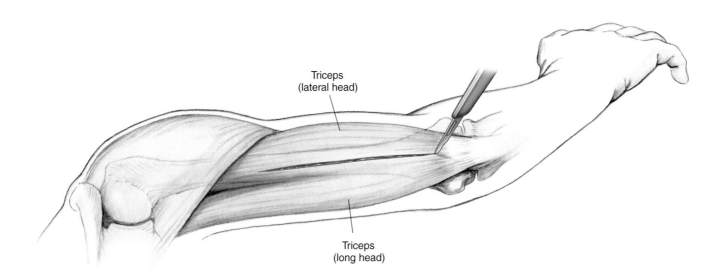

Triceps
(lateral head)

Triceps
(long head)

FIGURE SA-45   Posterior approach skin incision.

SUPERFICIAL DISSECTION

- ▨ Incise the fascia in line with the skin incision
- ▨ Identify and separate the lateral and long head of the triceps (Figure SA-46)
  - ● The interval is more obvious proximally as the tendons merge distally

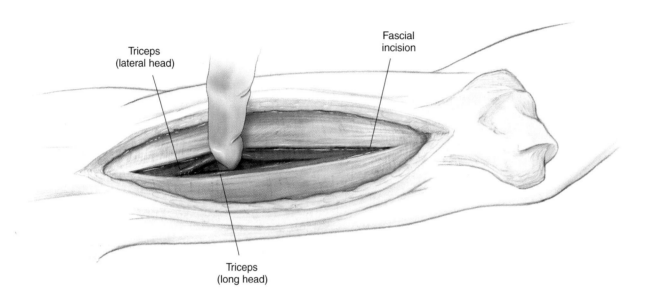

FIGURE SA-46 Identification and separation of the lateral and long heads of the triceps.

DEEP DISSECTION

- **The medial (deep) head is exposed and split (Figure SA-47)**
  - The radial nerve passes from medial to lateral in the upper/middle portion of the field and should be identified and protected

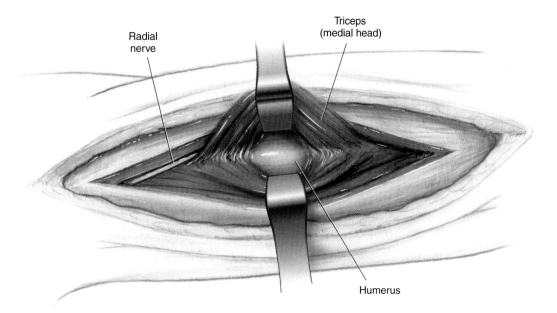

FIGURE SA-47   The medial (deep) head is split, and the humerus can be accessed.

CLOSURE

- Skin and subcutaneous tissues are closed in standard fashion

SHOULDER ARTHROSCOPY

- Indications: Rotator cuff disease, shoulder instability, adhesive capsulitis, loose body removal

POSITIONING

- Beach-chair position (see Figure SA-13)
- Lateral decubitus position (see Figure SA-22)

PORTALS (FIGURE SA-48)

- Posterior
  - Location: 2 cm distal and 2 cm medial to the posterolateral corner of the acromion
  - Use: primary viewing portal

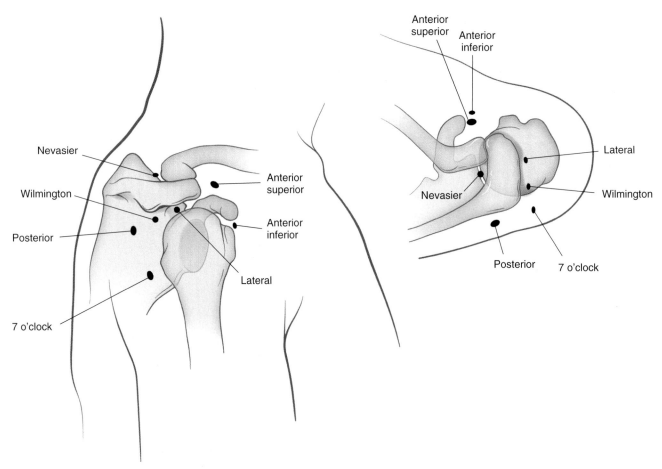

FIGURE SA-48   Arthroscopic shoulder portals.

● Anterior Superior

- ■ Location: superior and lateral to coracoid
  - ● Typically localized with a spinal needle from outside-in just anterior to the biceps adjacent to the superior glenoid (Figure SA-49)
  - ● Can be moved more medially for cases requiring distal clavicle resection

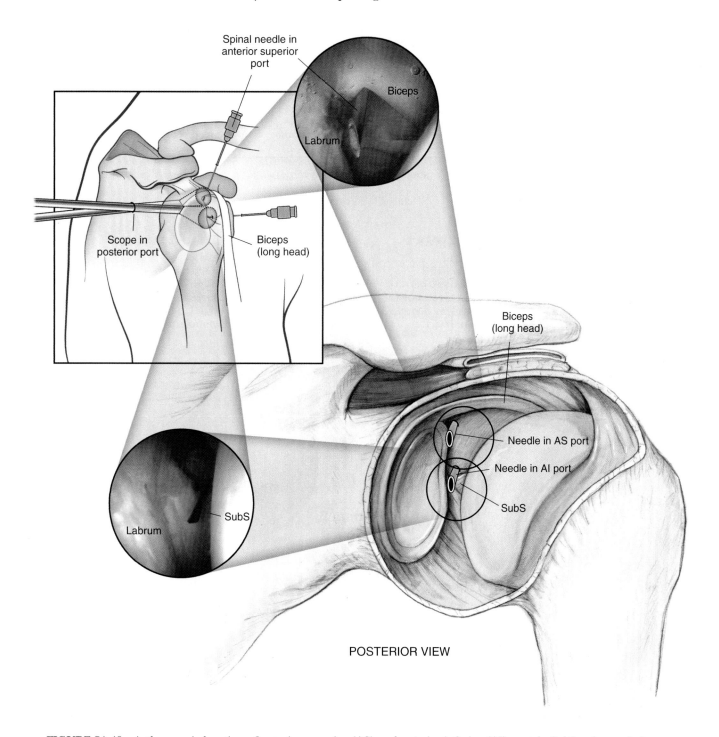

FIGURE SA-49 Arthroscopic location of anterior superior (AS) and anterior inferior (AI) portals. SubS, subscapularis.

■ Use: primary instrument portal

    ● Also can be used for visualization—especially to view the anterior glenoid and labrum (Figure SA-50)

● **Anterior Inferior**

    ■ Location: inferior and lateral to coracoid

        ● Typically localized with a spinal needle from outside-in just superior to the top of the subscapularis (see Figure SA-49)

    ■ Use: primarily for suture anchor placement and repair of anterior Bankart's lesions

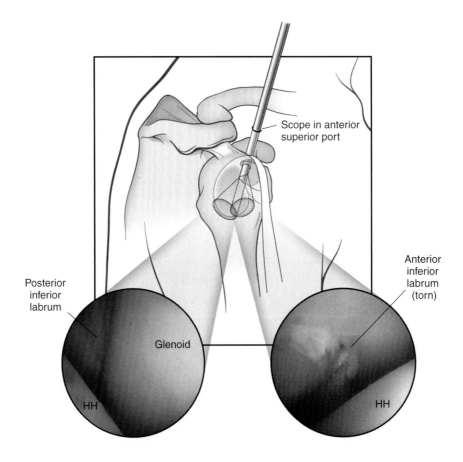

FIGURE SA-50   Visualization through anterior superior portal. **A,** Anterior view. **B,** Posterior view.

- ## Port of Wilmington
  - Location: 1 cm anterior and 1 cm distal to posterolateral corner of the acromion
    - Localized with a spinal needle while viewing the superior labrum (Figure SA-51).
  - Use: posterior superior labrum anterior to posterior (SLAP) repair

- ## Supraspinatus (Nevasier)
  - Location: corner of supraspinatus fossa
    - Localized with a spinal needle under visualization
  - Use: SLAP and rotator cuff repair (see Figure SA-51)

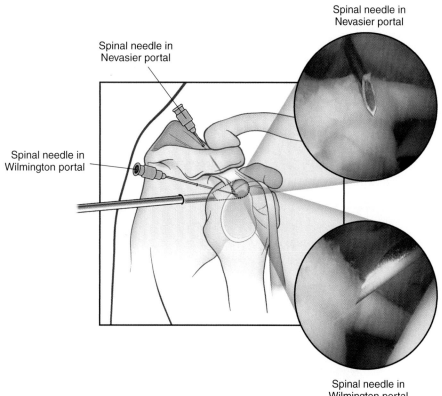

Spinal needle in
Nevasier portal

Spinal needle in
Nevasier portal

Spinal needle in
Wilmington portal

Spinal needle in
Wilmington portal

FIGURE SA-51 Arthroscopic localization of the Nevasier portal and port of Wilmington (used for SLAP repairs).

- **Lateral**
  - Location: 1-2 cm distal to the lateral acromion
    - Usually localized with a spinal needle while viewing in the subacromial space (Figure SA-52)
  - Use: subacromial decompression and rotator cuff repair
    - Arthroscopic repair, or can be extended for mini-open deltoid splitting approach

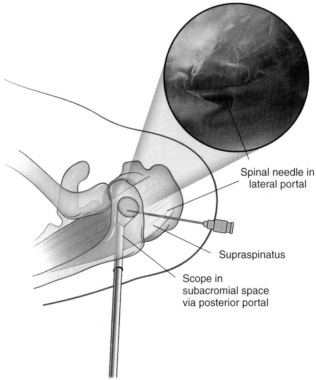

Spinal needle in
lateral portal

Supraspinatus

Scope in
subacromial space
via posterior portal

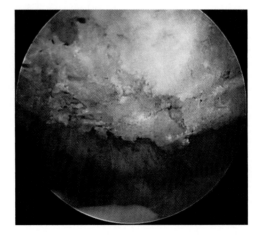

FIGURE SA-52   Arthroscopic localization of lateral portal. **A,** View in subacromial space. **B,** View through lateral portal medially.

VISUALIZATION OF STRUCTURES (FIGURE SA-53)

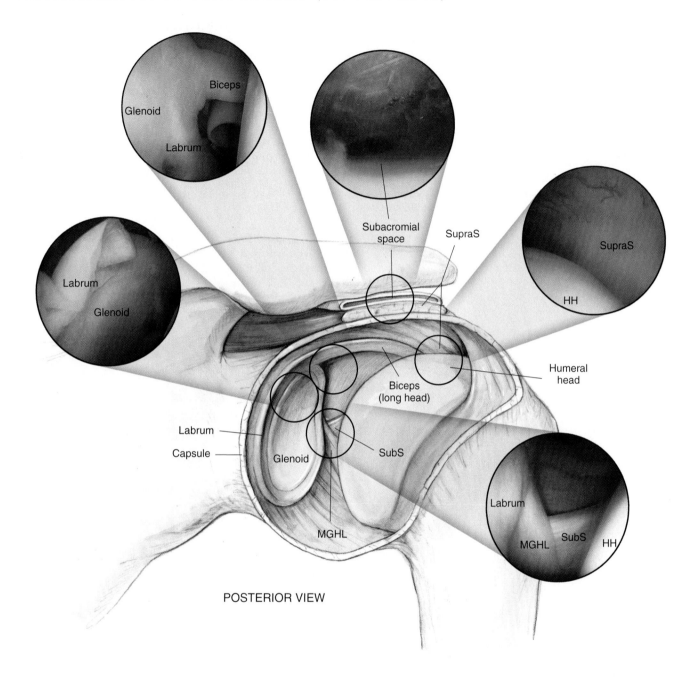

FIGURE SA-53 Visualization of the glenohumeral joint and subacromial space. HH, humeral head; MGHL, medial glenohumeral ligament; SubS, subscapularis; SupraS, suprascapularis.

REFERENCES

Cooper DE, O'Brien SJ, Warren RF: Supporting layers of the glenohumeral joint: An anatomic study. Clin Orthop 289:144-155, 1993.

Di Giacomo G, Costantini A: Arthroscopic shoulder anatomy: Basic to advanced portal placement. Op Tech Sports Med 12:64-74, 2004.

Lo IK, Burkhart SS, Parten PM: Surgery about the coracoid: neurovascular structures at risk. Arthroscopy 20:591-595, 2004.

Lo IK, Lind CC, Burkhart SS: Glenohumeral arthroscopy portals established using an outside-in technique: Neurovascular anatomy at risk. Arthroscopy 20:596-602, 2004.

McFarland EG, Caicedo JC, Guitterez MI, et al: The anatomic relationship of the brachial plexus and axillary artery to the glenoid: Implications for anterior shoulder surgery. Am J Sports Med 29:729-733, 2001.

Park JY, Levine WN, Marra G, et al: Portal-extension approach for the repair of small and medium rotator cuff tears. Am J Sports Med 28:312-316, 2000.

Shaffer BS, Conway J, Jobe FW, et al: Infraspinatus muscle-splitting incision in posterior shoulder surgery: An anatomic and electromyographic study. Am J Sports Med 22:113-120, 1994.

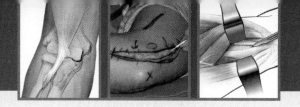

3

ELBOW AND FOREARM

—

A. BOBBY CHHABRA

REGIONAL ANATOMY

Osteology (Figures EF-1 and EF-2)

- Distal humerus

  - Widens and flattens distally into medial and lateral supracondylar ridges, then medial and lateral epicondyles
    - Extensor carpi radialis longus (ECRL) originates on lateral supracondylar ridge
    - Common flexor muscles and pronator teres originate on medial epicondyle
    - Common extensor muscles originate on lateral epicondyle
  - Capitulum articulates with radial head laterally
  - Trochlea articulates with ulnar trochlear notch medially
  - Coronoid fossa lies on anterior humerus
  - Olecranon fossa lies on posterior humerus
  - Radial fossa is anterolateral to accommodate radial head when the elbow is in flexion
  - Radial groove for radial nerve lies on posterior aspect of middle third of humerus
  - Groove for ulnar nerve lies between medial epicondyle and trochlea

- Proximal radius

  - Discoid radial head articulates with humeral capitulum and ulna radial notch
  - Radial neck
  - Radial tuberosity for insertion of biceps tendon
  - Has triangular shaft that widens distally

- Proximal ulna

  - Trochlear notch articulates with trochlea of the humerus
  - Olecranon process inserts into olecranon fossa of the humerus when the elbow is in extension
  - Coronoid process inserts into coronoid fossa on the humerus when the elbow is in flexion
  - Has triangular shaft that narrows distally

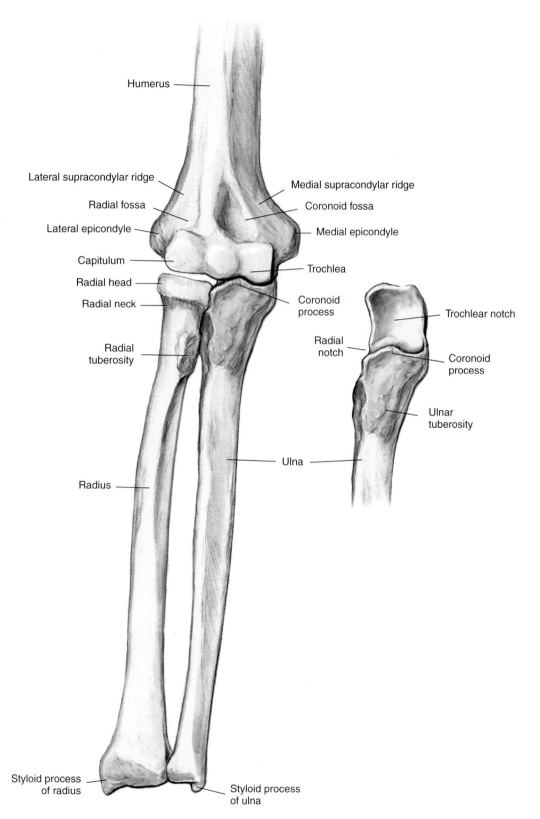

FIGURE EF-1   Elbow and forearm bony anatomy—volar view.

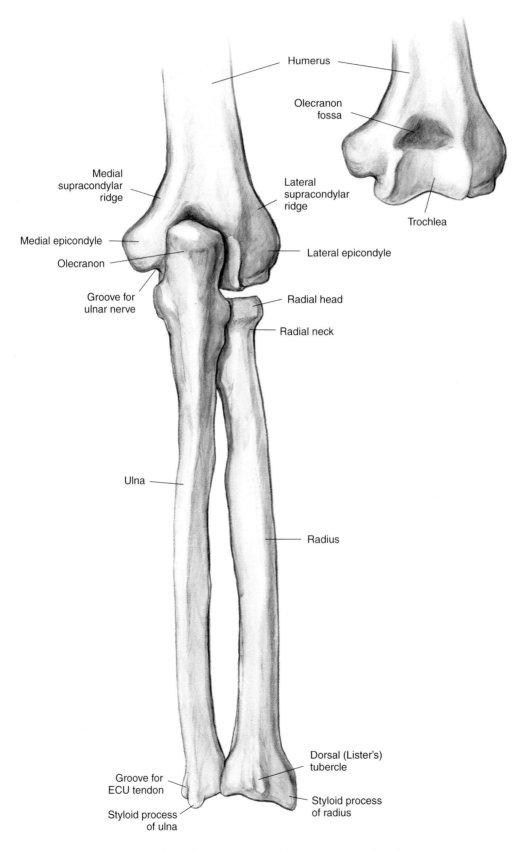

FIGURE EF-2   Elbow and forearm bony anatomy—dorsal view.

Arthrology (Figure EF-3)

- **Elbow joint**
  - Hinge joint that allows flexion and extension
  - Articulations are humeroulnar and humeroradial
  - Ligaments
    - Lateral collateral ligament
      - Fanlike ligament that extends from anteroinferior lateral epicondyle of the humerus and blends distally with annular ligament of the radius
      - Three parts
        - Annular ligament of radius
        - Radial collateral ligament
        - Lateral ulnar collateral ligament
          - From lateral epicondyle to ulna supinator crest
          - Deficiency leads to posterolateral rotatory instability
    - Medial collateral ligament
      - Triangular ligament consisting of 3 bands
        - Anterior band: inferior medial epicondyle to coronoid process
        - Posterior band: inferior medial epicondyle to olecranon process
        - Transverse band: olecranon process to coronoid process
    - Joint capsule
      - Thin fibrous capsule that attaches to ulna proximal to coronoid process and to radius proximal to radial head, and widens to reach medial and lateral epicondyles of the humerus
      - Posteriorly, capsule attaches to humerus proximal to olecranon fossa and to ulna olecranon process
    - Fat pads
      - Three pads located between joint capsule and synovial membrane
        - Olecranon fossa fat pad (largest)
        - Coronoid fossa fat pad
        - Radial fossa fat pad
    - Major stabilizers of elbow joint
      - Lateral ulnar collateral ligament
      - Medial collateral ligament
      - Coronoid
      - Olecranon fossa

- **Proximal radioulnar joint**
  - Pivot joint that allows pronation and supination
  - Articulations: radial head with ulna radial notch

- **Middle radioulnar joint**
  - The radial and ulnar shafts are connected by a syndesmosis
    - Oblique cord is a flat band of fascia on the deep head of the supinator muscle that originates proximally on the ulna and distally on the radius; its fibers run in an opposite direction of the interosseous membrane
    - Interosseous membrane begins 2-3 cm distal to radial tuberosity and runs the length of the forearm between radial and ulnar shafts

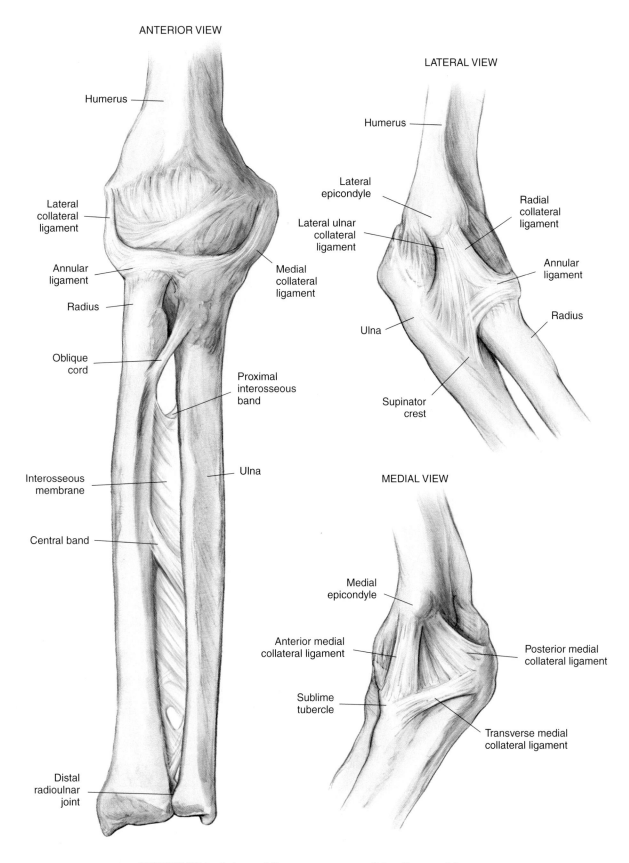

FIGURE EF-3   Joint and ligament anatomy of the elbow and forearm.

Muscles (Figures EF-4 and EF-5)

- Best considered in compartments (Table EF-1)

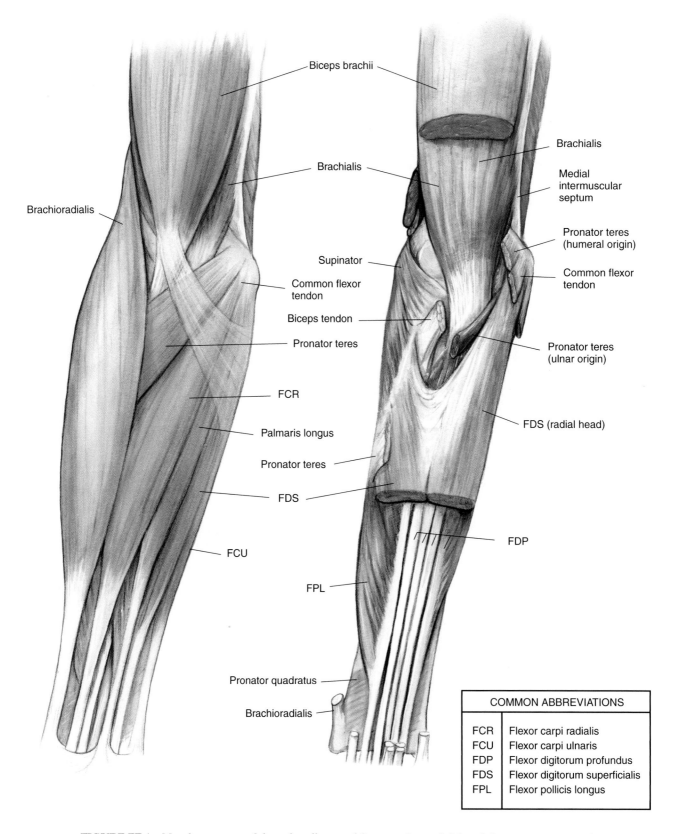

COMMON ABBREVIATIONS	
FCR	Flexor carpi radialis
FCU	Flexor carpi ulnaris
FDP	Flexor digitorum profundus
FDS	Flexor digitorum superficialis
FPL	Flexor pollicis longus

FIGURE EF-4 Muscle anatomy of the volar elbow and forearm (superficial and deep compartments).

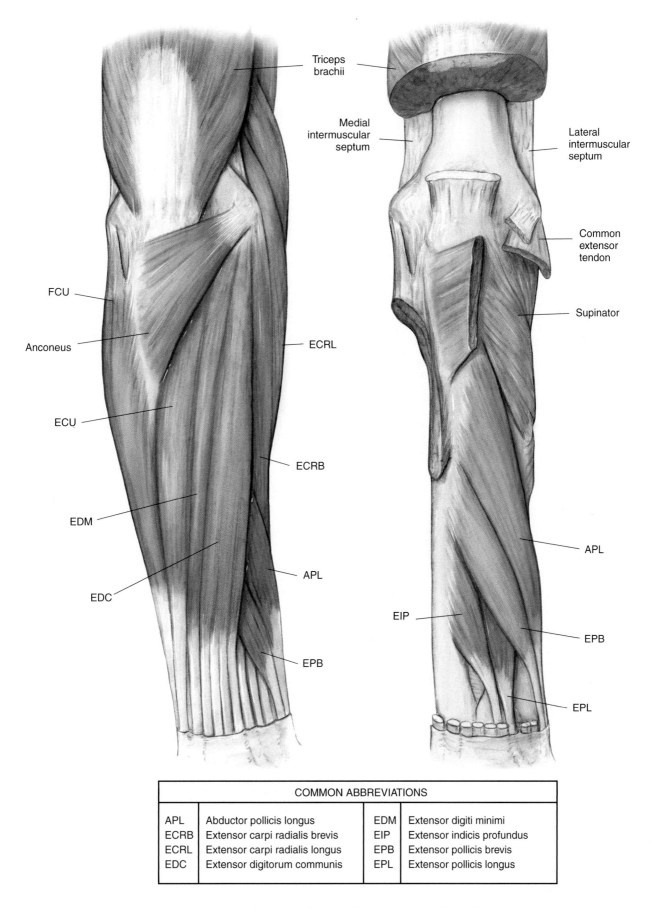

COMMON ABBREVIATIONS			
APL	Abductor pollicis longus	EDM	Extensor digiti minimi
ECRB	Extensor carpi radialis brevis	EIP	Extensor indicis profundus
ECRL	Extensor carpi radialis longus	EPB	Extensor pollicis brevis
EDC	Extensor digitorum communis	EPL	Extensor pollicis longus

FIGURE EF-5 Muscle anatomy of the dorsal elbow and forearm (superficial and deep compartments).

TABLE EF–1   Compartments and Muscles of the Elbow

Compartment	Muscle	Origin	Insertion	Innervation	Function
Anterior arm	Biceps brachii	Long head—supraglenoid tubercle Short head—coracoid process	Radial tuberosity	Musculocutaneous nerve	Supination of forearm; flexion of elbow
	Brachialis	Distal half of anterior humerus	Ulnar tuberosity	Musculocutaneous nerve	Flexion of elbow in pronation
Posterior arm	Triceps brachii	Long head—infraglenoid tubercle Lateral head—proximal lateral half of humerus Medial head—posterior humerus	Olecranon process	Radial nerve	Extension of elbow
Superficial forearm flexors	Pronator teres	Medial epicondyle and ulna coronoid process	Lateral middle surface of radius	Median nerve	Forearm pronation
	Flexor carpi radialis	Medial epicondyle	Base of 2nd and 3rd MC	Median nerve	Flexion of wrist
	Palmaris longus	Medial epicondyle	Palmar fascia	Median nerve	Weak flexion of wrist
	Flexor carpi ulnaris	Medial epicondyle and proximal posterior shaft and olecranon process of ulna	5th MC, pisiform, and hamate	Ulnar nerve	Wrist flexion and ulnar deviation
	Flexor digitorum superficialis	Medial epicondyle, ulna coronoid process, and anterior oblique line of radius	Splits at level of proximal phalanx and inserts onto volar middle phalanx	Median nerve	Finger flexion at PIP joints
Deep forearm flexors	Flexor digitorum profundus	Proximal interosseous membrane and anterior ulna	Volar aspect of distal phalanges	Lateral half—AIN Medial half—ulnar nerve	Finger flexion at DIP joints
	Flexor pollicis longus	Anterior shaft of radius and interosseous membrane	Volar aspect of thumb distal phalanx	AIN	Flexion of thumb IP joint
	Pronator quadratus	Distal anterior ulna	Distal anterior radius	AIN	Forearm pronation
Superficial forearm extensors	Brachioradialis	Lateral supracondylar ridge	Radial styloid process	Radial nerve	Flexion of elbow
	Extensor carpi radialis longus	Lateral supracondylar ridge of humerus and lateral epicondyle	Dorsal base of 2nd MC	Radial nerve	Wrist extension and some radial deviation
	Extensor carpi radialis brevis	Lateral epicondyle	Dorsal base of 3rd MC	PIN	Wrist extension and some radial deviation
	Extensor digitorum	Lateral epicondyle	Extensor hood of digits 2-5	PIN	Finger extension
	Extensor digiti minimi	Lateral epicondyle	Extensor hood of 5th digit	PIN	5th finger extension
	Extensor carpi ulnaris	Lateral epicondyle	Dorsal 5th MC	PIN	Wrist extension and ulnar deviation; stabilizes wrist in grip
	Anconeus	Posterior lateral epicondyle	Lateral olecranon process and posterior ulna shaft	Radial nerve	Weakly extends elbow
Deep forearm extensors	Supinator	Lateral epicondyle and proximal ulna	Proximal lateral radius	PIN	Forearm supination
	Abductor pollicis longus	Posterior ulna shaft and interosseous membrane	Dorsal base of 1st MC and trapezium	PIN	Thumb abduction

TABLE EF–1   Compartments and Muscles of the Elbow—cont'd

Compartment	Muscle	Origin	Insertion	Innervation	Function
	Extensor pollicis brevis	Posterior radial shaft and interosseous membrane	Dorsal proximal phalanx of thumb	PIN	Extends thumb at MC joint
	Extensor pollicis longus	Posterior ulnar shaft and interosseous membrane	Dorsal distal phalanx of thumb	PIN	Extends thumb at IP joint
	Extensor indicis	Posterior ulnar shaft and interosseous membrane	Ulnar side of extensor digitorum communis tendon to 2nd digit at level of MCP joint	PIN	Assists in extension of 2nd digit

AIN, anterior interosseous nerve; DIP, distal interphalangeal; IP, interphalangeal; MC, metacarpal; MCP, metacarpophalangeal; PIN, posterior interosseous nerve; PIP, proximal interphalangeal.

Nerves (Figures EF-6 and EF-7)

- **Musculocutaneous nerve C5, C6, C7**

  - Lies between biceps brachii and brachialis in the arm
  - Emerges from beneath biceps brachii on lateral side of biceps tendon
  - After crossing the antebrachium, the nerve pierces through the deep fascia and becomes the lateral antebrachial cutaneous nerve
  - Lateral antebrachial cutaneous nerve continues into forearm, crossing under cephalic vein and running **superficial** to brachioradialis
  - The nerve branches in the upper third of the forearm into the anterior and posterior branches, which provide sensation to the lateral aspect of the forearm

- **Radial nerve C5, C6, C7, C8 (T1)**

  - Travels in radial groove on posterior middle third of humerus, then enters lateral intramuscular septum between medial and lateral heads of the triceps
  - Emerges from intramuscular septum between brachialis and brachioradialis muscles and approaches the elbow anterolaterally between brachialis and ECRL
  - Anterior to the lateral epicondyle it branches into
    - **Superficial** sensory branch
      - In proximal forearm, the nerve lies superficial to the supinator muscle and continues into lateral middle forearm deep to brachioradialis
      - Approximately 9 cm proximal to the wrist, the nerve emerges through antebrachial fascia between the brachioradialis tendon and ECRL tendons and **superficially** crosses the abductor pollicis longus (APL) and extensor pollicis brevis (EPB) muscles as it descends to the hand
      - Provides sensation to posterior aspect of thumb, index finger, and middle finger
    - **Deep motor branch** or posterior interosseous nerve (PIN)
      - Provides motor innervation to forearm extensor muscles
      - After bifurcating from the radial nerve, the PIN turns toward the posterior forearm and gives off 3 short branches to the ECRL, extensor carpi radialis brevis (ECRB), and extensor carpi ulnaris (ECU) muscles, then pierces the proximal supinator muscle
      - After traveling within supinator fibers, the PIN exits distal end of supinator and continues distally in the forearm deep to extensor digitorum communis (EDC) and EDM muscle bellies; the nerve continues to give off multiple branches to APL, EPB, extensor pollicis longus, and EIP
      - The terminal portion of the nerve dives between extensor pollicis longus and EPB to the interosseous membrane, where it descends to the wrist and provides innervation to the wrist capsule

- **Median nerve C5, C6, C7, C8 (T1)**

  - Crosses elbow anteriorly, just medial to brachial artery
  - Gives off muscular branches to pronator teres, flexor carpi radialis (FCR), and palmaris longus

- Passes between the heads of pronator teres; anterior interosseous nerve branches off here and has terminal branches that supply flexor pollicis longus (FPL), lateral half of flexor digitorum profundus (FDP), and pronator quadratus
- Median nerve and anterior interosseous nerve travel distally through the forearm toward the wrist between muscle bellies of flexor digitorum superficialis (FDS) and FDP

- ## Ulnar nerve C7, C8 (T1)

  - Approaches elbow posteromedially, travels in medial intermuscular septum of triceps, and travels beneath arcade of Struthers
    - Crosses elbow in cubital tunnel posterior to medial epicondyle
    - At distal end of cubital tunnel, the nerve passes beneath Osbourne's ligament, then descends through flexor carpi ulnaris (FCU) fascia and passes between 2 heads of FCU
  - Travels distally in forearm between FCU and ulnar side of FDP, supplying both
  - At approximately the level of the midforearm, the nerve gives off the dorsal palmar cutaneous branches, which continue to the hand
  - Ulnar nerve continues toward wrist and emerges just radial to FCU tendon into Guyon's canal

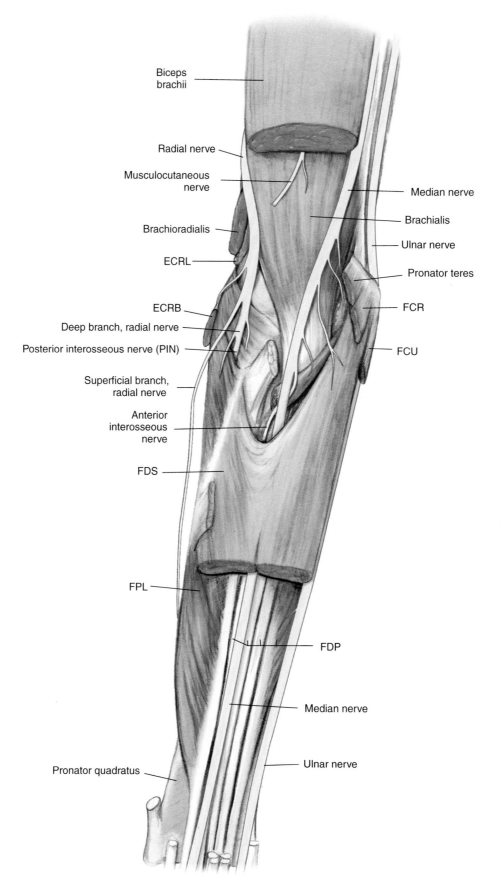

Biceps brachii

Radial nerve

Musculocutaneous nerve

Brachioradialis

ECRL

ECRB

Deep branch, radial nerve

Posterior interosseous nerve (PIN)

Superficial branch, radial nerve

Anterior interosseous nerve

FDS

FPL

Pronator quadratus

Median nerve

Brachialis

Ulnar nerve

Pronator teres

FCR

FCU

FDP

Median nerve

Ulnar nerve

FIGURE EF-6 Course of peripheral nerves at level of the elbow and the volar forearm.

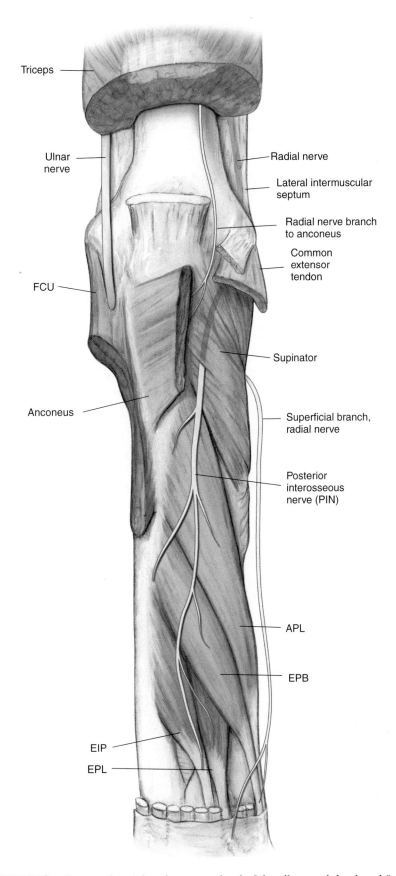

Triceps

Ulnar nerve

FCU

Anconeus

EIP

EPL

Radial nerve

Lateral intermuscular septum

Radial nerve branch to anconeus

Common extensor tendon

Supinator

Superficial branch, radial nerve

Posterior interosseous nerve (PIN)

APL

EPB

FIGURE EF-7 Course of peripheral nerves at level of the elbow and the dorsal forearm.

Surgical intervals are commonly between internervous planes allowing for safest exposure of desired structures; the internervous planes for common approaches to the elbow and forearm are depicted in Figures EF-8 through EF-11

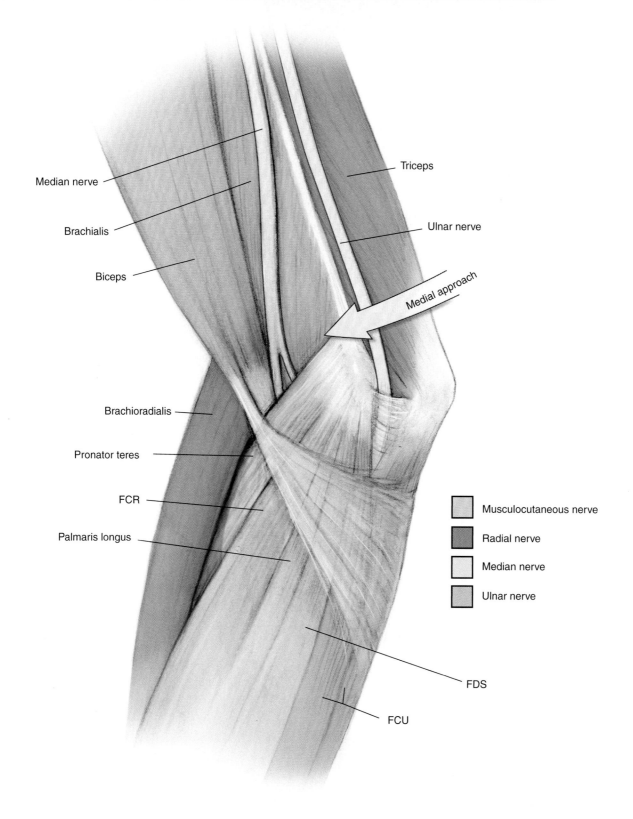

Median nerve

Brachialis

Biceps

Brachioradialis

Pronator teres

FCR

Palmaris longus

Triceps

Ulnar nerve

Medial approach

Musculocutaneous nerve

Radial nerve

Median nerve

Ulnar nerve

FDS

FCU

FIGURE EF-8 Internervous planes for medial approaches to the elbow.

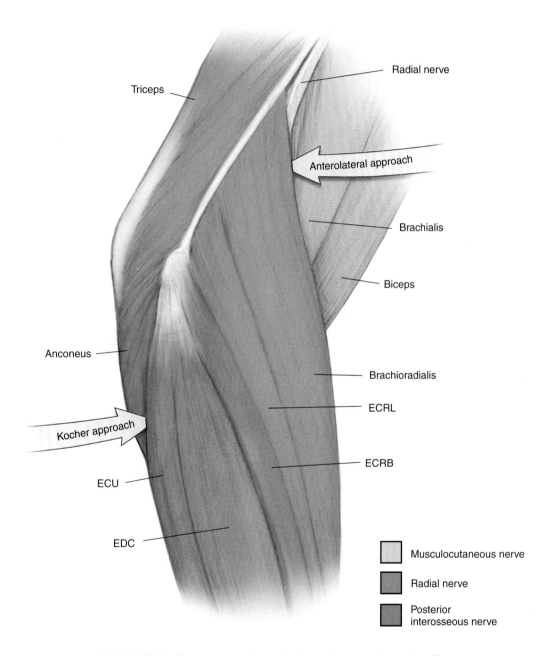

FIGURE EF-9 Internervous planes for lateral approaches to the elbow.

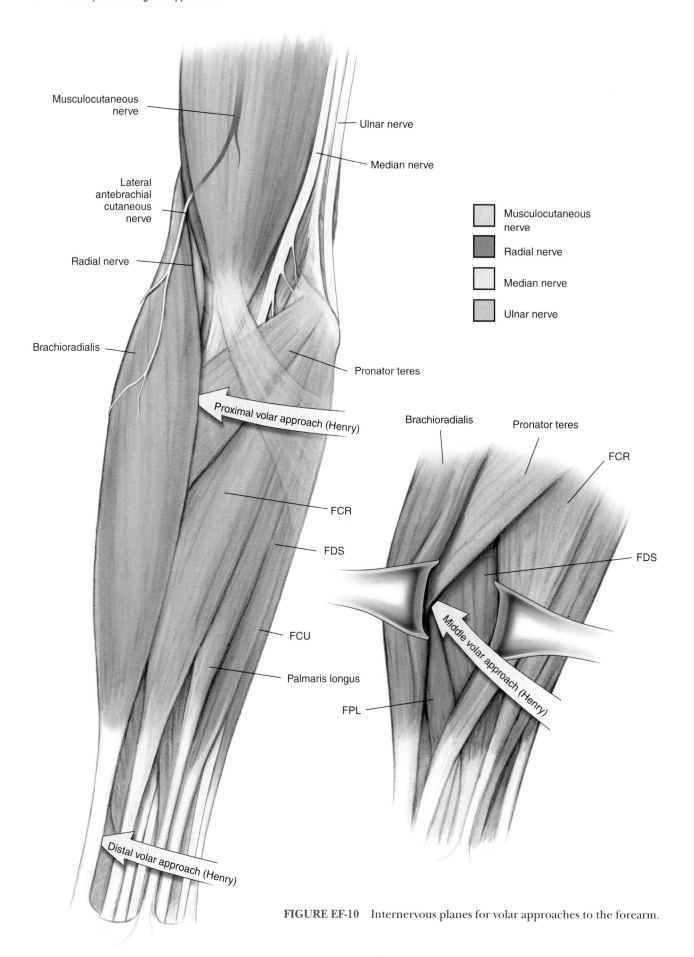

Musculocutaneous nerve

Ulnar nerve

Median nerve

Lateral antebrachial cutaneous nerve

Radial nerve

Brachioradialis

Pronator teres

Musculocutaneous nerve

Radial nerve

Median nerve

Ulnar nerve

Proximal volar approach (Henry)

Brachioradialis

Pronator teres

FCR

FCR

FDS

FDS

FCU

FPL

Palmaris longus

Middle volar approach (Henry)

Distal volar approach (Henry)

FIGURE EF-10   Internervous planes for volar approaches to the forearm.

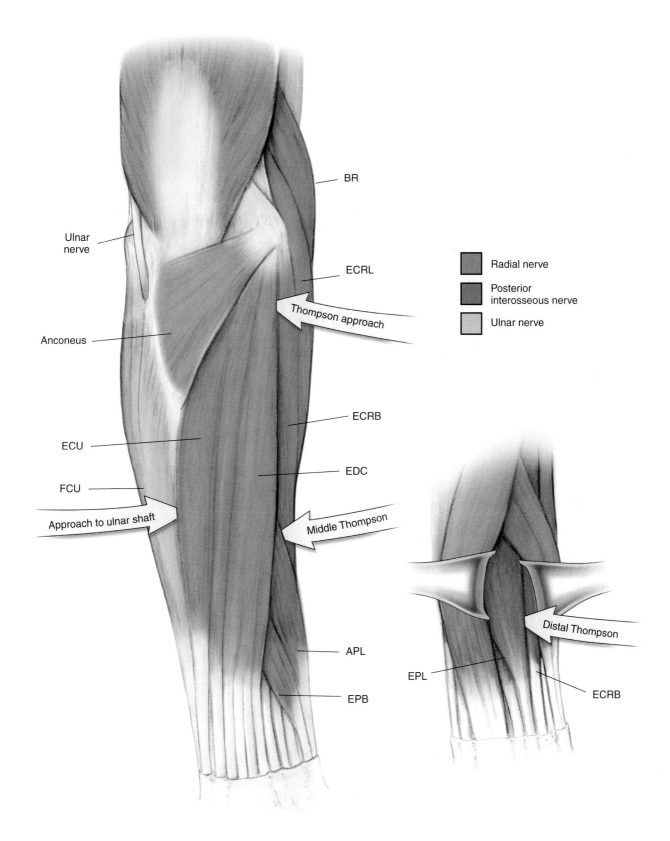

FIGURE EF-11 Internervous planes for dorsal approaches to the forearm.

Vascular (Figure EF-12)

- **Brachial artery**

  - Approaches anterior elbow on medial side of biceps brachii muscle; median nerve lies medial to artery
  - Artery branches at approximately the level of the radial neck
    - Radial artery
      - Passes under bicipital aponeurosis
      - Gives off radial recurrent artery as first branch
      - Continues into forearm under brachioradialis muscle belly and emerges between brachioradialis and FCR tendons before entering wrist and hand
    - Ulnar artery
      - Larger of the 2 branches
      - Gives off ulnar anterior or posterior recurrent artery, or both, as first branch
      - Continues into forearm with ulnar nerve between FDS and FDP muscle bellies and emerges in distal forearm between FDS and FCU tendons before entering wrist and hand
      - Common interosseous artery branches at a level just distal to the radial tuberosity, then divides into
        - Anterior interosseous artery: lies anterior to interosseous membrane between FDP and FPL in the forearm; travels with anterior interosseous nerve
        - Posterior interosseous artery: passes to posterior arm between oblique cord and proximal border of interosseous membrane and emerges from under the inferior border of the supinator and continues down the posterior forearm supplying the superficial extensor muscles; travels with PIN
        - Anterior and posterior interosseous arteries reanastomose at the distal end of interosseous membrane

- **Basilic and cephalic veins**

  - Basilic vein lies medially in arm
  - Cephalic vein lies laterally in arm
  - Anastomose via the median cubital vein in cubital fossa superficial to biceps brachii tendon
  - Continue superficially in forearm

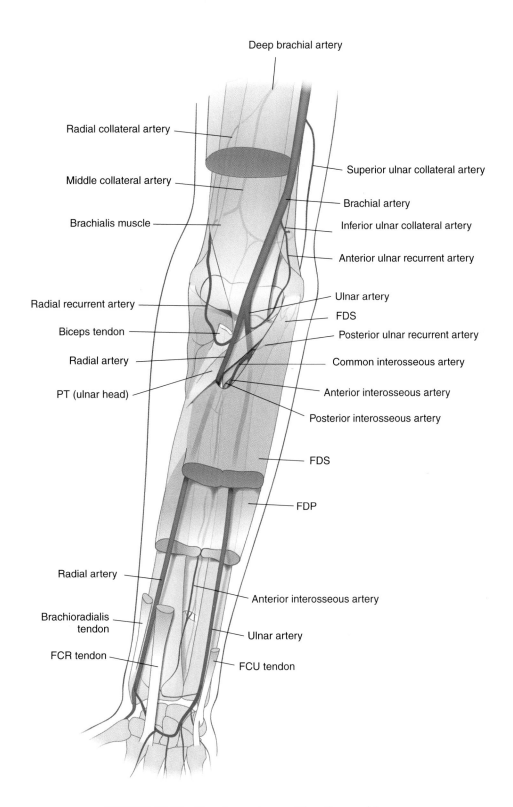

FIGURE EF-12   Vascular anatomy of the elbow and forearm.

Cross-sectional anatomy at proximal, middle, and distal portions of the forearm

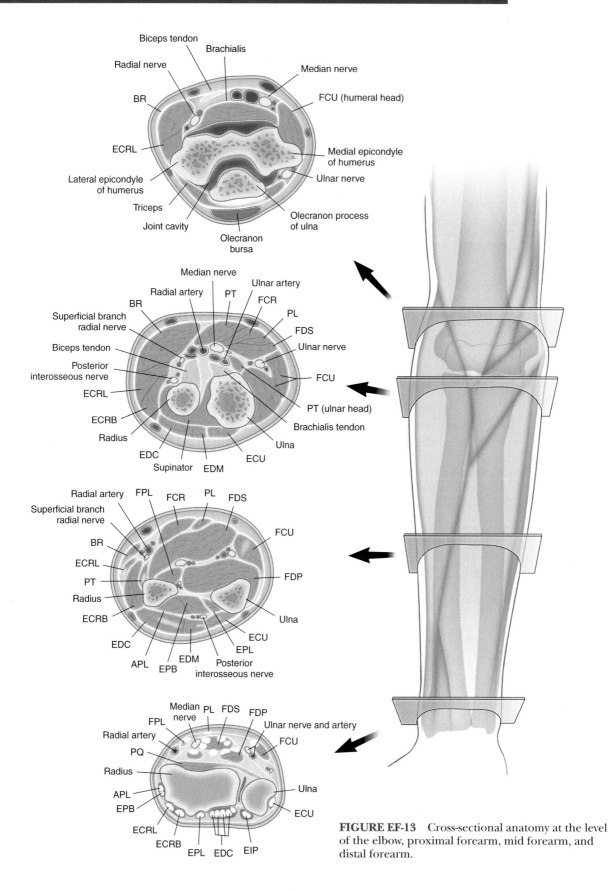

FIGURE EF-13 Cross-sectional anatomy at the level of the elbow, proximal forearm, mid forearm, and distal forearm.

Palpable anatomical landmarks for surgical incisions and approaches

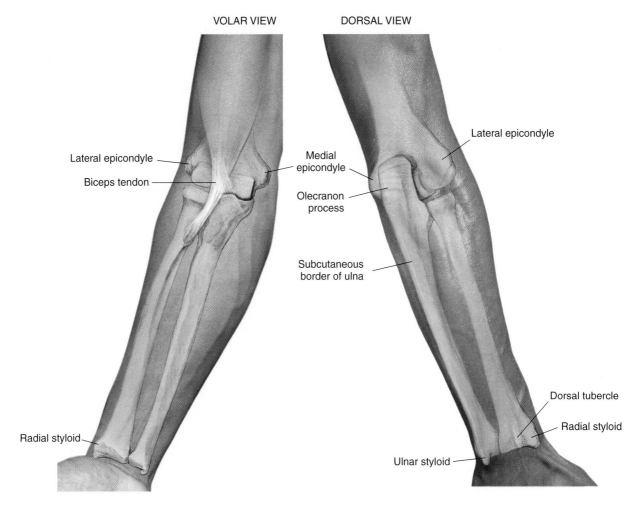

VOLAR VIEW

DORSAL VIEW

Lateral epicondyle

Biceps tendon

Medial epicondyle

Olecranon process

Lateral epicondyle

Subcutaneous border of ulna

Dorsal tubercle

Radial styloid

Radial styloid

Ulnar styloid

FIGURE EF-14   Palpable anatomical landmarks for surgical incisions and approaches.

Hazards

- **Nerves**

  - ▧ Radial nerve
    - During posterior approach to humerus, lateral approach to humerus, and Kocher approach
  - ▧ PIN
    - Vulnerable to compression or traction injury as it travels around radial neck between the 2 origins of the supinator muscle; vulnerable to injury during the Kocher approach, antecubital approach, and dorsal approach to the forearm
  - ▧ Lateral antebrachial cutaneous nerve
    - Retract with skin flap in anterolateral approach to the elbow
    - Be cautious during anterior approach to the cubital fossa to avoid injury during incision of deep fascia
  - ▧ Ulnar nerve
    - Identify and isolate during medial approach to the elbow
    - Strip FCU off of ulna subperiosteally to avoid dissection into muscle to avoid injury to nerve
  - ▧ Median nerve
    - During medial approach to the elbow, avoid traction of nerve during distal dissection; identify during antecubital approach to the elbow

- **Vascular**

  - ▧ Brachial artery
    - Identify and protect during anterior approach to the elbow
  - ▧ Radial artery
    - Ligate recurrent branches of radial artery during mobilization of the brachioradialis to prevent postoperative bleeding
    - During anterior approach to the elbow be cautious while incising bicipital aponeurosis because radial artery courses directly underneath
    - Be cautious when mobilizing brachioradialis muscle during anterior approach to the forearm because the artery lies directly under the muscle belly

ANTERIOR APPROACH TO ELBOW (ANTECUBITAL FOSSA)

Indications: Median or radial nerve repairs, brachial artery repair, biceps tendon repair, capsular release, tumor or mass excision

POSITIONING (FIGURE EF-15)

● Supine, arm in supination on hand table, exsanguinate limb, and elevate tourniquet

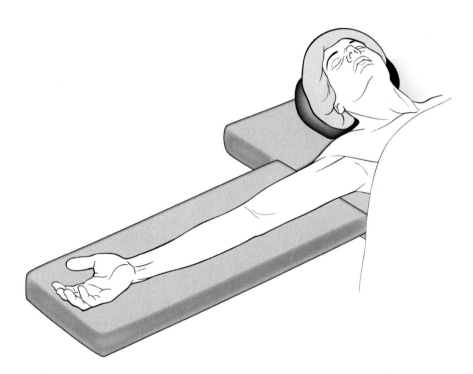

FIGURE EF-15   Positioning for anterior approach to the elbow.

INCISION (FIGURE EF-16)

● Curved incision beginning transversely in flexion crease, extending proximally along medial border of biceps muscle, and extending distally along radial border of brachioradialis muscle

● Avoid creating 90-degree angles when crossing flexion crease

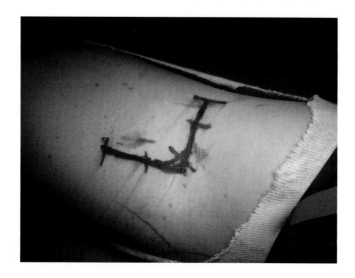

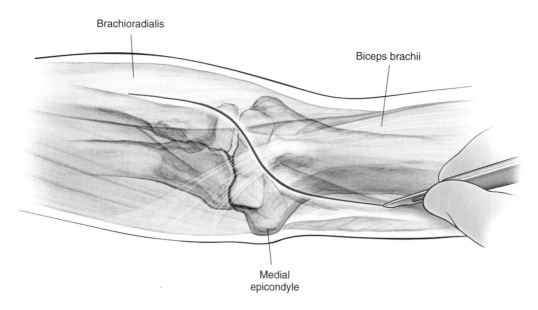

FIGURE EF-16   Surgical incision for anterior approach to the elbow.

SUPERFICIAL DISSECTION (FIGURES EF-17 AND EF-18)

- Incise skin and subcutaneous tissues carefully to avoid violating medial or lateral antebrachial cutaneous nerves, which lie in close proximity

- Incise fascia overlying muscles, and identify and protect lateral cutaneous nerve to forearm, which lies just lateral to biceps muscle

- Carefully incise and reflect biceps aponeurosis (lacertus fibrosus) near its origin on biceps tendon

- Identify several structures—brachial artery lies directly under aponeurosis and bifurcates just distal to this point to become the radial and ulnar arteries; median nerve and brachial vein also are in this area

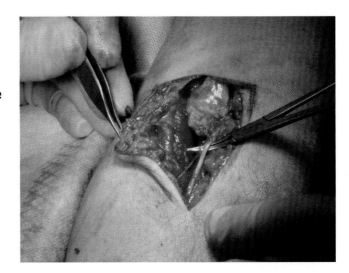

- The median nerve is the most medial structure

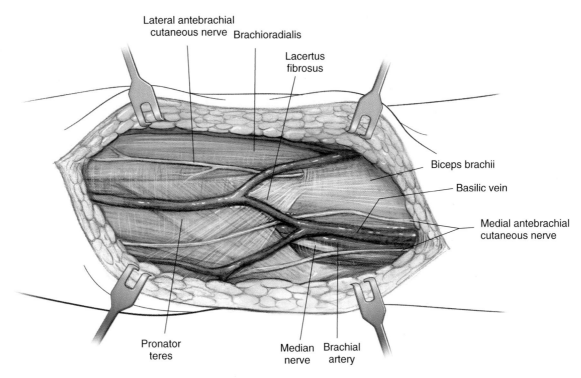

FIGURE EF-17 Anterior approach to elbow. Superficial dissection with exposure of the lateral antebrachial cutaneous nerve, superficial veins, lacertus fibrosus, and fascia.

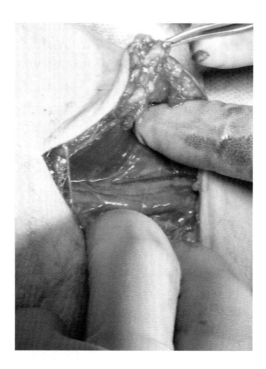

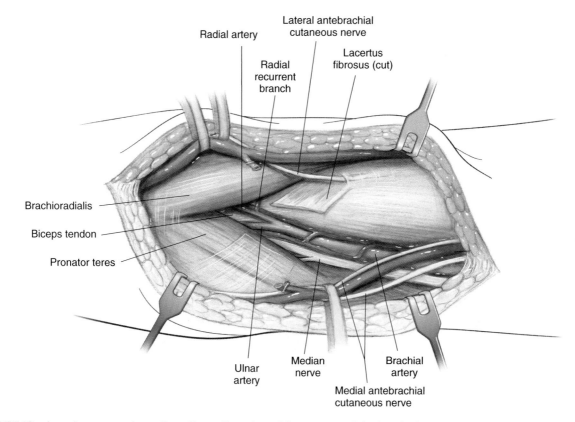

FIGURE EF-18   Anterior approach to elbow. Deep dissection with exposure of the brachial artery and median nerve. The interval between the brachioradialis and pronator teres is identified. Supinate the forearm to protect PIN.

DEEP DISSECTION (FIGURES EF-19 AND EF-20)

- Retract brachioradialis muscle laterally and pronator teres muscle medially; fully supinate forearm to protect PIN

- Identify recurrent branches of radial artery, and ligate them to allow for deeper dissection

- Identify and carefully incise supinator muscle from its origin, and subperiosteally dissect on radius to expose anterior elbow joint capsule

- Carefully identify and protect PIN and superficial sensory nerve branches in anterior elbow

- Incise joint capsule to expose anterior elbow joint

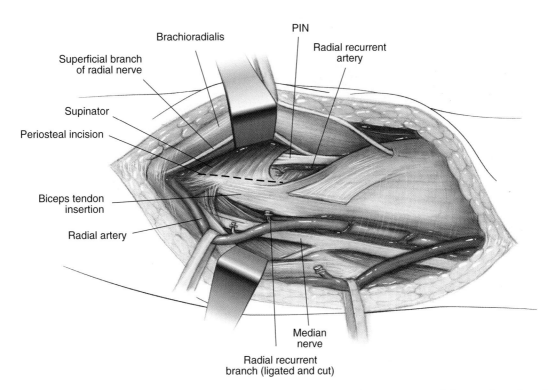

FIGURE EF-19 Anterior approach to elbow. Deep dissection and ligation of the recurrent radial artery branches. Subperiosteally reflect the supinator muscle, protecting PIN, to expose the anterior joint capsule.

CLOSURE

- Close subcutaneous tissue and skin with suture after hemostasis is obtained

HAZARDS

- Medial and lateral antebrachial cutaneous nerves
- Median nerve
- Brachial artery and vein and their branches, including radial and ulnar arteries
- PIN

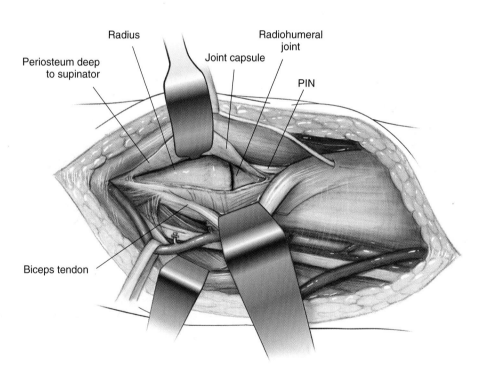

FIGURE EF-20   Anterior approach to elbow. Exposure of the anterior elbow joint.

MEDIAL APPROACH TO ELBOW AND HUMERUS

Indications: Transposition of ulnar nerve, medial epicondyle débridement, open reduction and internal fixation (ORIF) of coronoid process fractures or medial epicondyle and condyle fractures, contracture release, heterotopic ossification excision, medial collateral ligament reconstruction

POSITIONING (FIGURE EF-21)

- Supine, arm in supination on hand table
- Can flex elbow and bring across patient's body after exposure

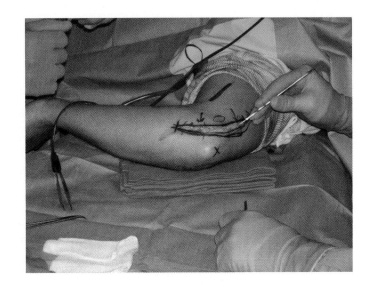

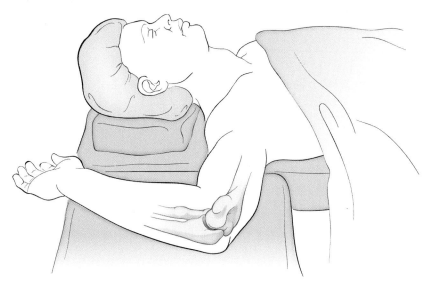

FIGURE EF-21   Positioning for medial approach to the elbow.

INCISION (FIGURE EF-22)

- 8-10 cm longitudinally centered between olecranon tip and medial epicondyle

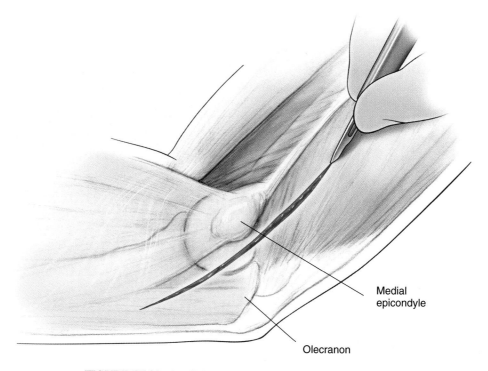

Medial
epicondyle

Olecranon

FIGURE EF-22   Medial approach to elbow. Surgical incision.

SUPERFICIAL DISSECTION (FIGURES EF-23, EF-24, AND EF-25)

- Skin and subcutaneous tissues are carefully dissected; medial antebrachial nerve branches are identified distal to the medial epicondyle and protected; ulnar nerve is identified within fascia posterior to medial epicondyle

- Incise fascia and all points of compression over ulnar nerve to isolate and protect nerve during exposure

- Resect medial intermuscular septum, and decompress sites of ulnar nerve compression if ulnar nerve transposition is planned

- Epicondyle and medial column can be exposed for ORIF after ulnar nerve is transposed

- Incise fascia over superficial flexor muscles, and retract this anteriorly to expose common flexor tendon origin on medial epicondyle

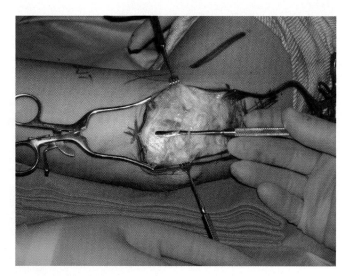

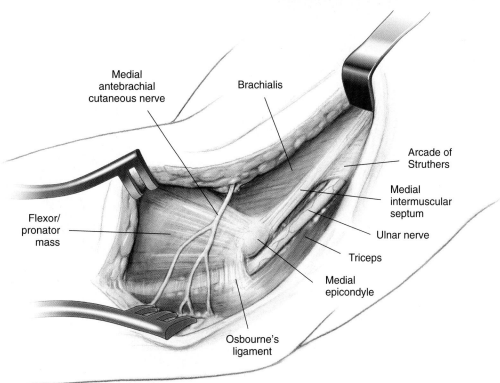

FIGURE EF-23 Medial approach to elbow. Superficial dissection with exposure of the medial antebrachial cutaneous nerves, ulnar nerve, and flexor pronator fascia.

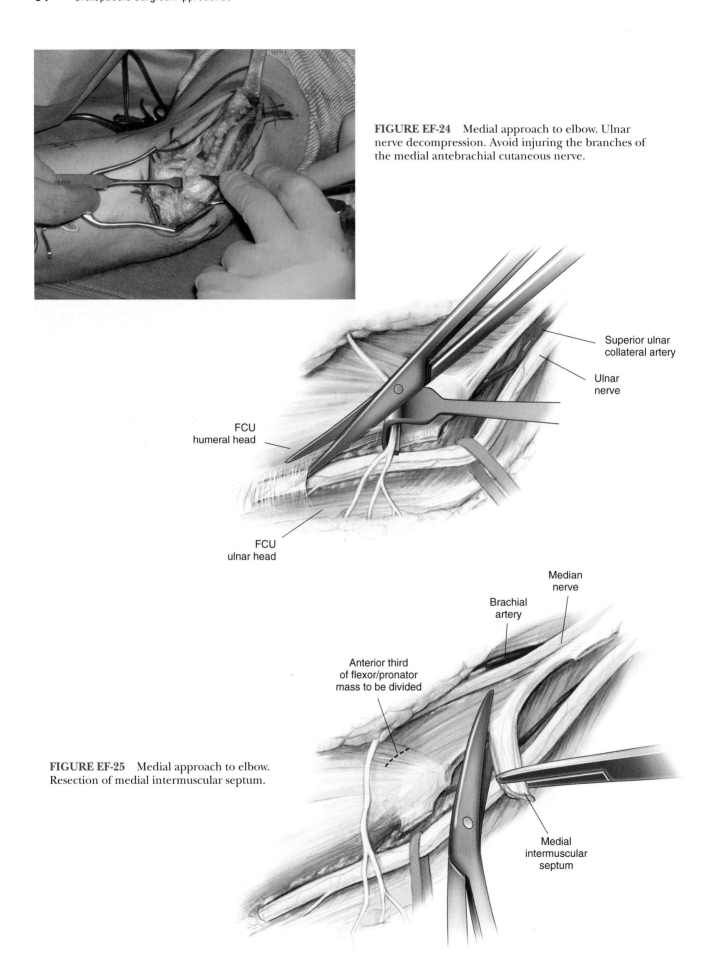

FIGURE EF-24 Medial approach to elbow. Ulnar nerve decompression. Avoid injuring the branches of the medial antebrachial cutaneous nerve.

Superior ulnar collateral artery

Ulnar nerve

FCU humeral head

FCU ulnar head

Median nerve

Brachial artery

Anterior third of flexor/pronator mass to be divided

Medial intermuscular septum

FIGURE EF-25 Medial approach to elbow. Resection of medial intermuscular septum.

DEEP DISSECTION (FIGURES EF-26 AND EF-27)

- Visualize and protect the ulnar nerve at all times

- Incise anterior one third of flexor pronator fascia and underlying muscle, and divide proximally leaving a cuff of tendon for repair

- Elevate underneath flexor pronator muscle, and expose elbow capsule; place Homan retractor under brachialis muscle to protect median nerve and brachial artery

- Capsulectomy can be performed at this time to expose elbow joint; coronoid fractures can be exposed and ORIF performed with this exposure

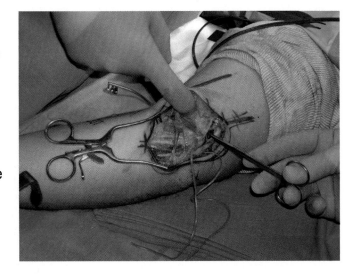

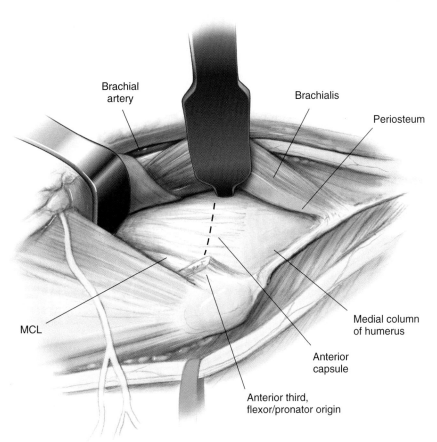

FIGURE EF-26 Medial approach to elbow. Deep dissection with protection of the ulnar nerve. Incise the anterior one third of the flexor pronator fascia, and elevate the flexor pronator muscle mass to expose the elbow capsule.

EXTENSION

- Proximal extension can be performed along medial supracondylar ridge

- Take care to prevent injury to medial collateral ligament origin on posterior aspect of medial epicondyle

- Dissection can be followed proximally in subperiosteal manner to expose medial condyle and humeral shaft for ORIF of medial column fractures

- Distal extension is limited by ulnar nerve and flexor pronator mass

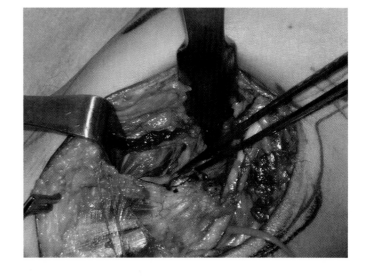

CLOSURE

- Transpose ulnar nerve if indicated

- Close subcutaneous tissue and skin with suture

HAZARDS

- Medial antebrachial cutaneous nerve

- Ulnar nerve

- Median nerve

- Brachial artery

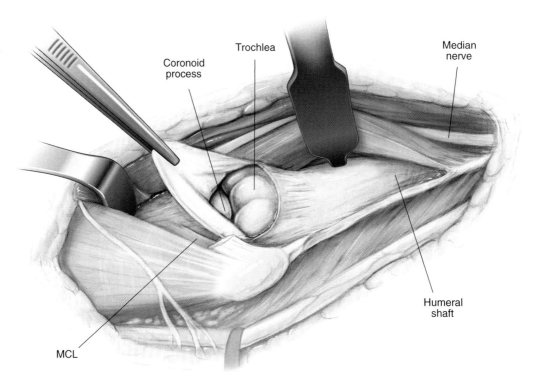

FIGURE EF-27 Medial approach to elbow. Deep dissection. Incise the capsule to expose the elbow joint.

KOCHER APPROACH (LATERAL ELBOW)

INDICATIONS: Radial head ORIF, radial head arthroplasty, capsular release, ORIF of capitulum, ORIF of radial column of humerus

POSITIONING (FIGURE EF-28)

- Patient supine, arm on hand table; exsanguinate limb, and elevate tourniquet
- Keep forearm pronated to protect PIN (Figure EF-29)

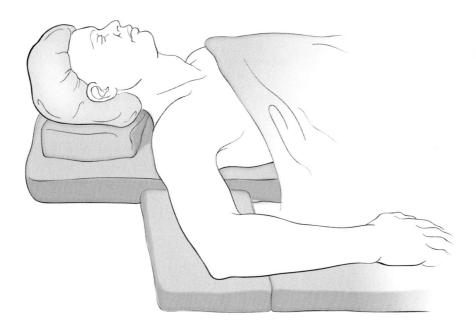

FIGURE EF-28   Positioning for lateral approach to elbow (Kocher).

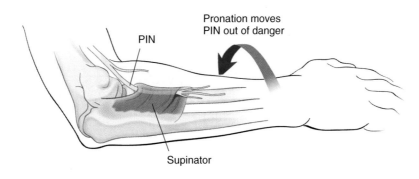

PIN

Pronation moves
PIN out of danger

Supinator

FIGURE EF-29   Pronate forearm to protect PIN.

INCISION (FIGURE EF-30)

- Anterior to lateral epicondyle at an oblique angle centered on level of radial head

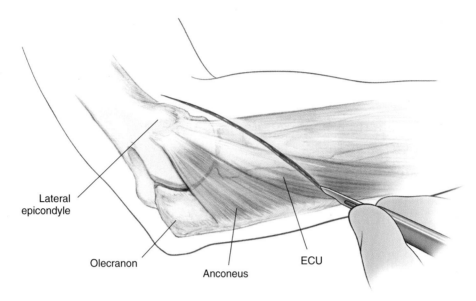

FIGURE EF-30   Incision for Kocher approach to elbow.

SUPERFICIAL DISSECTION (FIGURE EF-31)

- Skin and subcutaneous dissection to expose fascia overlying anconeus and ECU

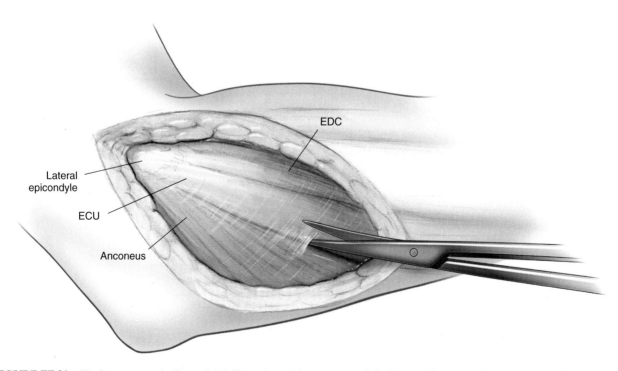

FIGURE EF-31   Kocher approach. Superficial dissection with exposure of the interval between the anconeus and ECU.

DEEP DISSECTION

- Interval is between ECU (PIN innervated) and anconeus (proper radial nerve innervated); divide fascia between these muscles, and split this interval bluntly to expose underlying annular ligament and joint capsule

- Keep forearm pronated to protect PIN (Figure EF-32)

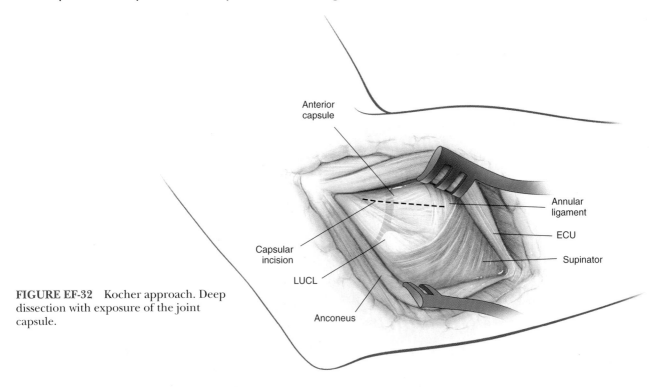

FIGURE EF-32 Kocher approach. Deep dissection with exposure of the joint capsule.

- Divide capsule and annular ligament longitudinally to expose radiocapitellar joint

- Limit distal dissection to distal extent of annular ligament to avoid injuring PIN (Figure EF-33)

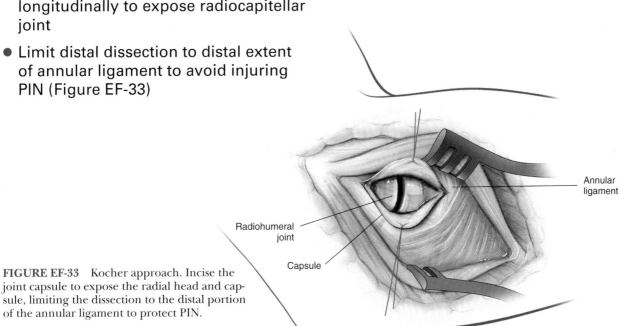

FIGURE EF-33 Kocher approach. Incise the joint capsule to expose the radial head and capsule, limiting the dissection to the distal portion of the annular ligament to protect PIN.

EXTENSION (FIGURES EF-34 AND EF-35)

- Proximal extension can be performed along lateral supracondylar ridge with subperiosteal exposure of anterior humerus and lateral column

- Place retractor underneath brachialis to protect radial nerve

- Lateral collateral ligament reconstructions and ORIF of distal humerus and lateral column fractures can be performed with this proximal extension

- Distal extension is limited by PIN, and dissection should be limited to level of annular ligament

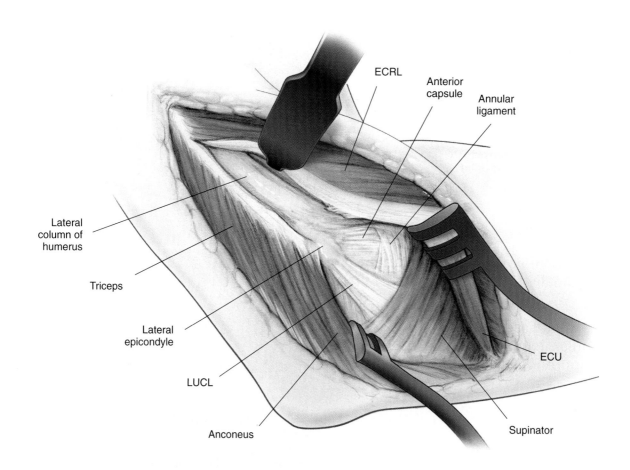

FIGURE EF-34 Kocher approach. Proximal extension along the lateral supracondylar ridge.

CLOSURE

● Subcutaneous tissue and skin are closed with suture after hemostasis

HAZARDS

● PIN
● Radial nerve
● Lateral collateral ligament complex

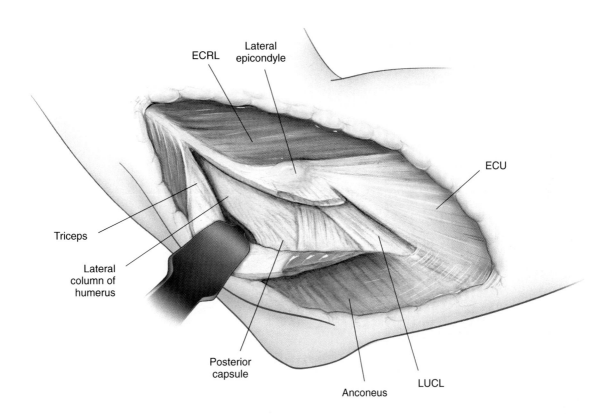

FIGURE EF-35 Kocher approach. Subperiosteally elevate the triceps and the brachialis to expose the lateral column of the humerus.

BRYAN-MORREY APPROACH (TRICEPS SPARING APPROACH)

Indications: ORIF of supracondylar and intercondylar humerus fractures, total elbow arthroplasty, removal of loose bodies

POSITIONING (FIGURE EF-36)

- Patient in lateral decubitus position with operative arm across chest and elbow in flexion

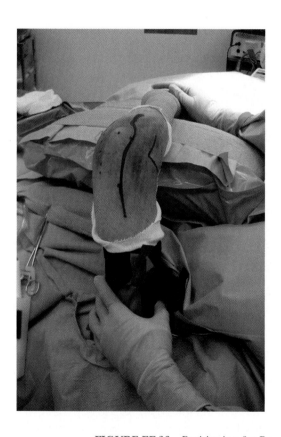
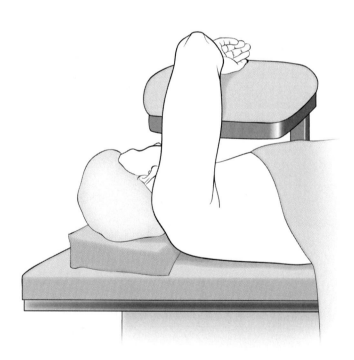

FIGURE EF-36   Positioning for Bryan-Morrey approach (triceps sparing) to the posterior elbow.

INCISION

- Identify surface anatomy, including medial epicondyle, lateral epicondyle, olecranon, and ulnar nerve within cubital tunnel
- Longitudinal incision is made at posterior aspect of humerus beginning 10 cm proximal to olecranon, curving medially or laterally around olecranon, and continuing distally over ulna border (Figure EF-37)

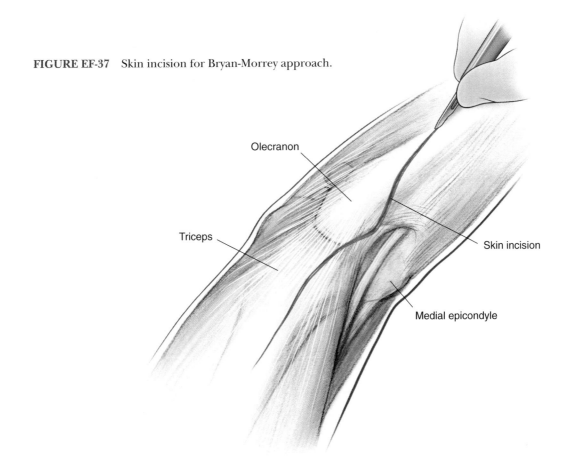

FIGURE EF-37   Skin incision for Bryan-Morrey approach.

Olecranon

Triceps

Skin incision

Medial epicondyle

SUPERFICIAL DISSECTION (FIGURES EF-38 AND EF-39)

- Incise skin and subcutaneous tissues
- Identify and isolate ulnar nerve as it emerges from medial intramuscular septum and enters cubital tunnel
- Transpose ulnar nerve anteriorly after decompression and excision of medial intermuscular septum

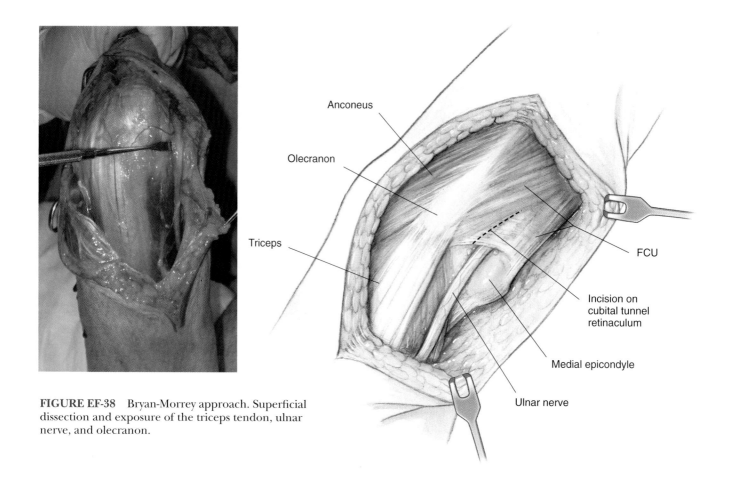

Anconeus

Olecranon

Triceps

FCU

Incision on cubital tunnel retinaculum

Medial epicondyle

Ulnar nerve

FIGURE EF-38 Bryan-Morrey approach. Superficial dissection and exposure of the triceps tendon, ulnar nerve, and olecranon.

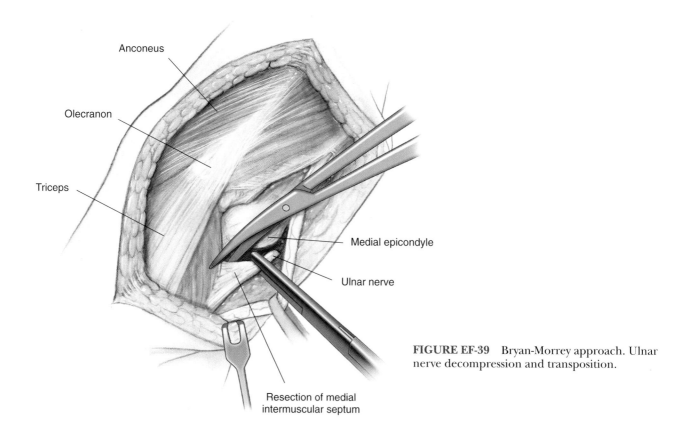

Anconeus

Olecranon

Triceps

Medial epicondyle

Ulnar nerve

Resection of medial intermuscular septum

FIGURE EF-39 Bryan-Morrey approach. Ulnar nerve decompression and transposition.

DEEP DISSECTION (FIGURES EF-40 AND EF-41)

- Identify medial aspect of triceps muscle, and bluntly release fascia to reflect muscle laterally; release triceps from entire distal humerus, taking care to avoid releasing too proximally and injuring radial nerve within radial groove

- Incise the forearm fascia and ulna periosteum on medial aspect of ulna, and reflect laterally

- Sharply incise triceps tendon insertion from olecranon process, and begin retracting triceps laterally

- Identify and subperiosteally incise insertion site of anconeus on ulna, and reflect laterally with triceps tendon

- Elevate entire triceps insertion and periosteal expansion of ulna to expose distal humerus; take care so that triceps mechanism is not disrupted transversely

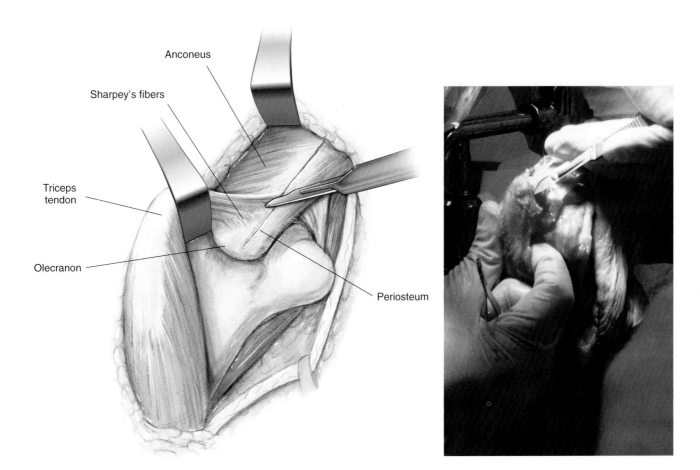

FIGURE EF-40 Bryan-Morrey approach. Elevation of the triceps mechanism from medial to lateral with subperiosteal elevation off the olecranon tip and the proximal ulna. Do not disrupt the triceps mechanism transversely.

- Bring elbow into full flexion to identify lateral ulnar collateral ligament and medial collateral ligament; protect ligaments during fracture fixation

- With elbow extensor mechanism reflected laterally, entire ulnohumeral joint can be exposed

- If more exposure is needed, olecranon process (tip) can be osteotomized

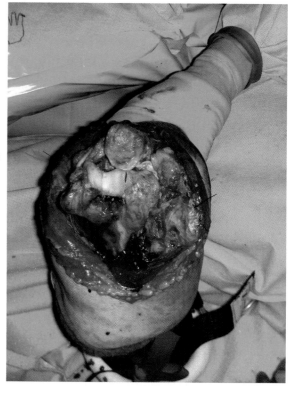

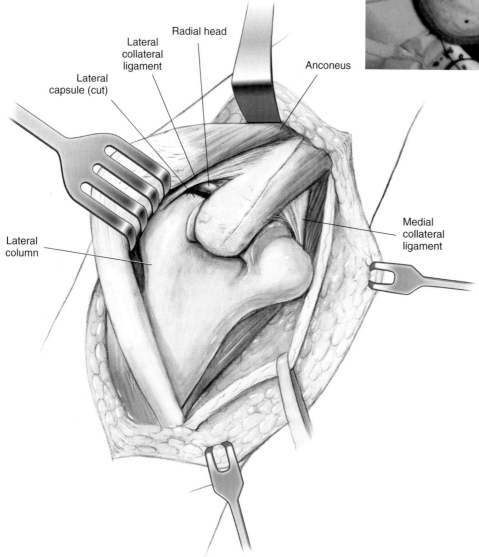

FIGURE EF-41 Bryan-Morrey approach. Exposure of the elbow joint.

CLOSURE (FIGURE EF-42)

- Reapproximate all intervals, and repair insertion site of triceps

- Drill 2 holes in a cruciate manner across olecranon; reapproximate triceps tendon over olecranon, and pass a suture from distal to proximal through one hole, up the triceps tendon using a Bunnell-type technique, and pass back through olecranon from proximal to distal using opposite drill hole

- Transpose ulnar nerve

- Close skin and subcutaneous tissue with suture or staples

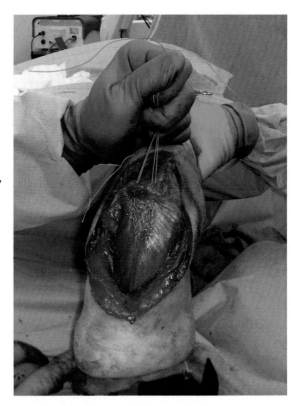

HAZARDS

- Radial nerve running in radial groove of humerus when elevating medial triceps

- Ulnar nerve during initial exposure

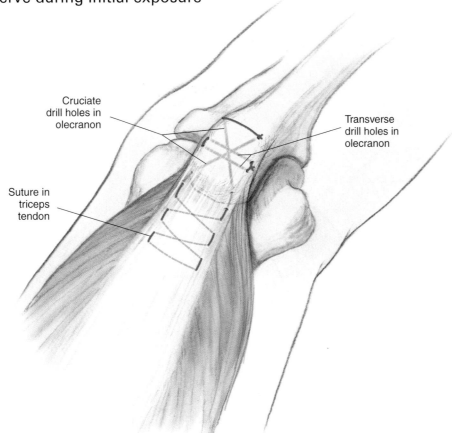

FIGURE EF-42 Bryan-Morrey approach. Repair of the triceps mechanism.

TRICEPS SPLITTING APPROACH

Indications: ORIF of distal third humerus fractures, synovectomy, total elbow arthroplasty, ulnohumeral arthroplasty

POSITIONING (SEE FIGURE EF-36)

- Patient in lateral decubitus position with operative arm across chest, elbow in flexion

INCISION (FIGURE EF-43)

- Identify medial epicondyle, lateral epicondyle, olecranon, and ulnar nerve within cubital tunnel
- Perform longitudinal incision at posterior aspect of the humerus beginning 8 cm proximal to olecranon and extend to just past olecranon tip

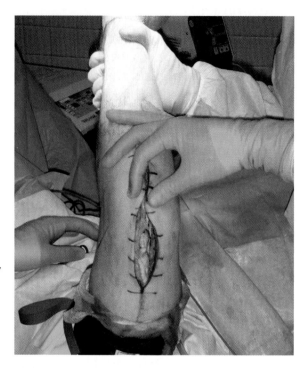

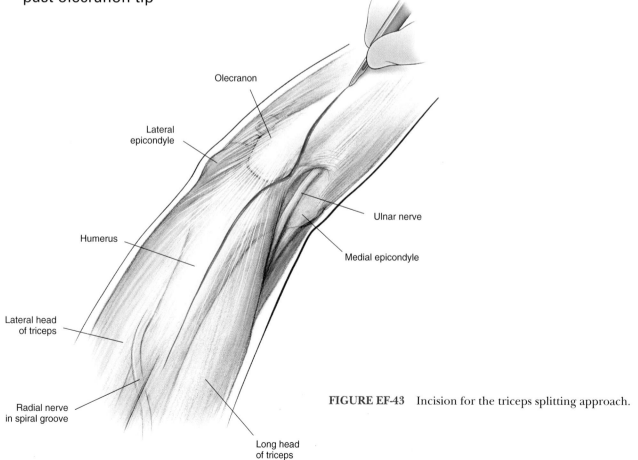

FIGURE EF-43 Incision for the triceps splitting approach.

SUPERFICIAL DISSECTION (FIGURE EF-44)

- Incise the skin and subcutaneous tissues

- Identify and protect the ulnar nerve

- Split the triceps tendon midline to the olecranon tip; do not disrupt the triceps insertion

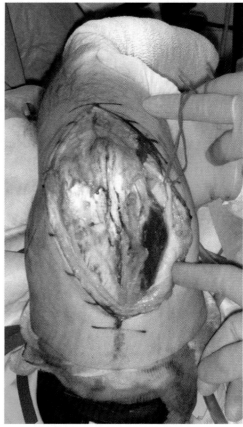

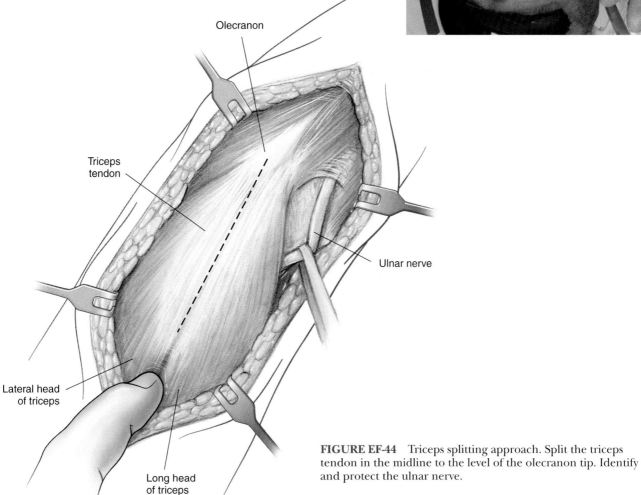

FIGURE EF-44 Triceps splitting approach. Split the triceps tendon in the midline to the level of the olecranon tip. Identify and protect the ulnar nerve.

DEEP DISSECTION (FIGURE EF-45)

- Triceps split is extended proximally between the interval of the long and lateral head of the triceps; it is often easier to find this interval and proceed distally

- Medial head of the triceps is identified, and radial nerve is identified and protected proximally; proximal extension is limited by the course of the radial nerve

- Medial head of the triceps is identified and split after radial nerve is identified proximally

- Humeral shaft is exposed in subperiosteal manner

CLOSURE

- Interval between the long and lateral heads is approximated

- Split in the triceps tendon is closed with nonabsorbable suture

- Close the skin and subcutaneous tissue with suture or staples

HAZARDS

- Radial nerve in spiral groove of humerus during exposure

- Ulnar nerve during superficial dissection

- Proximal dissection limited by radial nerve

- Distal dissection limited to triceps insertion on olecranon tip

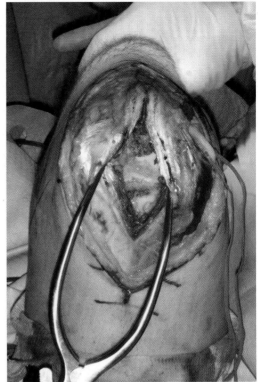

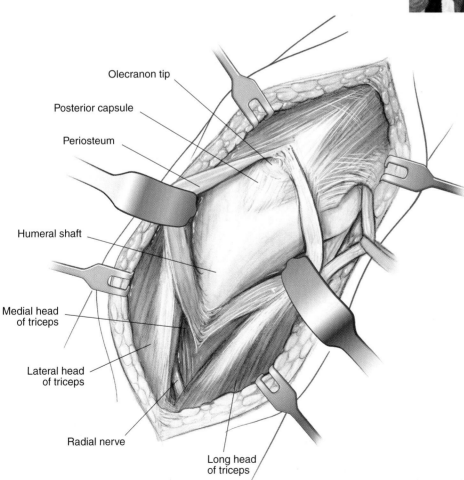

Olecranon tip

Posterior capsule

Periosteum

Humeral shaft

Medial head
of triceps

Lateral head
of triceps

Radial nerve

Long head
of triceps

FIGURE EF-45 Triceps sparing approach. Identify the interval between the long and lateral heads of the triceps. Identify the radial nerve proximally, and divide and subperiosteally elevate the medial head of the triceps to expose the distal humerus shaft.

OLECRANON OSTEOTOMY

Indications: ORIF of intra-articular distal humerus fractures

POSITIONING (SEE FIGURE EF-36)

- Prone versus supine on the table, arm across the patient's body
- Exsanguinate the limb, and elevate tourniquet

INCISION

- Identify olecranon process and medial and lateral epicondyles
- Begin posterior incision midline 5 cm above the olecranon process, and curve to lateral side of the olecranon process; extend incision distally remaining on the lateral aspect of the posterior forearm

SUPERFICIAL DISSECTION (FIGURE EF-46)

- Incise skin and subcutaneous tissue
- Bluntly release the overlying fascia, and identify the ulnar nerve
- Carefully incise the fascia over the ulnar nerve for exposure, and place vessel loops around the nerve for easy identification throughout procedure
- Gently retract nerve away from the osteotomy site
- Osteotomize the olecranon process in the shape of a "V" approximately 2 cm from the tip of the olecranon

DEEP DISSECTION (FIGURE EF-47)

- Reflect the olecranon tip, and elevate triceps muscle off of the humerus to widen the exposure
- Avoid dissecting too proximal on the humerus to avoid damage to the radial nerve as it courses in the spiral groove and toward the lateral intermuscular septum
- Entire distal humerus is exposed in this fashion

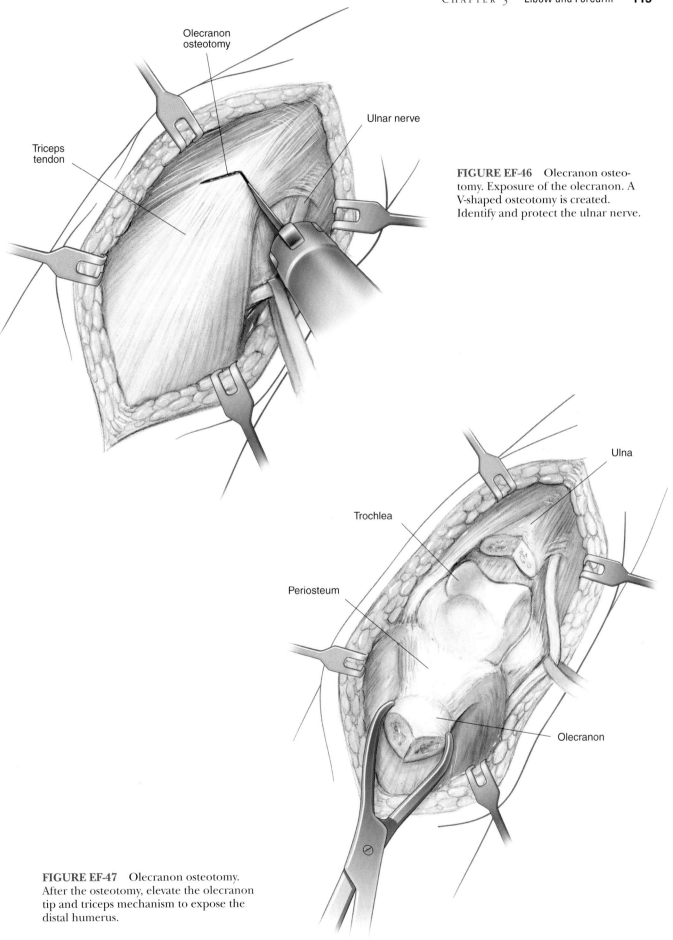

Olecranon
osteotomy

Ulnar nerve

Triceps
tendon

FIGURE EF-46   Olecranon osteo-
tomy. Exposure of the olecranon. A
V-shaped osteotomy is created.
Identify and protect the ulnar nerve.

Ulna

Trochlea

Periosteum

Olecranon

FIGURE EF-47   Olecranon osteotomy.
After the osteotomy, elevate the olecranon
tip and triceps mechanism to expose the
distal humerus.

CLOSURE (FIGURE EF-48)

● Repair olecranon with tension band technique

● Transpose the ulnar nerve before closure, particularly if hardware is placed along the medial column of the humerus

● Close subcutaneous tissues with absorbable suture

● Close skin with staples or suture

HAZARDS

● Ulnar nerve

  ▪ Be cautious during exposure and osteotomy to protect nerve and avoid traction injury

● Radial nerve

  ▪ At risk during stripping of triceps muscle from humerus

  ▪ Nerve runs through lateral intramuscular septum of triceps in distal third of muscle

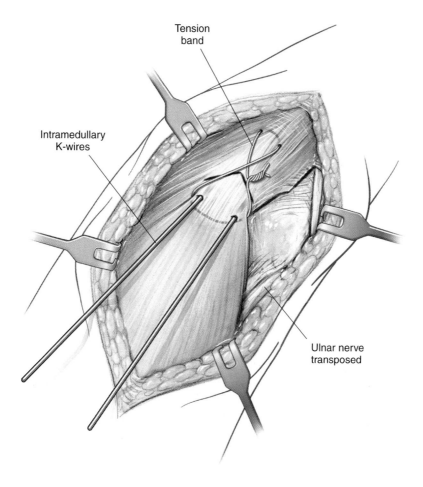

FIGURE EF-48 Repair of the olecranon osteotomy with a tension band technique.

ELBOW ARTHROSCOPY

Indications: Diagnostic evaluation of elbow, loose body removal, osteochondritis dissecans treatment, capsular and contracture release, lateral epicondylitis débridement, olecranon tip and fossa débridement, synovectomy

POSITIONING (FIGURE EF-49)

- Prone versus lateral decubitus (surgeon's preference) with arm in arm-holder
- Tourniquet may be used
- Gravity flow for joint

INCISION

- Draw anatomical landmarks, including olecranon, medial and lateral epicondyles, and ulnar nerve
- Mark all portals

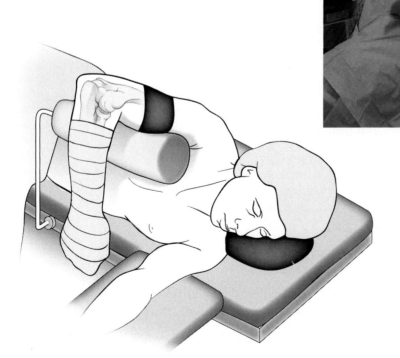

FIGURE EF-49   Positioning for elbow arthroscopy.

PORTALS (FIGURE EF-50)

- **Proximal anterolateral portal**
  - ▨ 2 cm proximal and 1 cm anterior to lateral epicondyle
    - Lateral gutter, capitulum, coronoid, trochlea, and radial head are visualized
    - Commonly used as a visualization portal
    - Radial nerve and PIN at risk

- **Anterolateral**
  - ▨ 3 cm distal and 1 cm anterior to lateral epicondyle
    - View distal humerus, trochlear ridges, coronoid process, and medial radial head
    - Use caution to avoid injury to the anterior branch of the posterior antebrachial cutaneous nerve and PIN
    - This portal is rarely used

- **Midlateral portal**
  - ▨ In soft area between radial head, olecranon tip, and lateral epicondyle
    - Use this portal as a working portal
    - PIN is at risk

- **Proximal anteromedial portal**
  - ▨ 2 cm proximal to medial epicondyle, just anterior to medial intramuscular septum
  - ▨ Anterior capsule, capitulum, trochlea, radial head, and medial and lateral gutters are visualized
  - ▨ Commonly used as a visualization portal
  - ▨ Ulnar nerve, median nerve, and brachial artery are at risk

- **Anteromedial portal**
  - ▨ 2 cm distal and 2 cm anterior to medial epicondyle—create under direct visualization using a blunt trochar
  - ▨ Capitulum, trochlea, coronoid, and radial head are seen when forearm is in pronation

- **Proximal posterolateral portal**
  - ▨ 2-3 cm proximal to olecranon process just lateral to triceps tendon
    - Olecranon tip and fossa are visualized

- **Central posterior portal**
  - ▨ 3 cm proximal to the olecranon tip, midline on the triceps tendon
    - Use this portal as a working portal for posterior compartment procedures

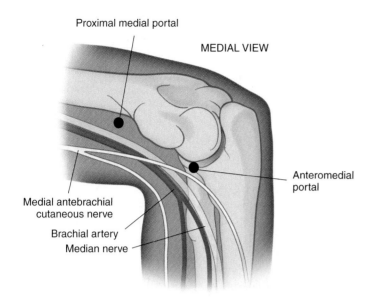

Proximal medial portal

MEDIAL VIEW

Anteromedial portal

Medial antebrachial cutaneous nerve

Brachial artery

Median nerve

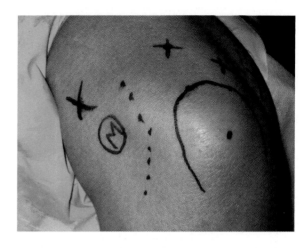

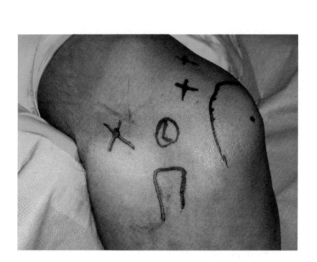

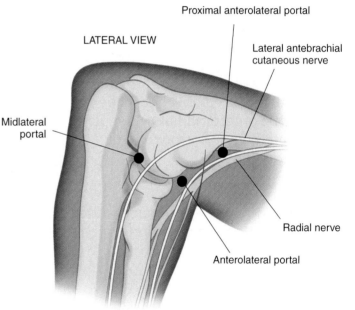

Proximal anterolateral portal

Lateral antebrachial cutaneous nerve

LATERAL VIEW

Midlateral portal

Radial nerve

Anterolateral portal

POSTERIOR VIEW

Posterior antebrachial cutaneous nerve

Proximal posterolateral portal

Central posterior portal

Distal posterolateral portal

Ulnar nerve

Triceps tendon

Midlateral portal

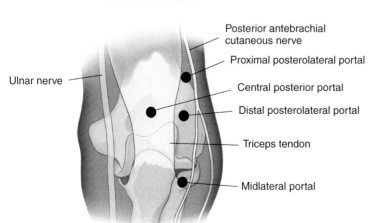

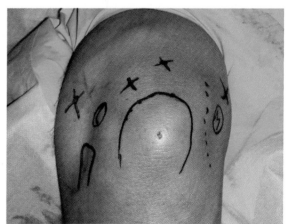

FIGURE EF-50 Portals for elbow arthroscopy with relationship to neurovascular structures.

TECHNIQUE (FIGURES EF-51 THROUGH EF-56)

- Patient is positioned, and anatomic landmarks are drawn
    - Ulnar nerve, medial intermuscular septum, and lateral intermuscular septum are palpated and marked
    - Beware of subluxating ulnar nerve
    - Sterile tourniquet is applied to the arm, and the patient is prepared and draped

- Portals are identified and marked, including proximal anterolateral, proximal anteromedial, proximal posterolateral, and midlateral portals

- Tourniquet is inflated, and 30 mL of saline is injected into the elbow joint at the elbow soft spot

- Proximal anteromedial portal is identified, and skin and subcutaneous tissues are incised with a no. 11 blade
    - Arthroscope is introduced into the joint via a blunt trocar
    - Gravity inflow is established

- Proximal anterolateral portal or anterolateral portal is identified and established under direct visualization from the proximal anteromedial portal using a blunt trocar; diagnostic evaluation is performed

- Proximal posterolateral portal is established next, and evaluation of the posterior compartment is performed

- Remaining portals are made under direct visualization depending on the pathology encountered and the procedure indicated

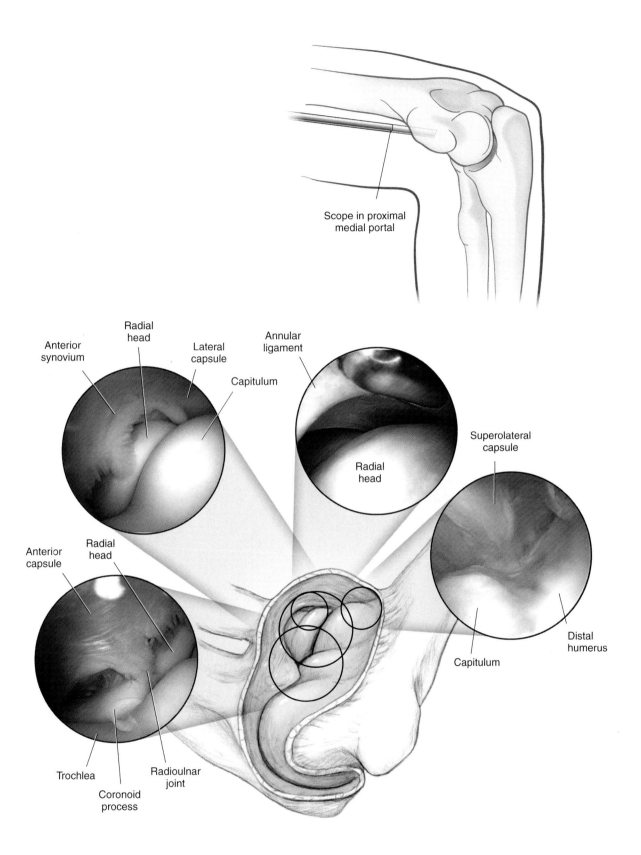

FIGURE EF-51   Visualization from the proximal medial portal.

CLOSURE

● After removal of all instruments, close each portal with sutures

HAZARDS

● Lateral portals: lateral antebrachial cutaneous nerve, radial nerve, PIN

● Median antebrachial cutaneous nerve, median nerve and brachial artery when establishing proximal anteromedial portal

● Medial and posterior antebrachial cutaneous nerves when establishing proximal posterolateral portal

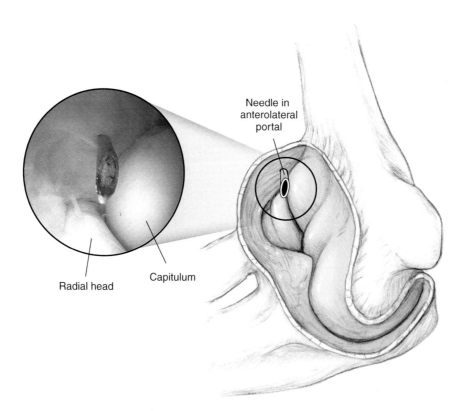

Needle in anterolateral portal

Radial head

Capitulum

FIGURE EF-52 Anterolateral portal.

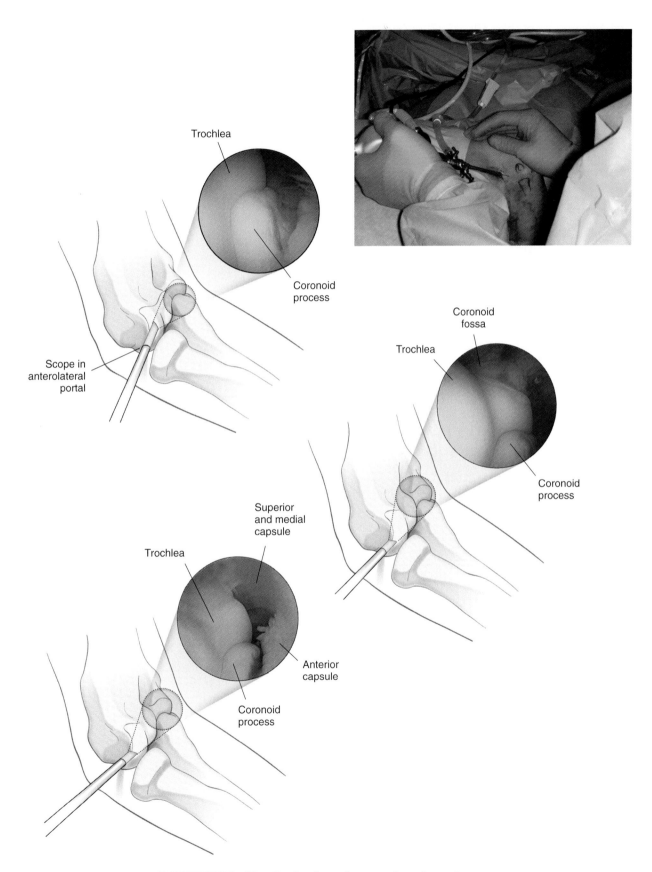

FIGURE EF-53   Visualization from the anterolateral portal.

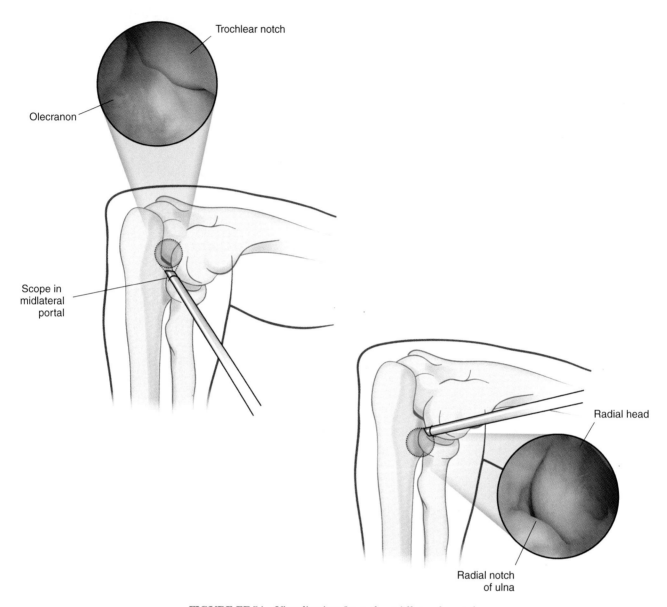

FIGURE EF-54 Visualization from the midlateral portal.

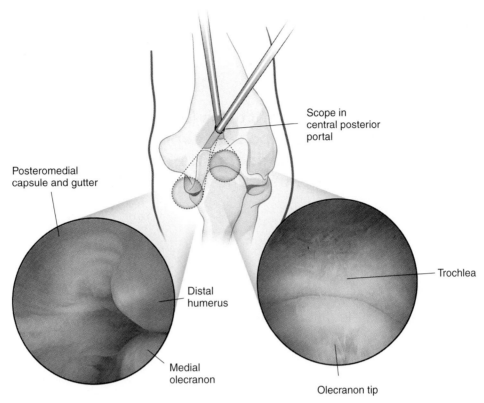

Scope in central posterior portal

Posteromedial capsule and gutter

Distal humerus

Medial olecranon

Trochlea

Olecranon tip

FIGURE EF-55   Visualization from the central posterior portal.

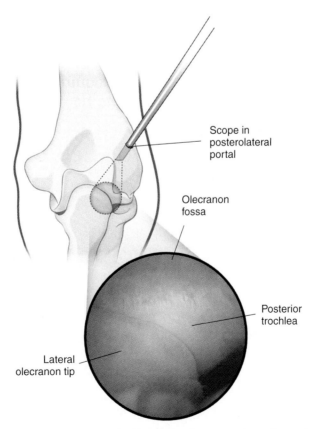

Scope in posterolateral portal

Olecranon fossa

Posterior trochlea

Lateral olecranon tip

FIGURE EF-56   Visualization from the posterolateral portal.

HENRY APPROACH (VOLAR APPROACH TO FOREARM)

Indications: ORIF of radial shaft fractures (middle and distal portions of radial shaft can be exposed), exposure of tumors and forearm masses, débridement of radial shaft osteomyelitis, distal exposure used for volar plating of distal radius fractures

POSITIONING (SEE FIGURE EF-15)

- Patient supine and arm supine on the hand table
- Exsanguinate limb, and elevate tourniquet

INCISION (FIGURE EF-57)

- Depends on how much of radial shaft or volar forearm needs to be exposed
- Mark radial styloid and lateral aspect of biceps tendon, and draw a line along brachioradialis along these 2 points
- Adjust incision length based on what structures require exposure or which portion of radial shaft needs to be exposed

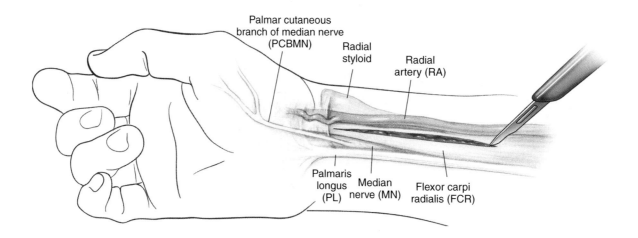

FIGURE EF-57   Surgical incision for volar approach to the distal forearm (Henry approach).

INTERVAL

- Between brachioradialis (radial nerve innervated) and pronator teres (median nerve innervated) (middle interval)
- Between brachioradialis (radial nerve innervated) and FCR (median nerve innervated) distally

SUPERFICIAL DISSECTION

- Incise skin and subcutaneous tissues; avoid lateral antebrachial cutaneous nerve as it runs on the anterolateral forearm
- Identify brachioradialis muscle, and bluntly find the interval between it and FCR
- Identify superficial radial nerve and radial artery directly beneath brachioradialis
- Divide fascia based on level of exposure of radial shaft required

DISTAL APPROACH

- Deep dissection (Figures EF-58 and EF-59)
  - Identify FCR, and open its sheath and retract it radially to protect radial artery
  - Divide floor of FCR tendon, and identify FPL tendon; retract FPL ulnarly to protect the median nerve

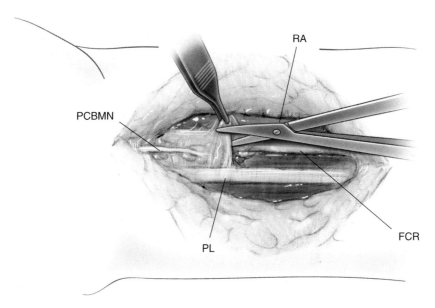

FIGURE EF-58   Henry approach. Exposure of the FCR tendon sheath. Dissect through the floor of the FCR tendon to expose the FPL.

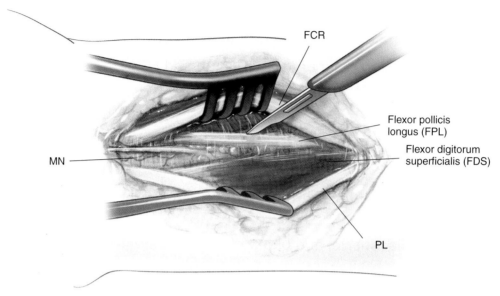

FIGURE EF-59 Henry approach. Retract the FCR radially to protect the radial artery. Identify and protect the median nerve.

- Slightly supinate forearm, and identify origin of FPL and insertion of pronator quadratus on distal third of radius
- Remove these muscles subperiosteally from radius, and retract medially to expose distal third of radius (Figures EF-60 and EF-61)

- **Closure**

  - Radial attachments of FPL and pronator quadratus can be approximated
  - Close skin and subcutaneous tissues with suture

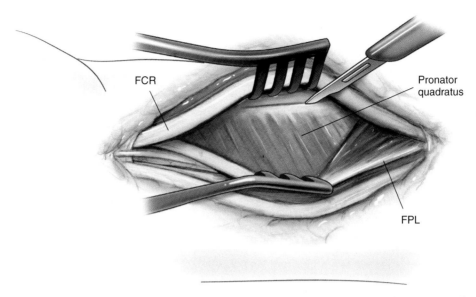

FIGURE EF-60   Henry approach. Expose the pronator quadratus, and elevate it subperiosteally to expose the distal radial shaft.

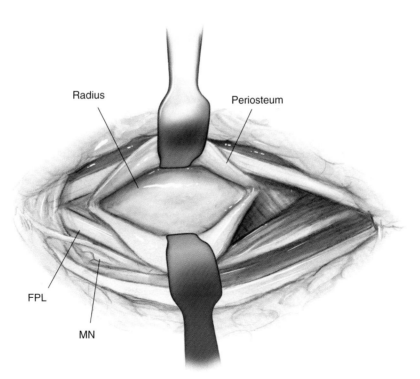

FIGURE EF-61   Henry approach. Exposure of the distal radial shaft.

MIDDLE APPROACH

● Deep dissection (Figure EF-62)

  ▪ Identify pronator teres, and pronate forearm to identify its insertion onto lateral aspect of radius

  ● The origin of FDS also can be identified just anterior to this area on the radius

  ▪ Incise insertion point of pronator teres subperiosteally

  ● Part of FDS muscle origin also is incised

  ● Retract these radially to expose middle third of radial shaft

● Closure

  ▪ Radial attachments of FDS and pronator teres can be approximated

  ▪ Close skin and subcutaneous tissues with suture

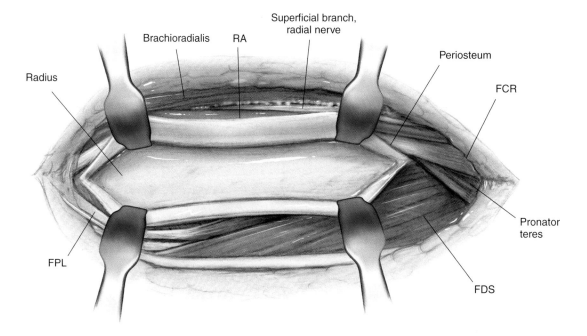

FIGURE EF-62 Henry approach. Proximal extension of the approach to the midshaft radius.

PROXIMAL VOLAR APPROACH

- Deep dissection
  - Identify biceps tendon, and deepen incision on its lateral aspect to avoid injury to the radial artery, which is located medial to the tendon
  - Fully supinate forearm, and identify supinator muscle as it inserts onto anterior radius
    - Subperiosteally incise insertion site of supinator, and retract muscle posterolaterally to expose proximal third of radius
    - Avoid excessive traction of supinator muscle and placement of retractors behind radius because these may cause subsequent PIN palsy
  - For proximal radial shaft fractures, PIN is at risk with this exposure; dorsal approach to proximal radial shaft is recommended

- Closure
  - Radial attachment of supinator can be approximated
  - Close skin and subcutaneous tissues with suture

HAZARDS

- Lateral antebrachial cutaneous nerves during superficial dissection
- Superficial radial nerve during retraction of brachioradialis
- Radial artery during retraction of brachioradialis and proximal approach as it courses medial to biceps tendon
- PIN can be injured during deep dissection and subperiosteal incision of supinator muscle with proximal exposure of radial shaft; take care during retraction to avoid neurapraxia

THOMPSON APPROACH (DORSAL APPROACH TO FOREARM)

Indications: ORIF of proximal and middle radial shaft fractures, radial osteotomy, exposure of tumors and masses in forearm, PIN decompression and exposure

POSITIONING

- Patient supine with forearm in pronation
- Exsanguinate limb, and elevate tourniquet

INCISION (FIGURE EF-63)

- Identify and mark lateral epicondyle of humerus and Lister's tubercle on distal radius
- Draw line beginning just anterior to lateral epicondyle and ending on ulnar side of Lister's tubercle

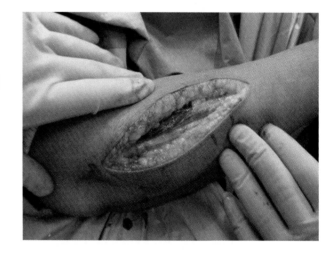

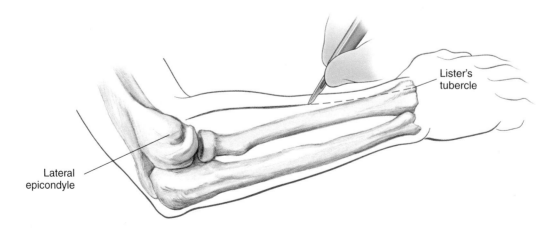

FIGURE EF-63 Positioning for dorsal approach to the forearm (Thompson approach).

INTERVAL

- Between ECRB and EDC (both PIN innervated)

SUPERFICIAL DISSECTION (FIGURE EF-64)

- Incise skin and subcutaneous tissues
- Identify ECRB and EDC, and incise fascia at this interval
- Retract these muscles to expose supinator and APL; use caution, and identify PIN as it exits supinator and continues distally in forearm on top of APL

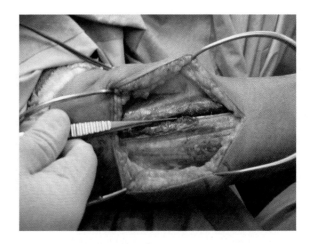

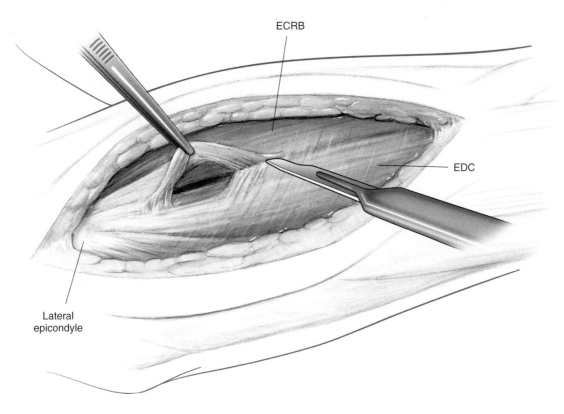

FIGURE EF-64   Thompson approach. Develop the interval between the ECRB and EDC to expose the underlying supinator muscle belly.

PROXIMAL DORSAL

● Deep dissection (Figures EF-65 and EF-66)

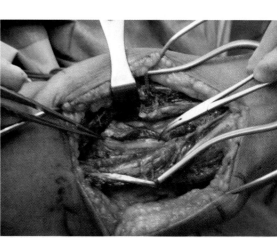

FIGURE EF-65 Thompson approach. Identify PIN as it exits the supinator.

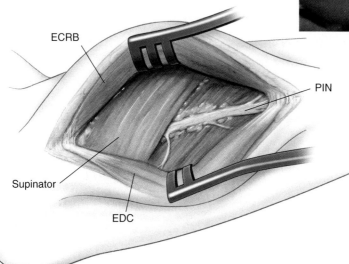

ECRB

PIN

Supinator

EDC

FIGURE EF-66 Thompson approach. Decompress PIN, and visualize and protect the nerve and all its branches.

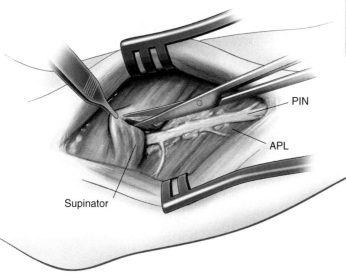

PIN

APL

Supinator

- Identify PIN as it exits the supinator (1 cm distal to muscle belly), and carefully divide supinator from distal to proximal, carefully visualizing and protecting PIN at all times
  - Be careful to identify distal branches, and visualize and protect these at all times
  - If PIN is difficult to identify distally, it can be located proximally as it enters supinator, and muscle belly can be divided in a proximal-to-distal fashion
- Fully supinate forearm, and identify supinator on anterior surface of radius (Figure EF-67)
- Subperiosteally strip supinator muscle from radius, and reflect it to expose proximal radius (Figure EF-68)

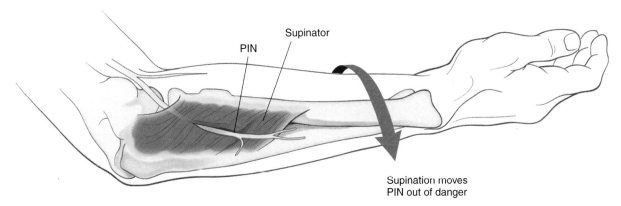

FIGURE EF-67 Thompson approach. When PIN is identified and protected, supinate the forearm and palpate the radial shaft.

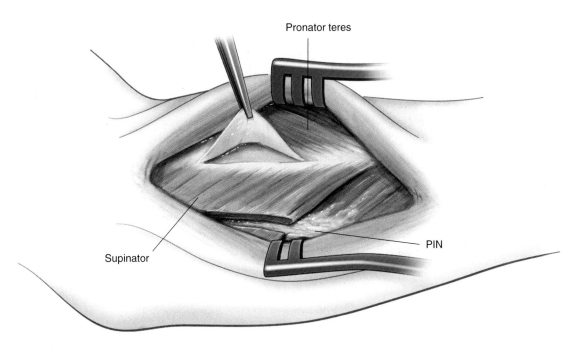

FIGURE EF-68 Thompson approach. With PIN visualized and protected, elevate the supinator in a subperiosteal fashion to expose the proximal radial shaft.

MIDDLE DORSAL

- ● Deep dissection (Figure EF-69)

   ▪ After visualization of PIN and its distal branches, identify APL and EPB

   ▪ Subperiosteally free superior border of APL and inferior border of EPB from radius, and retract these to expose middle third of radius

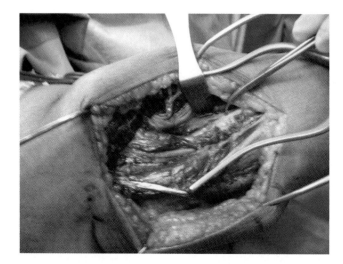

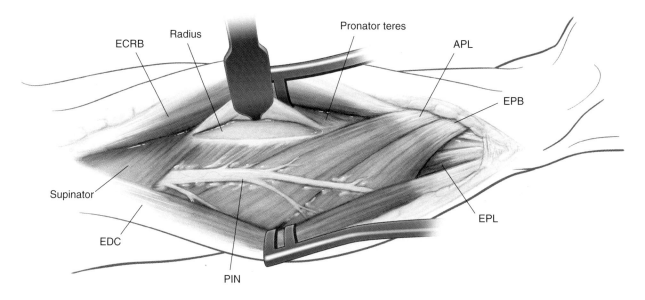

FIGURE EF-69   Thompson approach. Exposure of the midshaft of the radius.

DISTAL DORSAL

- ● Deep dissection (Figure EF-70)
  - ■ Subperiosteally dissect interval between ECRB and EDC distally
  - ■ Retract to expose distal third of radius

CLOSURE

- ● Close skin and subcutaneous tissue after hemostasis

HAZARDS

- ● PIN

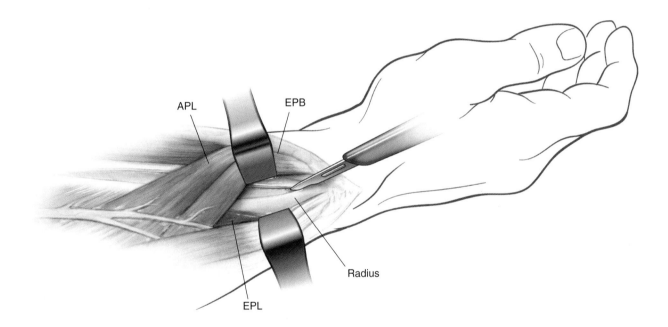

FIGURE EF-70   Thompson approach. Exposure of the distal third shaft of the radius.

Approach to Ulnar Shaft

Indications: ORIF of ulna shaft fractures, tumor or forearm mass excision, ulnar osteotomy

POSITIONING (FIGURE EF-71)

- Supine on table, arm in prontation across patient's body
- Exsanguinate limb, and elevate tourniquet

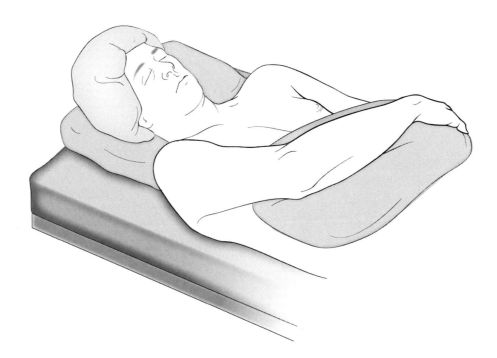

FIGURE EF-71   Positioning for exposure of the ulnar shaft.

INCISION (FIGURE EF-72)

● Linear incision along posterior ulnar shaft; length of incision depends on how much exposure is needed.

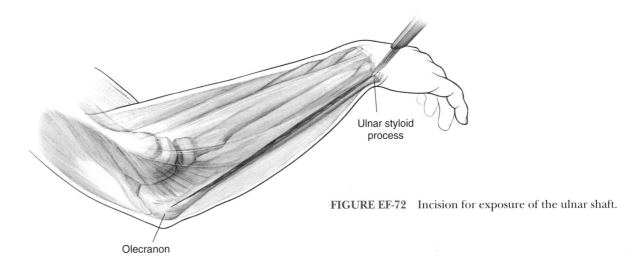

FIGURE EF-72 Incision for exposure of the ulnar shaft.

SUPERFICIAL DISSECTION (FIGURE EF-73)

● Incise skin and subcutaneous tissues
● Define interval between ECU (PIN innervated) and FCU (ulnar nerve innervated)

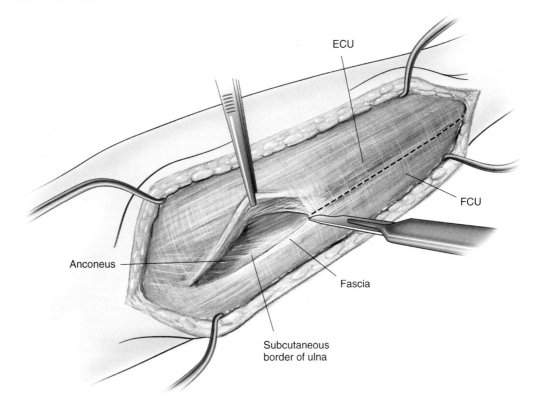

FIGURE EF-73 Exposure of the ulnar shaft. Define the interval between the ECU and FCU.

DEEP DISSECTION (FIGURE EF-74)

● Expose ulnar shaft by retracting ECU and FCU, and widen exposure by stripping muscles from ulna shaft periosteally to protect ulnar nerve lying volar to FDP muscle

CLOSURE

● Close skin and subcutaneous tissues with suture

HAZARDS

● Ulnar nerve and artery

  ▪ Take care to strip FCU muscle off of ulna in subperiosteal fashion to avoid injury to these structures

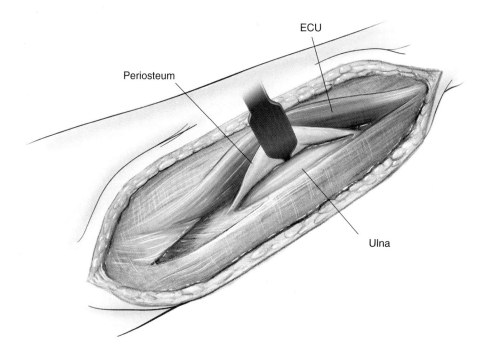

FIGURE EF-74   Exposure of the ulnar shaft. Subperiosteal elevation of the ECU and FCU to expose the ulnar shaft.

FOREARM COMPARTMENT RELEASE

Volar

Indications: Forearm compartment syndrome

POSITIONING

- Patient supine, arm in supination on hand table

INCISION (FIGURE EF-75)

- Use curvilinear incision to expose underlying fascia

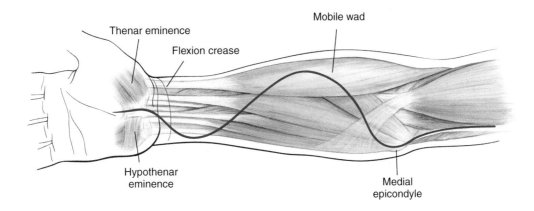

FIGURE EF-75   Incision for volar forearm compartment release.

SUPERFICIAL DISSECTION (FIGURE EF-76)

- Incise skin and subcutaneous tissues; avoid lateral antebrachial cutaneous nerve as it runs on the anterolateral forearm

- Incise fascia overlying mobile wad and the superficial flexor muscles, including FCR, pronator teres, and palmaris longus

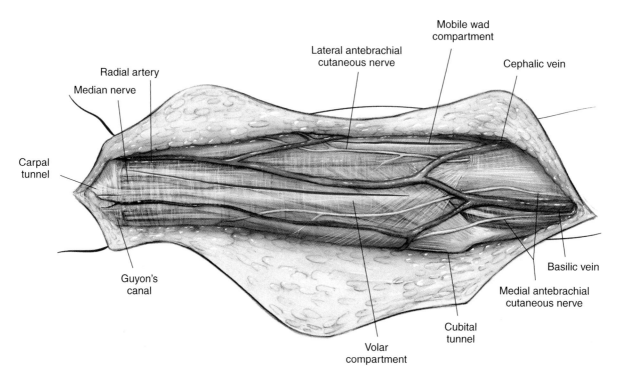

FIGURE EF-76 Volar forearm compartment release. Exposure of the fascia. Carefully avoid superficial cutaneous nerve branches.

DEEP DISSECTION (FIGURE EF-77)

- Identify and bluntly divide interval between brachioradialis and FCR taking care to identify superficial radial nerve and radial artery directly beneath brachioradialis

- Through this interval, incise fascia overlying deep flexors of the forearm, including FDS, FDP, and FPL

- All volar muscle compartments and mobile wad should be released

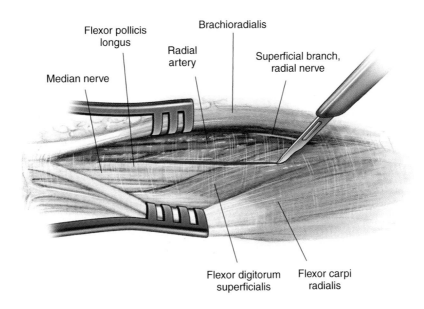

FIGURE EF-77   Volar forearm compartment release. Incision of fascia of superficial and deep muscle compartments.

CLOSURE

- Leave skin incision and fascia open
- Delayed closure or skin grafting often indicated

HAZARDS

- Lateral antebrachial cutaneous nerve during skin incision
- Superficial sensory radial nerve and radial artery under brachioradialis during exposure of deep muscles
- Median nerve in forearm between FDS and FDP

Dorsal

Indications: Forearm compartment syndrome

POSITIONING

- Patient supine, arm in supination on hand table

INCISION (FIGURE EF-78)

- Linear incision along dorsal forearm

SUPERFICIAL DISSECTION

- Incise skin and subcutaneous tissues over dorsal forearm in longitudinal manner

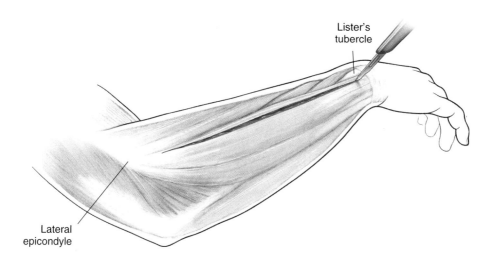

Lister's tubercle

Lateral epicondyle

FIGURE EF-78 Incision for dorsal forearm compartment release.

DEEP DISSECTION (FIGURE EF-79)

- Incise fascia overlying extensor muscle bellies

CLOSURE

- Leave skin incision and fascia open
- Delayed closure or skin grafting often indicated

HAZARDS

- Superficial sensory nerves

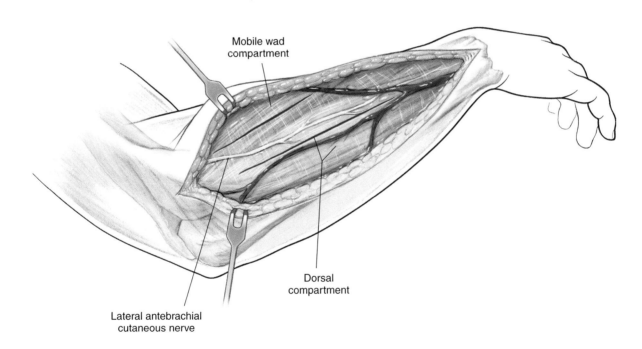

FIGURE EF-79 Dorsal forearm compartment release. Incision of fascia of extensor muscle compartments. See TABLE EF-1, Compartments and Muscles of the Elbow.

REFERENCES

Doyle JR, Botte MJ: Surgical Anatomy of the Hand and Upper Extremity. Philadelphia, Lippincott Willams & Wilkins, 2003.

Hoppenfeld S, deBoer P: Surgical Exposures in Orthopedics, 3rd ed. Philadelphia, Lippincott Williams & Wilkins, 2003, pp 147-214.

Morrey B: The Elbow and Its Disorders, 3rd ed. Philadelphia, Saunders, 2000, pp 109-134.

Morrey B: Master Techniques in Orthopedic Surgery: The Elbow, 2nd ed. Philadelphia, Lippincott Williams & Wilkins, 2002.

Netter F: Atlas of Human Anatomy, 4th ed. Philadelphia, Saunders, 2006, plates 418-484.

Standring S: Gray's Anatomy, 38th ed. Philadelphia, Churchill Livingstone, 1995, pp 635-659, 841-867, 1269-1274.

Triceps Splitting Approach to the Elbow. Duke Orthopaedics presents Wheeless' Textbook of Orthopaetics Website, 2007. Available at: http://www.wheelessonline.com/ortho/triceps_splitting_approach_to_the_elbow.

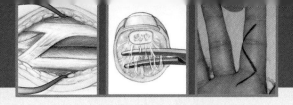

4

WRIST AND HAND

—

A. BOBBY CHHABRA

REGIONAL ANATOMY

Osteology (Figure HW-1)

- ● Distal radius

  - ▪ Radial styloid process
  - ▪ Two fossae for carpal articulation
    - ● Scaphoid fossa
    - ● Lunate fossa
  - ▪ Sigmoid notch—articulation with distal ulna
  - ▪ Lister's tubercle between the 2nd and 3rd extensor compartments; acts as a pulley for extensor pollicis longus (EPL) tendon

- ● Distal ulna

  - ▪ Ulna styloid process
  - ▪ Fovea—depression at base of ulnar styloid process, attachment for triangular fibrocartilage cartilage complex (TFCC)
  - ▪ Groove for extensor carpi ulnaris (ECU) tendon

- ● Scaphoid

  - ▪ Largest bone in proximal row
  - ▪ Divided into proximal pole, waist, and distal pole
  - ▪ Tenuous blood supply to proximal pole; most of the blood supply enters distal tubercle in a dorsal retrograde fashion
  - ▪ Flexor retinaculum and abductor pollicis brevis attach on palmar surface; radial collateral ligament attaches on dorsal surface
  - ▪ Joint capsule attaches on dorsal tubercle/waist

- ● Lunate

  - ▪ Semilunar shape
  - ▪ Articulates with radius in lunate fossa

- ● Triqu etrum

  - ▪ Has attachment for ulnar collateral ligament
  - ▪ Articulates with pisiform

- ● Pisiform

  - ▪ Pea-shaped
  - ▪ Situated on palmar surface of triquetrum
  - ▪ Insertion for flexor carpi ulnaris (FCU)
  - ▪ Origin of flexor digiti minimi

- Trapezoid
  - Oblong shape
  - Articulates with 2nd metacarpal, scaphoid, trapezium, and capitate

- Trapezium
  - Has groove for flexor carpi radialis (FCR) tendon
  - Has attachment of thenar muscles, opponens pollicis, flexor pollicis brevis, and abductor pollicis brevis
  - Articulates with distal pole of scaphoid, trapezoid, and 1st and 2nd metacarpals

- Capitate
  - Central, largest carpal bone
  - Articulates with trapezoid; hamate; lunate; scaphoid; and 2nd, 3rd, and 4th metacarpal bases

- Hamate
  - Has hamulus (hook)
  - Flexor retinaculum attaches to hook of hamate
  - Deep branch ulnar nerve courses around the hook of the hamate

- Metacarpals
  - Five metacarpals
    - 1st—abductor pollicis longus inserts on base
    - 2nd—extensor carpi radialis longus inserts on dorsal base; FCR has shared insertion on volar base
    - 3rd—extensor carpi radialis brevis inserts on dorsal base; FCR has shared insertion on volar base
    - 4th—no insertions on base
    - 5th—insertion of ECU on ulnar base and FCU on volar radial base

- Phalanges
  - Proximal
    - No tendinous insertions
  - Middle
    - Insertion of flexor digitorum superficialis (FDS) on volar surface at base
    - Insertion of central slip of extensor hood on dorsal surface
  - Distal
    - Insertion of flexor digitorum profundus (FDP) on volar surface
    - Insertion of terminal extensor tendon on dorsal surface

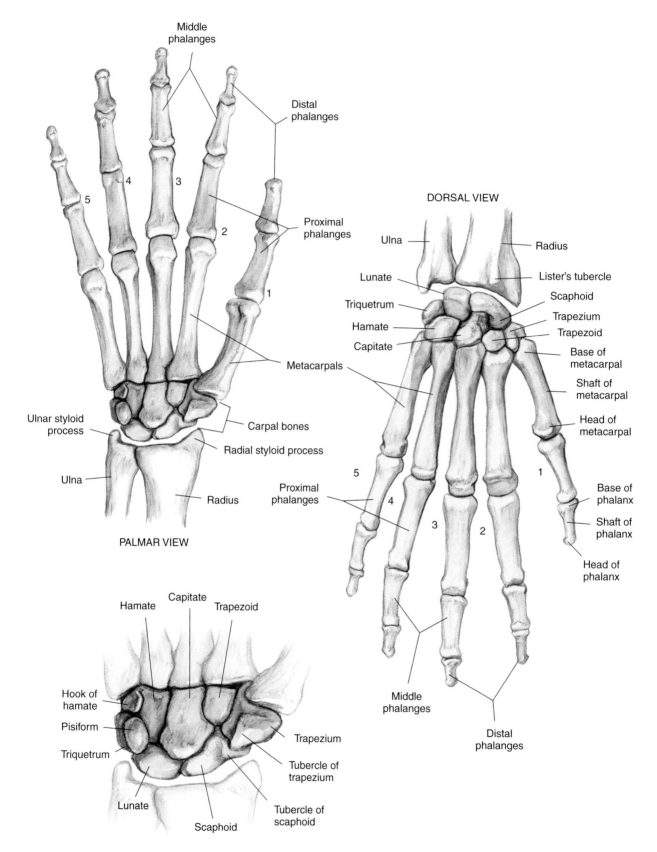

FIGURE HW-1 Hand and wrist bony anatomy (palmar and dorsal views).

Arthrology

- **Radiocarpal joint (Figure HW-2A and B)**
  - Distal radius articulates with proximal carpal row
  - Extrinsic volar and dorsal ligaments
  - Radioscaphocapitate, long and short radiolunate, ulnar collateral ligaments (part of TFCC)
  - Dorsal ligaments (dorsal intercarpal and dorsal radiocarpal)

- **Distal radioulnar joint**
  - Uniaxial pivot joint
  - Ulna articulates with radius in sigmoid notch
  - Distal radioulnar ligaments of the TFCC are the major stabilizers of the distal radioulnar joint
  - TFCC (see Figure HW-2D)
    - Triangular fibrocartilage
      - A meniscus homologue
      - Located on articular surface of distal ulna and the very ulnar aspect of distal radius
      - Central portion of triangular fibrocartilage is thin and avascular
      - Periphery is vascularized and amenable to repair
    - Volar and dorsal distal radioulnar ligaments
      - Volar and dorsal distal radioulnar ligaments attach to dorsal and volar sides of radial sigmoid notch, surround the triangular fibrocartilage, and converge at the ulnar styloid
      - Volar distal radioulnar ligament inserts into the ulna fovea, and dorsal distal radioulnar ligament attaches to ulna styloid
    - Ulnar collateral ligament
    - Ulnocarpal ligaments
      - Ulnolunate ligament
      - Ulnocapitate ligament
      - Ulnotriquetral ligament
    - Lunotriquetral ligament
    - Short radiolunate ligament
    - ECU subsheath

- **Midcarpal joint**
  - Proximal row—scaphoid, lunate, triquetrum
  - Distal row—trapezium, trapezoid, capitate, hamate, pisiform

- **Interosseous joints/ligaments (see Figure HW-2C and D)**
  - Between carpal bones
  - Scapholunate ligament
    - Strongest dorsally
  - Lunotriquetral ligament
    - Strongest volarly

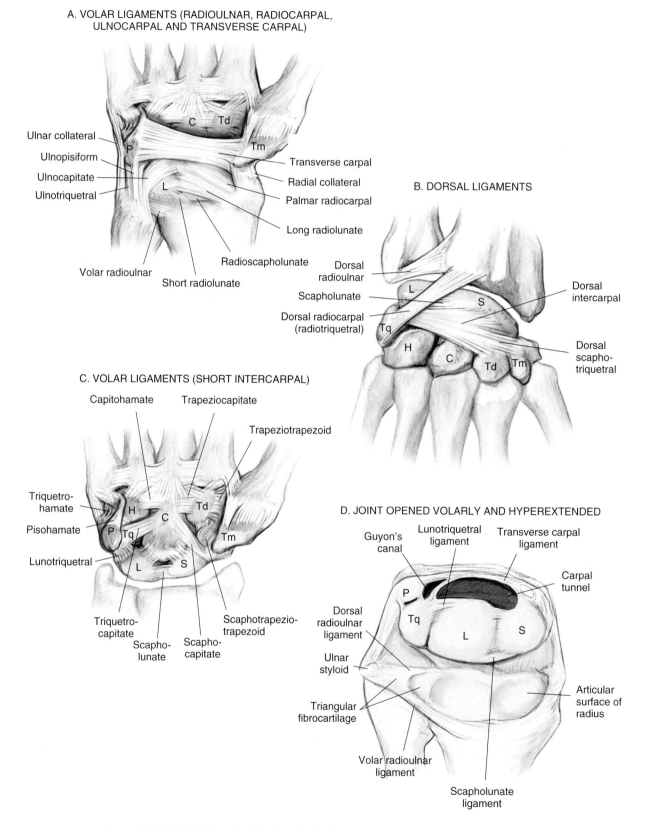

A. VOLAR LIGAMENTS (RADIOULNAR, RADIOCARPAL, ULNOCARPAL AND TRANSVERSE CARPAL)

Ulnar collateral

Ulnopisiform

Ulnocapitate

Ulnotriquetral

C Td

P

Tm

Transverse carpal

Radial collateral

Palmar radiocarpal

Long radiolunate

Radioscapholunate

Volar radioulnar

Short radiolunate

L

B. DORSAL LIGAMENTS

Dorsal radioulnar

Scapholunate

Dorsal radiocarpal (radiotriquetral)

L

S

Tq

H

C

Td Tm

Dorsal intercarpal

Dorsal scapho-triquetral

C. VOLAR LIGAMENTS (SHORT INTERCARPAL)

Capitohamate   Trapeziocapitate

Trapeziotrapezoid

Triquetro-hamate

Pisohamate

Lunotriquetral

H

P Tq

Td

C

Tm

L S

Triquetro-capitate

Scapho-lunate

Scapho-capitate

Scaphotrapezio-trapezoid

D. JOINT OPENED VOLARLY AND HYPEREXTENDED

Guyon's canal

Lunotriquetral ligament

Transverse carpal ligament

Carpal tunnel

Dorsal radioulnar ligament

Ulnar styloid

Triangular fibrocartilage

Volar radioulnar ligament

Scapholunate ligament

P

Tq

L

S

Articular surface of radius

FIGURE HW-2   A-D, Hand and wrist ligamentous and articular anatomy.

- Carpal-metacarpal joints (Figure HW-3)
  - Metacarpophalangeal (MCP) joints
    - Five joints
  - Proximal interphalangeal (PIP) joints
  - Distal interphalangeal (DIP) joints
  - Tendons **(Figure HW-4)**
    - Flexor tendon relationship in carpal tunnel
      - FDS to digits 3 and 4 lie volar to tendons 2 and 5 **(Figure HW-6A and B)**
      - FDP lie dorsal to FDS in forearm
    - Camper's chiasm—crossing of the FDS and FDP tendons at the level of the proximal phalanx. From the forearm to the Camper's chiasm, FDS lies volar to FDP. In the finger, FDS splits and attaches onto the middle phalanx. FDP emerges from between the chiasm volarly and continues to its attachment on the distal phalanx (see Figure **HW-4A**)
    - Finger flexor pulley system (see Figure **HW-4B**)
      - Five annular ligaments, 4 cruciate ligaments
      - A2 and A4 are crucial and prevent bowstringing of the flexor tendon
    - Extensor tendon compartments (Table HW-1; see Figure **HW-6C and D**)

Muscles

Best considered in groups **(Table HW-2)**
  - Thenar muscles (see **Figure HW-5A**)
  - Hypothenar muscles (see **Figure HW-5B**)
  - Intrinsic muscles (see **Figure HW-4A and C**)

VOLAR VIEW

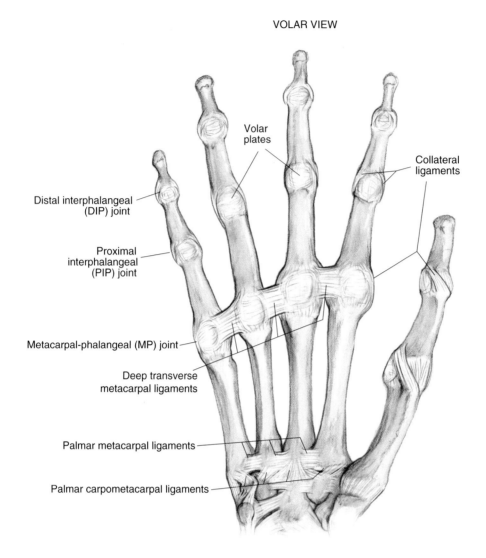

Volar plates

Collateral ligaments

Distal interphalangeal (DIP) joint

Proximal interphalangeal (PIP) joint

Metacarpal-phalangeal (MP) joint

Deep transverse metacarpal ligaments

Palmar metacarpal ligaments

Palmar carpometacarpal ligaments

FIGURE HW-3 Carpometacarpal, proximal interphalangeal, and distal interphalangeal joint anatomy.

TABLE HW–1 Extensor Tendon Compartments

Compartment	Tendons
1	EPB
	APL
2	ECRL
	ECRB
3	EPL
4	EIP
	EDC
5	EDM
6	ECU

Cross-sectional anatomy (see Figure HW-9) at the following levels: (1) distal radioulnar joint, (2) proximal carpal row, (3) distal carpal row, and (4) proximal metacarpal.

Landmarks (see Figure HW-10): palpable anatomic landmarks: pisiform, hook of the hamate, Lister's tubercle, palmaris.

APL, abductor pollicis longus; ECRB, extensor carpi radialis brevis; ECRL, extensor carpi radialis longus; ECU, extensor carpi ulnaris; EDC, extensor digitorum communis; EDM, extensor digiti minimi; EIP, extensor indicis proprius; EPB, extensor pollicis brevis; EPL, extensor pollicis longus.

TABLE HW–2   Hand Musculature

Group	Muscles	Origin	Insertion	Innervation	Action
Thenar	Opponens pollicis	Flexor retinaculum and tubercle of trapezium	Radial border of 1st metacarpal	Recurrent motor branch of median nerve	Thumb opposition
	Abductor pollicis brevis	Scaphoid tubercle and flexor retinaculum	Base of thumb proximal phalanx and tendon of EPL	Recurrent motor branch of median	Thumb abduction
	Flexor pollicis brevis	Flexor retinaculum and tubercle of trapezium	Base of thumb proximal phalanx	Dual innervation—deep head ulnar, superficial head median	Flexion of thumb MCP joint
	Adductor pollicis	Transverse head—3rd MC; oblique head—trapezium, trapezoid, capitate, and bases of 2nd and 3rd MC	Ulnar side of thumb proximal phalanx base	Deep branch of ulnar nerve	Thumb adduction
Hypothenar	Abductor digiti minimi	Pisiform and pisohamate ligament, flexor retinaculum	5th digit proximal phalanx base and extensor hood	Deep branch of ulnar nerve	Abducts 5th digit
	Flexor digiti minimi	Hook of hamate and flexor retinaculum	5th digit proximal phalanx base	Deep branch of ulnar nerve	Flexes 5th digit at MCP joint
	Opponens digiti minimi	Hook of hamate and flexor retinaculum	Ulnar border of 5th MC shaft	Deep branch of ulnar nerve	Opposes 5th finger
Intrinsic hand muscles	Lumbrical muscles	FDP tendons 1st and 2nd lumbricals are unipennate and arise on radial side of tendon; 3rd and 4th lumbricals are bipennate and arise from adjacent tendons	Radial side of extensor hood at level of proximal phalanx	1st and 2nd—median nerve; 3rd and 4th—deep branch of ulnar nerve	Flex MCP and extend PIP joints
	Dorsal interossei (DI) muscles	4 muscles—bipennate on metacarpal shafts	Proximal phalanges and extensor hood; 1st DI—radial side of index; 2nd DI—radial side of middle; 3rd DI—ulnar side of middle; 4th DI—ulnar side of ring	Deep branch of ulnar nerve	Abduct from axis of middle finger; flex MCP joints and extend PIP joints
	Palmar interossei (PI) muscles	3 muscles—unipennate on MC shafts; 1st PI—ulnar shaft of 2nd MC; 2nd PI—radial shaft of 4th MC; 3rd PI—radial shaft of 5th MC	Proximal phalanges and extensor hoods; 1st PI—ulnar side of index; 2nd PI—radial side of ring; 3rd PI—radial side of small	Deep branch of ulnar nerve	Adduct toward middle finger; flex MCP joints and extend PIP joints

EPL, extensor pollicis longus; FDP, flexor digitorum profundus; MC, metacarpal; MCP, metacarpophalangeal; PIP, proximal interphalangeal.

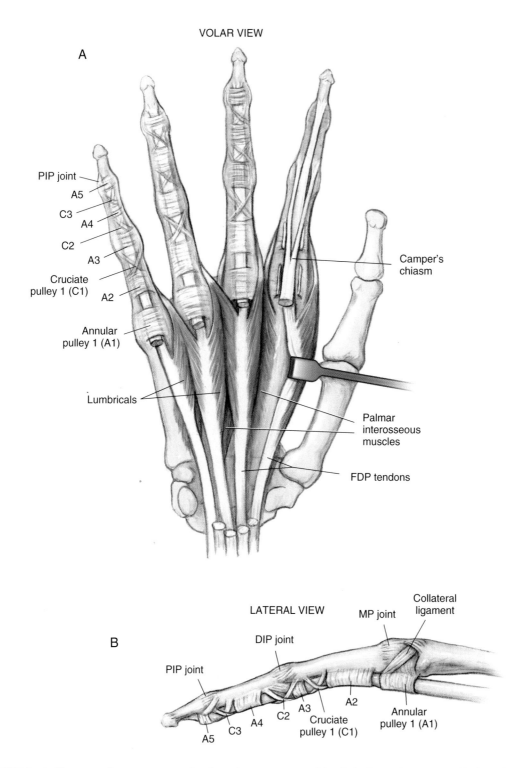

VOLAR VIEW

A

PIP joint

A5

C3

A4

C2

A3

Cruciate
pulley 1 (C1)

A2

Annular
pulley 1 (A1)

Camper's
chiasm

Lumbricals

Palmar
interosseous
muscles

FDP tendons

B

LATERAL VIEW

MP joint

Collateral
ligament

DIP joint

PIP joint

A5

C3

A4

C2

A3

Cruciate
pulley 1 (C1)

A2

Annular
pulley 1 (A1)

FIGURE HW-4 **A,** Flexor tendon anatomy and palmar interosseous and lumbrical muscle anatomy. **B,** Annular and cruciate pulley anatomy.

C   DORSAL VIEW

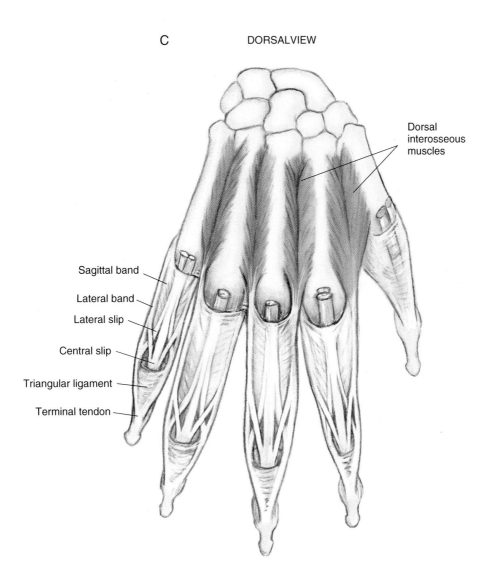

Dorsal interosseous muscles

Sagittal band

Lateral band

Lateral slip

Central slip

Triangular ligament

Terminal tendon

D   LATERAL VIEW

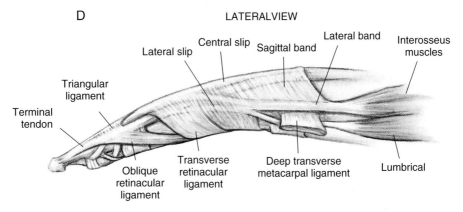

Lateral slip

Central slip

Sagittal band

Lateral band

Interosseus muscles

Triangular ligament

Terminal tendon

Oblique retinacular ligament

Transverse retinacular ligament

Deep transverse metacarpal ligament

Lumbrical

FIGURE HW-4, cont'd   **C** and **D,** Extensor tendon anatomy and dorsal interosseous muscle anatomy.

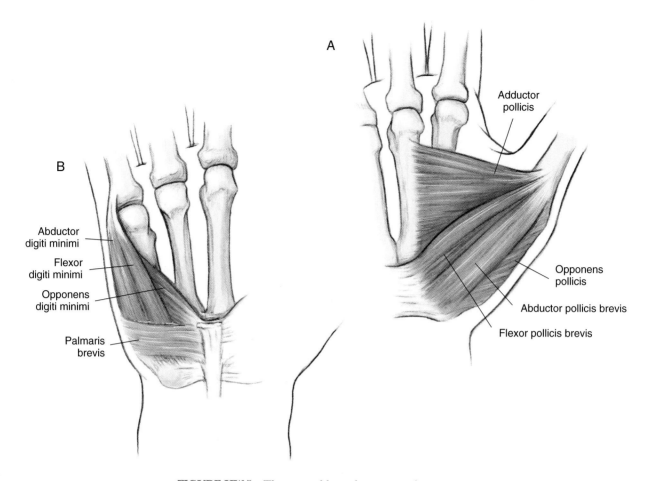

FIGURE HW-5 Thenar and hypothenar muscle anatomy.

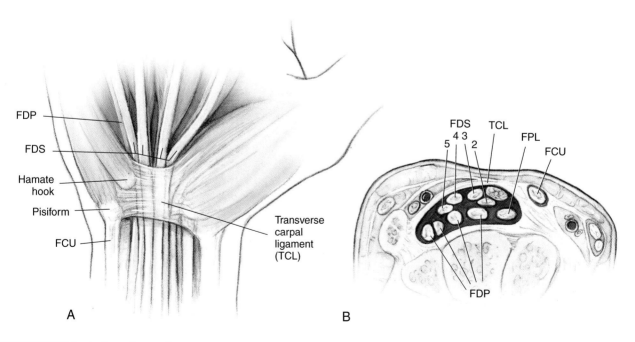

FIGURE HW-6 **A,** Carpal tunnel anatomy. **B,** Cross-sectional anatomy of the carpal tunnel. Note the relationship between the FDS and FDP tendons.

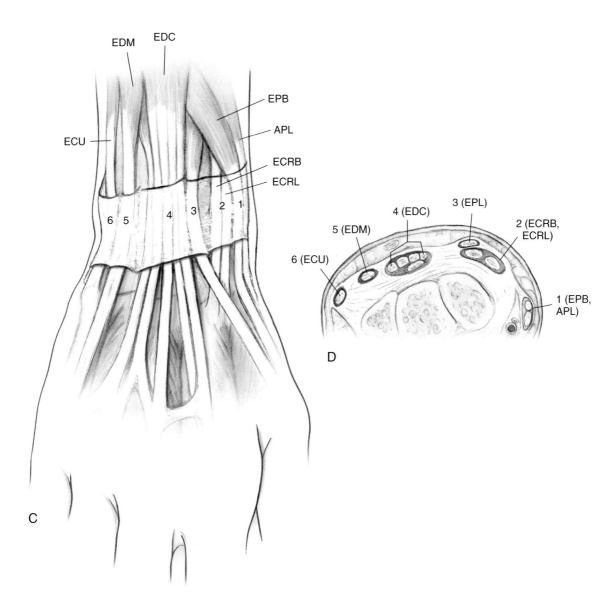

FIGURE HW-6, cont'd **C,** Extensor tendon compartments. **D,** Cross-sectional anatomy of the extensor tendon compartments.

Nerves (Figure HW-7A)

- **Median nerve**

  - Gives off sensory palmar branch approximately 6 cm proximal to radial styloid
  - Median nerve enters hand through carpal tunnel
  - Gives off recurrent motor branch with a variable course
    - 80% branch distal to transverse carpal ligament (TCL) and enter thenar musculature in a recurrent manner
    - 15% branch subligamentously
    - 5% branch transligamentously
  - Splits into common palmar digital nerves, which split into the digital nerves to thumb, index finger, middle finger, and radial side of ring finger

- **Ulnar nerve**

  - Dorsal cutaneous nerve branches approximately 7 cm proximal to wrist and provides sensation to dorsoulnar forearm and wrist
  - Main branch of ulnar nerve enters hand through Guyon's canal and divides in canal to deep motor branch and sensory branch
  - Deep motor branch courses around hook of hamate and crosses palm to supply intrinsic muscles
  - Sensory branch becomes common palmar digital nerves and proper palmar digital nerves, which supply sensation to small finger and ulnar side of ring finger

- **Radial nerve (Figure HW-7B)**

  - Terminal branch is superficial sensory branch, which lies on the radial aspect of distal radius and thumb and provides sensation to dorsum of hand

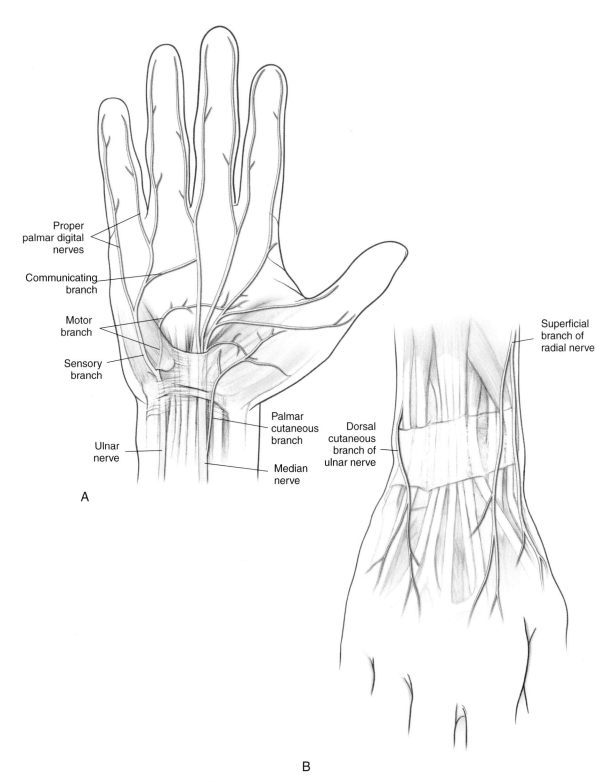

FIGURE HW-7 A and **B,** Peripheral anatomy of the hand and wrist.

Vascular (Figure HW-8)

- Radial artery branches
  - Dorsal branch
    - Deep palmar arch
    - Princeps pollicis artery
  - Volar branch
    - Anastomosis with superficial palmar arch in 80% of people

- Ulnar artery branches
  - Superficial palmar arch
  - Branch to 5th digit

- Common and proper digital arteries
- Superficial and deep arch have branches that communicate

Hazards

- Nerves
  - Recurrent motor branch of median nerve at risk during carpal tunnel release because of its variable course
  - Palmar cutaneous branch of median nerve at risk during Henry approach
  - Dorsal sensory ulnar nerve branch at risk during TFCC repairs
  - Superficial sensory radial nerve at risk during de Quervain's release and application of external fixator for distal radius fractures
  - Deep motor branch of ulnar nerve in Guyon's canal at risk during excision of the hook of hamate
  - Proper digital nerves at risk during trigger digit (A-1) pulley releases, and during volar and midlateral approaches to fingers

- Vascular
  - Radial artery at risk during distal volar Henry approach
  - Ulnar artery at risk during exposure of ulnar distal forearm and distal ulnar shaft
  - Superficial palmar arch at risk during carpal tunnel release and exposures in palm
  - Proper digital arteries at risk during midlateral approaches to finger and volar exposures

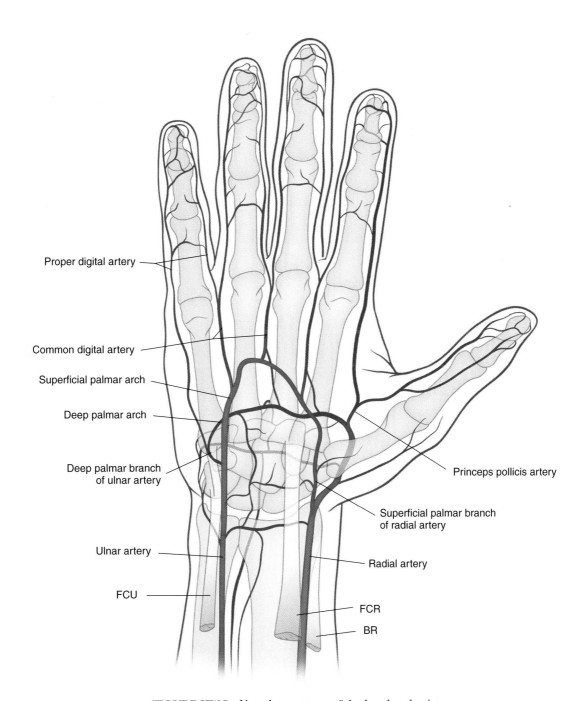

FIGURE HW-8 Vascular anatomy of the hand and wrist.

Cross-sectional Anatomy of the Distal Forearm, Carpal Tunnel, and Palm Is depicted in Figure HW-9

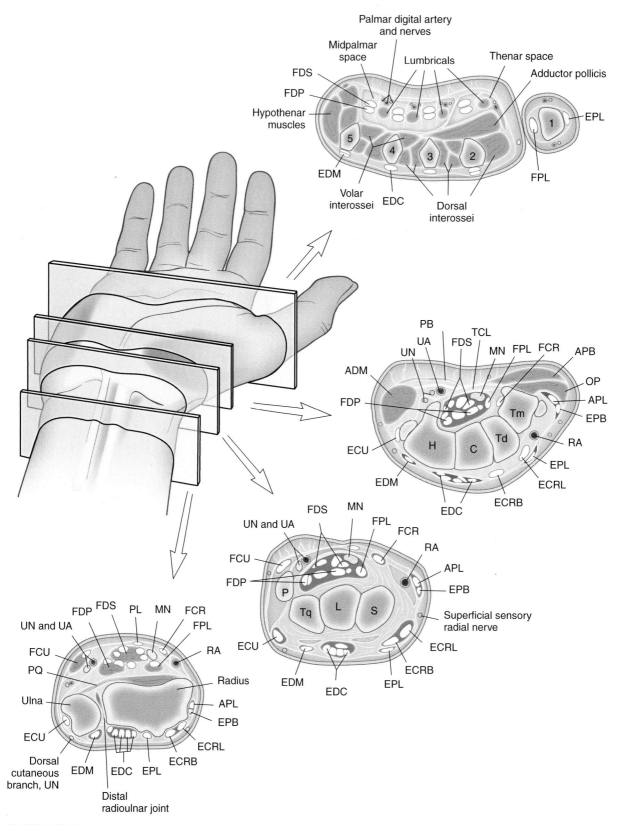

FIGURE HW-9 Cross-sectional anatomy of the hand and wrist. At the level of the (1) distal radioulnar joint, (2) proximal carpal row, (3) distal carpal row, and (4) proximal metacarpal.

Palpable Anatomic Landmarks of the Hand and Wrist (Figure HW-10)

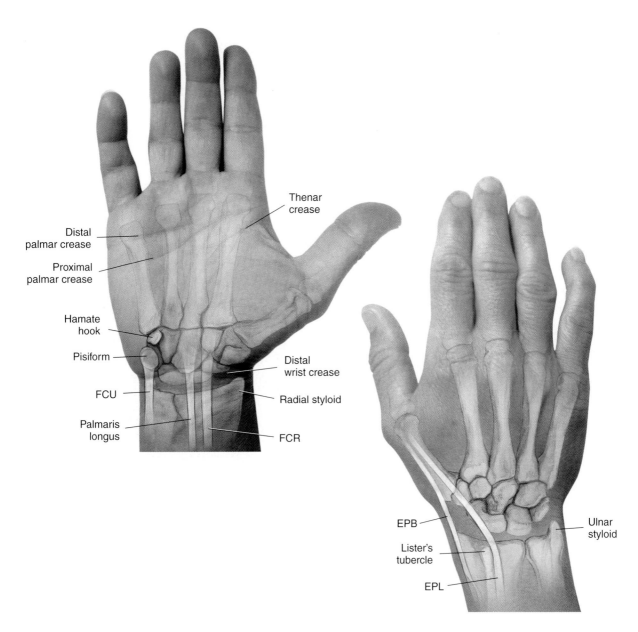

FIGURE HW-10 Palpable anatomical landmarks of the hand and wrist.

Dorsal Approach to the Forearm, Wrist, and Carpus

Indications: Synovectomy of extensor tendons, dorsal ganglion cyst excision, limited/total wrist arthrodesis, proximal row carpectomy, open reduction and internal fixation (ORIF) of distal radius fracture, scapholunate ligament repairs, extensor tendon repairs at level of distal forearm, vascularized bone grafting from distal radius, fixation of proximal pole scaphoid fractures, posterior interosseous nerve neurectomy

POSITIONING (FIGURE HW-11)

- Supine

  - Arm in pronation on hand table
  - Exsanguinate arm and elevate tourniquet, if indicated

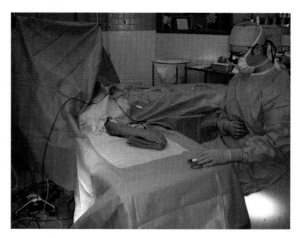

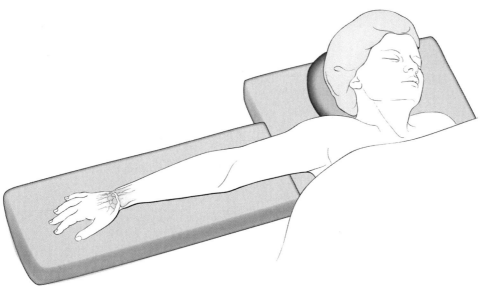

FIGURE HW-11 Positioning for the dorsal approach to the distal forearm and wrist.

INCISION (FIGURE HW-12)

- A 6-8 cm vertical incision centered on dorsal aspect of wrist between radius and ulna, just ulnar to Lister's tubercle

- Incision extends 3 cm proximal to wrist joint and 5 cm distal

- Length of incision depends on procedure being performed

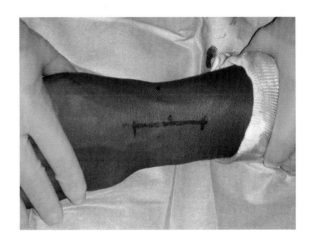

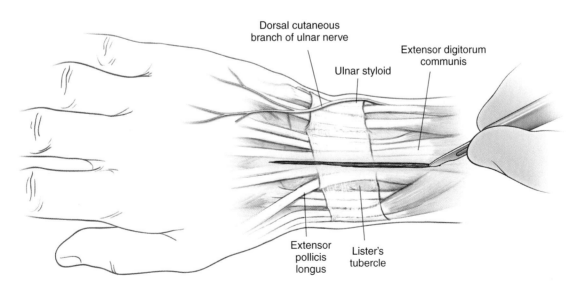

FIGURE HW-12 Incision for the dorsal approach to the distal forearm and wrist. Incision is just ulnar to Lister's tubercle.

SUPERFICIAL DISSECTION (FIGURE HW-13)

● Skin and subcutaneous tissues are dissected down to extensor retinaculum above 4th extensor compartment

DEEP DISSECTION

● Incise extensor retinaculum between 3rd and 4th compartments (see Figure HW-13)

● Transpose EPL and dissect under extensor compartments, but above joint capsule

   ■ Posterior interosseous nerve terminal branch is in floor of 4th extensor compartment

   ■ Posterior interosseous nerve neurectomy can be performed at this point if indicated (Figure HW-14)

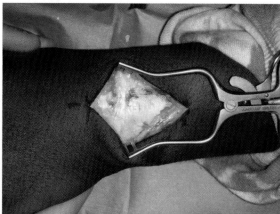

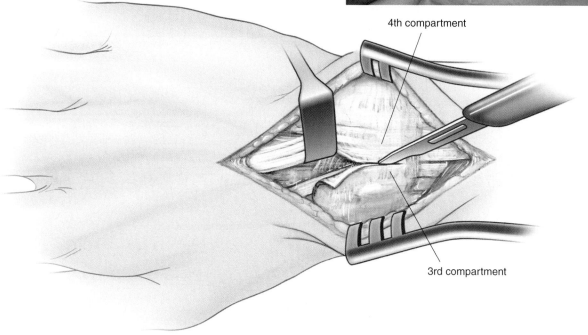

FIGURE HW-13 Dorsal approach to the distal forearm and wrist. Superficial dissection exposes the extensor retinaculum; the retinaculum is divided between the 3rd and 4th extensor compartments.

- Retract 3rd and 4th extensor compartments to expose dorsal extrinsic wrist ligaments and joint capsule (see Figure HW-14)

- Incise dorsal capsule over distal radius, and extend incision distally to expose distal radius, radiocarpal joint, and carpal bones (Figure HW-15; see Figure HW-14)

CLOSURE

- Repair capsule with suture

- Return EPL to 3rd compartment or keep it transposed and repair retinaculum

- Subcutaneous tissue and skin are approximated with suture

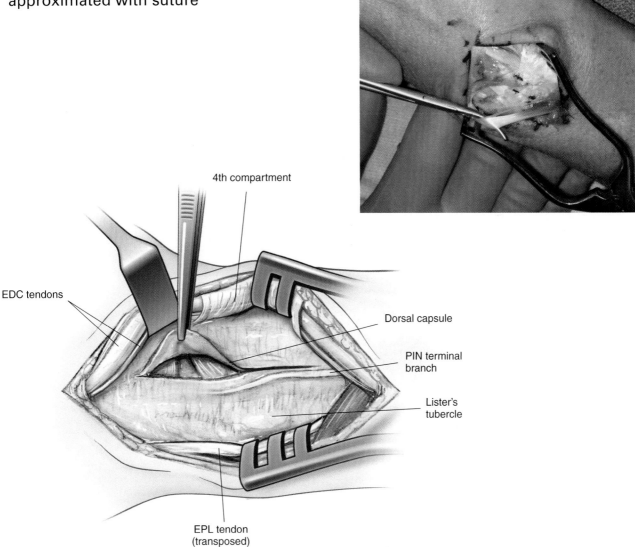

FIGURE HW-14 Dorsal approach to the distal forearm and wrist. The EPL is transposed radially, and the 4th compartment tendons are retraced ulnarly to expose the underlying dorsal capsule. The posterior interosseous nerve and artery are on the floor of the 4th extensor compartment.

HAZARDS

- **Superficial cutaneous nerve branches**
  - Superficial sensory radial nerve
  - Dorsal ulnar cutaneous nerve

- **Dorsal veins should be preserved if possible**
  - When dividing capsule, do not violate interosseous scapholunate ligament

PROXIMAL EXTENSION

- **Extension of approach can be performed proximally in subperiosteal manner along radial shaft**
  - Proximal exposure should be limited to level of outcropper muscles and musculotendinous junction of extensor muscles
  - Distal extension over metacarpal shafts can be performed in subperiosteal manner

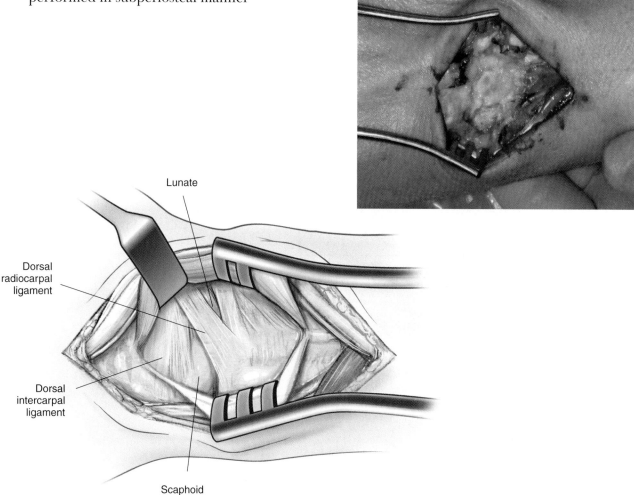

FIGURE HW-15 Dorsal approach to the distal forearm and wrist. The dorsal capsule is elevated to expose the dorsal carpal ligaments. Subperiosteal dissection is performed to expose the distal radius.

VOLAR (HENRY) APPROACH TO WRIST

Indications: Distal radius fractures, flexor tendon repair, vascular repair (radial artery), incision and drainage of infections, excision of masses or tumors, exposure of volar wrist capsule

POSITIONING (**FIGURE HW-16**)

- Supine
  - Hand in supination on hand table
  - Exsanguinate arm, and elevate tourniquet, if indicated

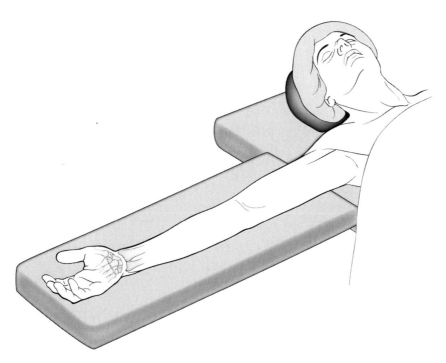

FIGURE HW-16   Positioning for the volar (Henry) approach to the wrist.

INCISION (**FIGURE HW-17**)

- This is the distal extension of the Henry approach in the forearm
- Incision is limited to just proximal to wrist crease along a line from radial styloid and lateral aspect of biceps tendon
  - Length of incision depends on exposure required

FIGURE HW-17 Incision for the volar approach to the wrist. Note the location of the radial artery, the FCR tendon, the palmaris tendon, and the median nerve and the palmar cutaneous branch.

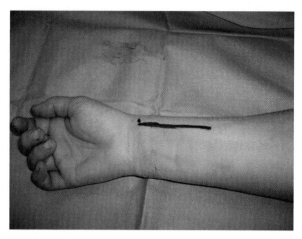

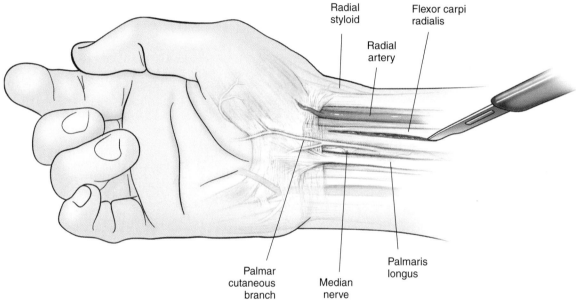

SUPERFICIAL DISSECTION (**FIGURE HW-18**)

- Incise skin and subcutaneous tissue
  - Identify FCR tendon and radial artery
  - Stay on radial side of FCR tendon to prevent injury to palmar cutaneous nerve branches
- Dissect through floor of FCR sheath to expose underlying tendons and identify median nerve deep to palmaris longus tendon (Figure HW-19)

DEEP DISSECTION (**SEE FIGURE HW-19**)

- Retract FCR radially to protect radial artery, and retract FPL and flexor tendons ulnarly to protect median nerve
  - FCR can be retracted ulnarly if exposure dictates this
- Sharply elevate pronator quadratus to expose subperiosteally volar wrist capsule and distal radius
  - Homan retractors are placed after exposure of radius (**Figure HW-20**)

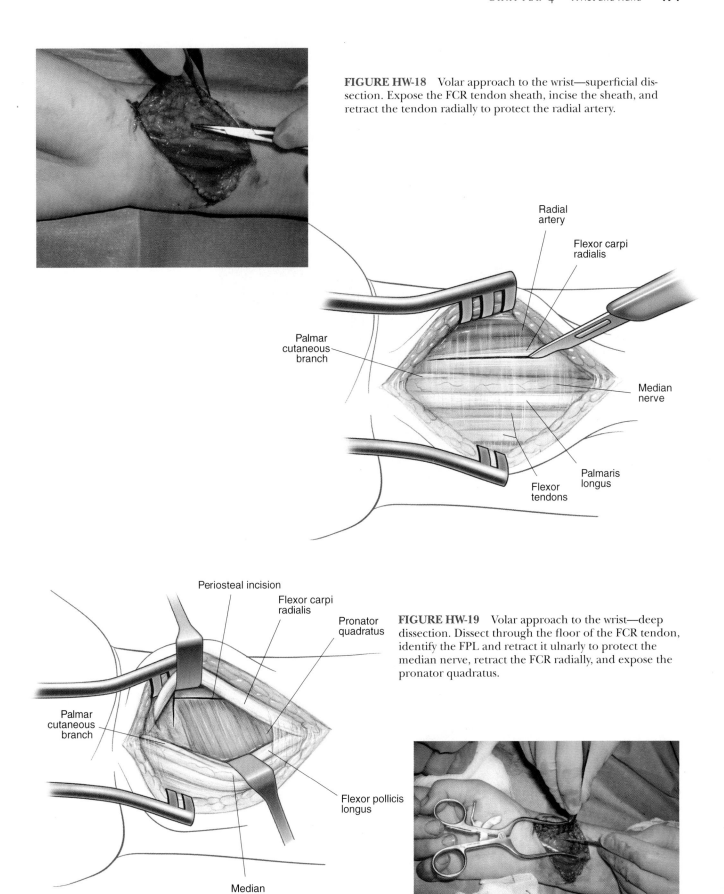

FIGURE HW-18   Volar approach to the wrist—superficial dissection. Expose the FCR tendon sheath, incise the sheath, and retract the tendon radially to protect the radial artery.

Radial artery

Flexor carpi radialis

Palmar cutaneous branch

Median nerve

Palmaris longus

Flexor tendons

Periosteal incision

Flexor carpi radialis

Pronator quadratus

Palmar cutaneous branch

Flexor pollicis longus

Median nerve

FIGURE HW-19   Volar approach to the wrist—deep dissection. Dissect through the floor of the FCR tendon, identify the FPL and retract it ulnarly to protect the median nerve, retract the FCR radially, and expose the pronator quadratus.

EXTENSILE APPROACH (FOR EXPOSURE OF MEDIAN NERVE, DISTAL RADIUS, AND CARPUS) (FIGURE HW-21)

- Incision is extended ulnarly at an angle across wrist crease
- Expose palmaris longus and palmar fascia (Figure HW-22)
- Palmaris longus tendon is identified
  - Release fascia of palmaris longus tendon, and retract tendons ulnarly to expose median nerve (**Figure HW-23**)

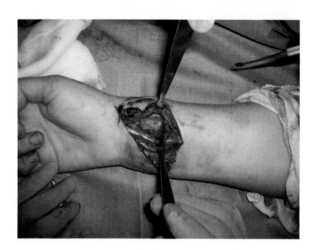

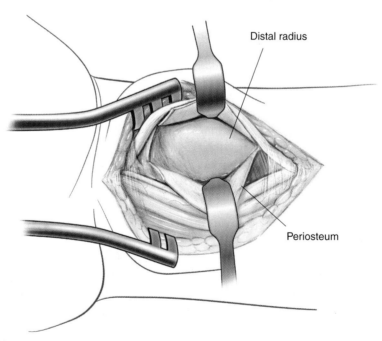

FIGURE HW-20 Sharply incise the radial border of the pronator quadratus, and elevate the muscle in a subperiosteal manner to expose the shaft of the radius. Limit the dissection to the distal radius volar ridge.

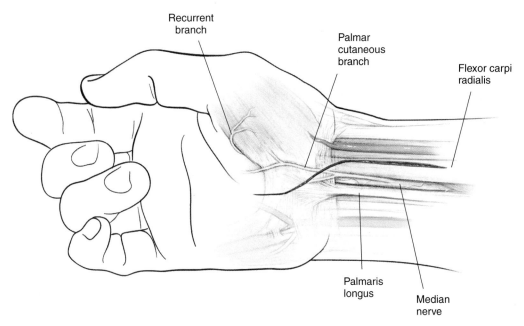

FIGURE HW-21   Incision for extension of the volar Henry approach distally.

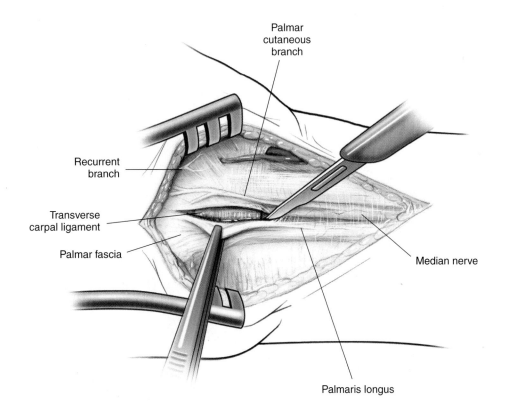

FIGURE HW-22   Extension of the volar Henry approach—superficial dissection. Identify the palmaris longus, incise the fascia, and identify the palmar cutaneous nerve branch and the median nerve.

- Remain on ulnar aspect of median nerve, and divide TCL protecting median nerve at all times (Figure HW-24)
- Identify palmar cutaneous nerve branch and recurrent motor branch, and protect them during exposure
  - Retraction of tendons provides access to volar ligaments and carpus **(Figure HW-25)**

CLOSURE

- Pronator is repaired loosely with absorbable sutures
- Subcutaneous tissue and superficial skin are closed with sutures

HAZARDS

- Radial artery and its branches
- Palmar cutaneous nerve
- Median nerve, recurrent branch

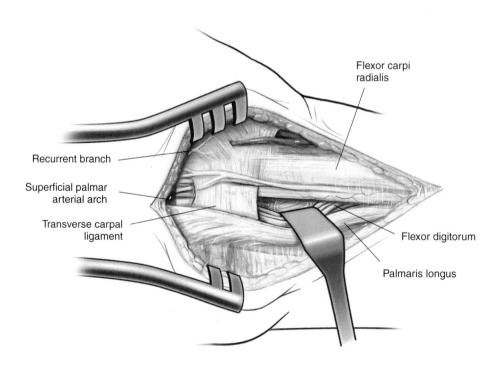

FIGURE HW-23 Extension of the volar Henry approach. Retract the palmaris tendon, and identify and protect the median nerve and the TCL.

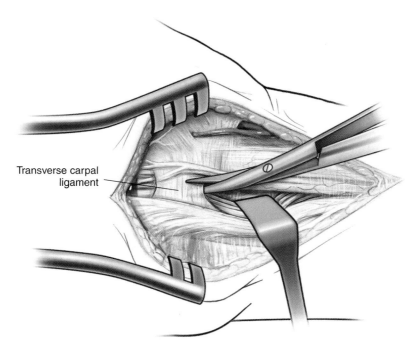

FIGURE HW-24　Remain on the ulnar side of the median nerve, and divide the TCL from a proximal to distal direction. Remain on the ulnar side of the nerve to prevent injury to the recurrent branch of the motor nerve.

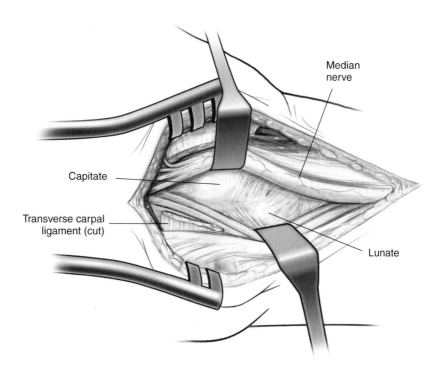

FIGURE HW-25　Retraction of the tendons after release of the TCL allows for access to the volar ligaments and carpus.

Exposure of the Median Nerve in the Palm and Distal Aspect of the Forearm

Indications: Median nerve decompression, synovectomy of flexor tendons, incision and drainage of midpalmar space infections

POSITIONING (FIGURE HW-26)

- Supine
  - Arm in supination on hand table, slight extension
  - Exsanguinate arm, and elevate tourniquet, if indicated

INCISION (FIGURE HW-27)

- Draw Kaplan's cardinal line from hook of hamate to first web space
- Locate incision site by drawing a line from radial aspect of ring finger to ulnar side of palmaris longus
- Hyperflex MCP joint of the ring finger past 90 degrees, and flex PIP and DIP joints to 90 degrees
  - The point at which finger touches palm marks distal end of incision and is approximate level of superficial palmar arch
  - From here, incision extends proximally approximately 2 cm
- Draw a line from radial aspect of middle finger
  - The point at which this intersects Kaplan's cardinal line is approximate location of recurrent motor branch of median nerve

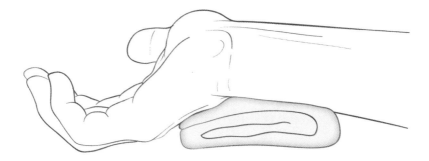

FIGURE HW-26   Positioning for exposure of the median nerve in the palm (carpal tunnel release).

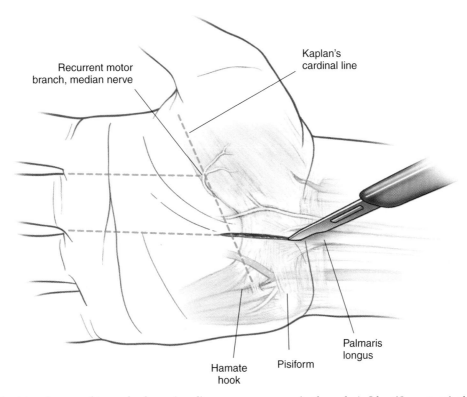

Recurrent motor
branch, median nerve

Kaplan's
cardinal line

Palmaris
longus

Pisiform

Hamate
hook

FIGURE HW-27   Incision for carpal tunnel release (median nerve exposure in the palm). Identify anatomical landmarks (pisiform, hook of the hamate, Kaplan's cardinal line). Incision is along the radial aspect of the ring finger.

SUPERFICIAL DISSECTION (FIGURE HW-28)

- Incise skin and subcutaneous tissue to expose palmar fascia
- Incise palmar fascia and retract to expose TCL

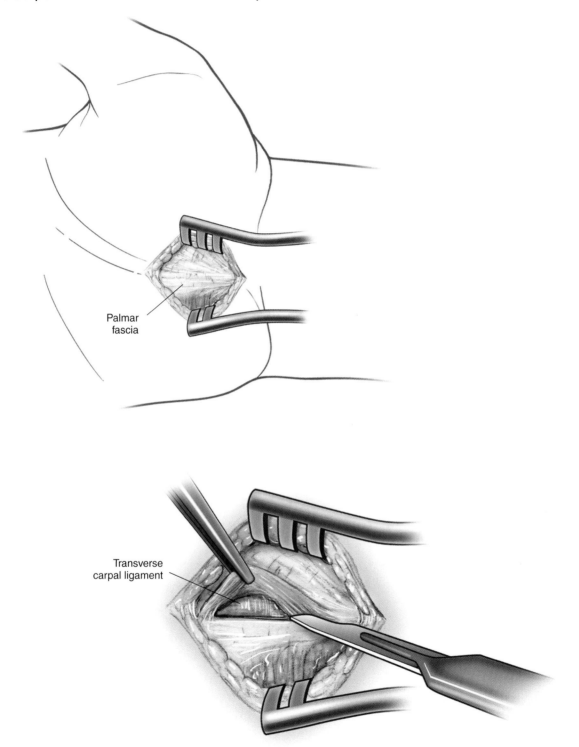

FIGURE HW-28   Exposure of the median nerve in the palm—superficial dissection. Incise the skin and subcutaneous tissue to expose the palmar fascia. Incise the palmar fascia along the radial aspect of the ring finger to expose the TCL.

DEEP DISSECTION (**FIGURE HW-29**)

- Small, sharp incision is made in distal aspect of TCL
  - Protect superficial palmar arch
  - Stay in line with the radial aspect of ring finger to avoid injury to recurrent motor branch
- Slide elevator into carpal tunnel beneath TCL to protect underlying median nerve (Figure HW-30)
- Sharply incise ligament while staying on top of elevator to expose median nerve and flexor tendons
- Using scissors with tips pointed ulnarly to protect median nerve, continue cutting TCL distal to proximal, then distally (see Figure HW-30)

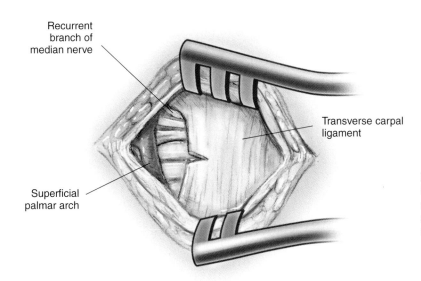

Recurrent branch of median nerve

Transverse carpal ligament

Superficial palmar arch

FIGURE HW-29 Exposure of the median nerve in the palm—deep dissection. Identify the distal aspect of the TCL. Protect the superficial palmar arch, which is just distal to the TCL. Divide the distal aspect of the TCL.

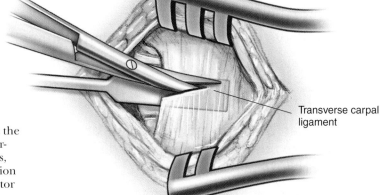

Transverse carpal ligament

FIGURE HW-30 Exposure of the median nerve in the palm—deep dissection. Place a Freer elevator underneath the TCL to protect the carpal tunnel contents, and divide the TCL from a distal to proximal direction on its ulnarmost aspect to protect the recurrent motor branch. Beware of variability in the anatomy of the recurrent motor branch.

● Visualize recurrent motor branch of the median nerve as it enters thenar musculature and superficial palmar arch to confirm that they are intact (Figure HW-31)

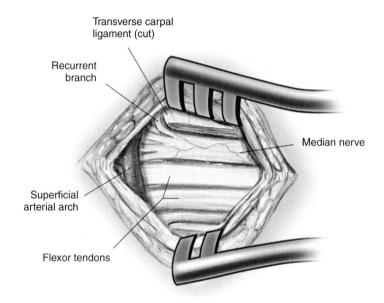

FIGURE HW-31 Exposure of the median nerve in the palm. After division of the TCL, identify the recurrent motor branch and the superficial palmar arch.

CLOSURE

● Skin is closed using sutures

HAZARDS

● Recurrent motor branch of median nerve has variable course
  ● 80% branch extraligamentously and are recurrent
  ● 15% branch subligamentously
  ● 5% branch transligamentously
● Superficial palmar arch
● Median nerve digital branches and carpal tunnel contents

PROXIMAL EXTENSION

● Incision can be extended proximally at an angle across wrist crease to expose median nerve in distal forearm (see Figures HW-23, HW-24, and HW-25)
  ▪ Stay on ulnar side of nerve to protect palmar cutaneous nerve
  ▪ Extension of incision in forearm can be used to perform fasciotomy of volar forearm

APPROACH TO THE ULNAR NERVE AND ARTERY IN THE DISTAL FOREARM AND PALM

Indications: Repair of ulnar nerve and artery injuries, decompression of ulnar nerve in Guyon's canal, hook of hamate excision

POSITIONING (SEE FIGURE HW-16)

- Supine
  - Hand supinated on the arm table
  - Exsanguinate and elevate tourniquet, if indicated

INCISION (FIGURE HW-32)

- Palpate hook of the hamate and pisiform
  - These two bones form boundaries of Guyon's canal in palm
  - Longitudinal incision along FCU tendon to level of wrist crease is marked
  - Bruner-type extension is made in palm between hamate hook and pisiform for distal extension of approach

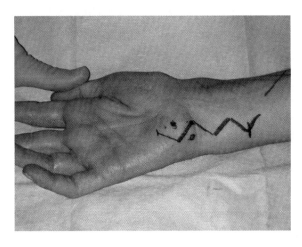

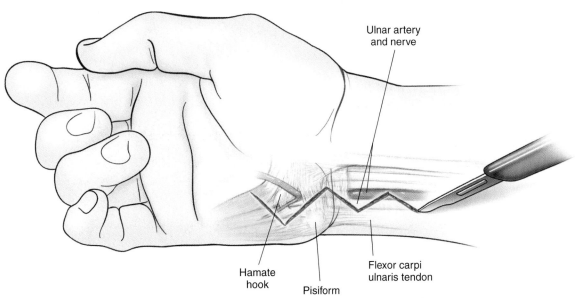

FIGURE HW-32   Incision for the approach to the ulnar nerve and artery in the distal forearm and palm.

SUPERFICIAL DISSECTION (**FIGURE HW-33**)

- Expose FCU tendon, and divide sheath of tendon so that it can be retracted ulnarly along with muscle belly

- Ulnar nerve and artery are deep to FCU tendon and identified in distal forearm

  ▪ Ulnar nerve is dorsal and ulnar to artery

- Identify artery and nerve, and slowly follow these structures into palm

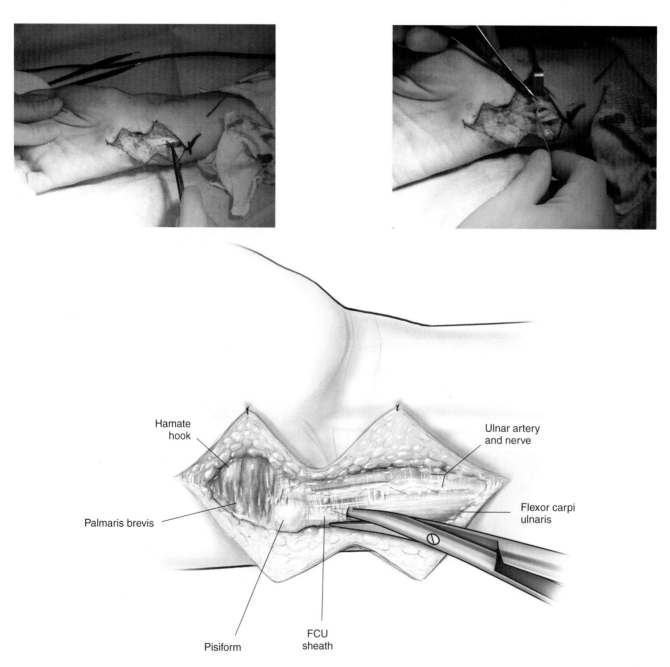

FIGURE HW-33 Approach to the ulnar nerve and artery in the distal forearm and palm—superficial dissection. Expose the FCU tendon, and divide the sheath. Retract the tendon ulnarly to expose the ulnar artery and nerve. Carefully follow the neurovascular bundle distally into Guyon's canal.

DEEP DISSECTION (FIGURE HW-34)

- Carefully divide palmar fascia over neurovascular structures
- By dissecting from a proximal-to-distal direction, branches of ulnar nerve are identified in palm
- Motor branch dives around hook of hamate to innervate intrinsic muscles
    - Sensory branch innervates radial aspect of ring finger and small finger
    - Ulnar artery makes a contribution to superficial palmar arch, and ulnar digital artery makes a contribution to small finger
- There is variability in the branching pattern, so careful dissection should be performed with loupe magnification
- For decompression of Guyon's canal, all branches of ulnar nerve should be decompressed
- The floor of Guyon's canal is TCL

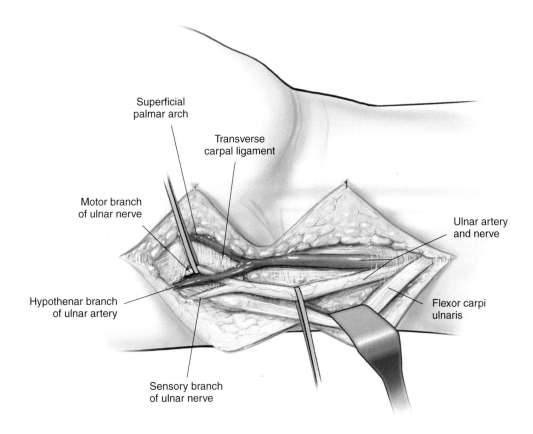

FIGURE HW-34   Approach to the ulnar nerve and artery in the distal forearm and palm—deep dissection. Carefully divide the palmar fascia over the neurovascular structures. Dissect in a proximal to distal direction, and identify the branches of the ulnar nerve. Decompress the ulnar nerve in Guyon's canal. The deep motor branch courses around the hook of the hamate and should be identified.

CLOSURE

- Obtain hemostasis
- Skin closure, no deep closure necessary

HAZARDS

- Ulnar nerve and artery
- Superficial palmar arch and digital arteries to small finger
- Deep branch of ulnar nerve as it passes around hook of hamate
- Dorsal ulnar nerve branch as it branches off ulnar nerve in mid to distal third of forearm

APPROACH TO APPLY AN EXTERNAL FIXATOR FOR THE WRIST

Indications: Treatment of distal radius fractures

POSITIONING

- Supine, arm in pronation

INCISION (FIGURE HW-35)

- Two 1 cm incisions are made on dorsal radial aspect of 2nd metacarpal
- A 4 cm incision also is made over distal radius, 8-12 cm proximal to wrist

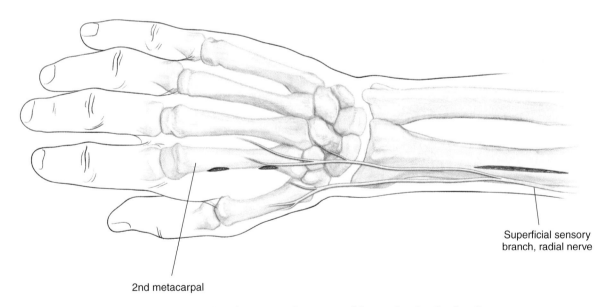

Superficial sensory
branch, radial nerve

2nd metacarpal

FIGURE HW-35   Incision for placement of an external fixator for the distal radius.

SUPERFICIAL DISSECTION (FIGURE HW-36)

- ● Skin and subcutaneous tissues overlying 2nd metacarpal are sharply incised
  - ▨ Blunt dissection is performed to expose metacarpal shaft
  - ▨ Extensor mechanism is protected

- ● Skin and subcutaneous tissues overlying distal radius are sharply incised
  - ▨ Blunt dissection is carried down to expose distal radius
  - ▨ Superficial sensory radial nerve should be identified and protected

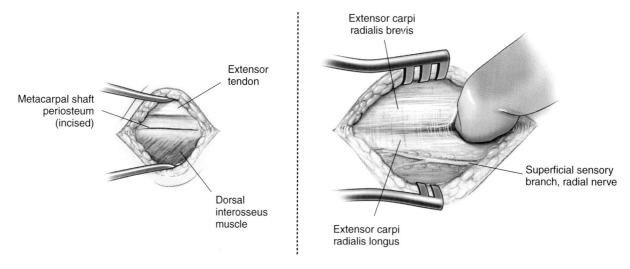

FIGURE HW-36   Superficial exposure of the 2nd metacarpal and radial shaft for placement of external fixator pins.

DEEP DISSECTION (FIGURE HW-37)

- ● Expose radial shaft for placement of external fixator pins
  - ▪ Place pins at 45 degrees to axis of forearm

- ● Expose index metacarpal shaft, and place appropriate external fixator pins in line with radial shaft pins
  - ▪ Pins should be placed in midportion of metacarpal

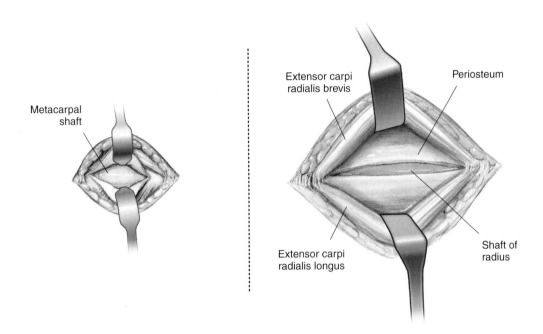

FIGURE HW-37 Deep dissection and exposure of metacarpal and radial shafts. Beware of the superficial sensory radial nerve.

CLOSURE

- ● Close skin around pin sites securely to limit pin tract infections

HAZARDS

- ● Superficial sensory radial nerve
- ● Index metacarpal fracture with inappropriately placed pins

WRIST ARTHROSCOPY

Indications: Diagnostic wrist arthroscopy for wrist pain, TFCC repair, ganglion cyst excision, wrist synovectomy, scapholunate ligament evaluation and débridement, arthroscopically assisted reduction of scaphoid and distal radius fractures

POSITIONING (FIGURE HW-38)

- Supine
    - Arm is secured to table just proximal to elbow
    - Elbow is bent to 90 degrees, and fingers are suspended from finger traps with 10-15 lb of traction in wrist arthroscopy traction tower
    - Wrist is flexed to 30 degrees, and all areas of compression are well padded

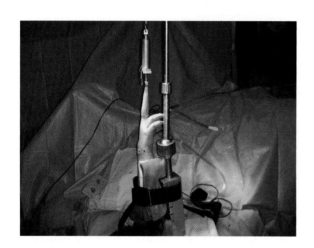
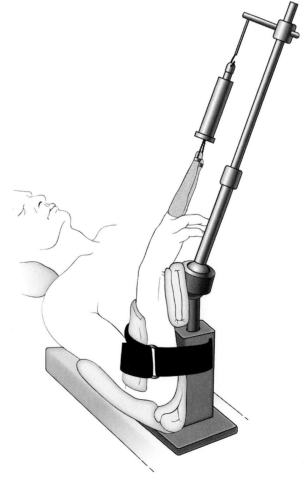

FIGURE HW-38   Positioning for wrist arthroscopy.

CHAPTER 4   Wrist and Hand   **189**

INCISIONS/PORTALS (FIGURE HW-39)

- ● Bony landmarks are palpated, and when wrist is secured in traction tower, portals are marked.

  - ■ All portals are named based on the extensor compartment of the hand: the 3-4 portal is between the 3rd and 4th extensor compartments (EPL and EDC)
  - ■ The 3-4, 4-5, 6R, radial midcarpal, and ulnar midcarpal portals are marked
  - ■ Most procedures can be performed through these portals

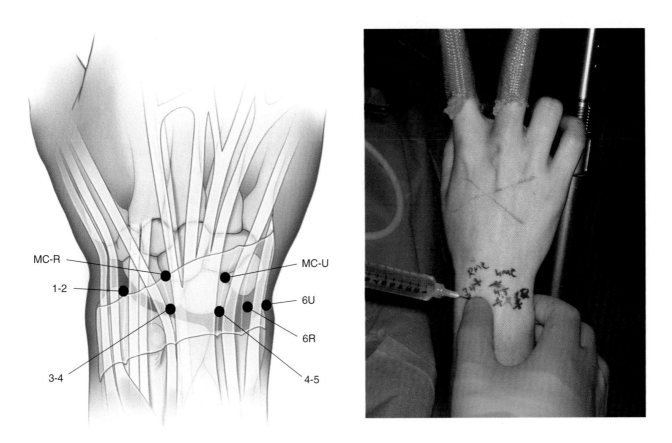

FIGURE HW-39   Wrist arthroscopy portals.

DISSECTION

- Longitudinal skin incisions are carefully made at 3-4 interval
  - Blunt cannula is carefully introduced into joint
  - Arthroscopic camera is placed, and inflow is connected
  - Spinal needle is placed at 6R interval for outflow
  - Diagnostic examination is initiated

- Begin examination radially and progress ulnarly
  - Evaluate radial recess, radial styloid **(Figure HW-40)**, volar ligaments, scaphoid articular surface, distal radius articular surface **(see Figure HW-40)**, scapholunate ligament, long and short radiolunate ligaments, lunate **(see Figure HW-40)**, TFCC, ulnar ligament complex, and dorsal capsule for ganglions **(see Figure HW-40)**

- The 4-5 portal is created under direct visualization
  - Blunt cannula is gently placed, making sure not to injure the carpal bones
  - Probe and shaver are placed through the portal
  - Arthroscopic portal can be switched, and the shaver and probe can be placed into the 3-4 portal if needed

- Radial midcarpal portal is created 1 cm distal to 3-4 portal in line with radial aspect of base of 3rd metacarpal

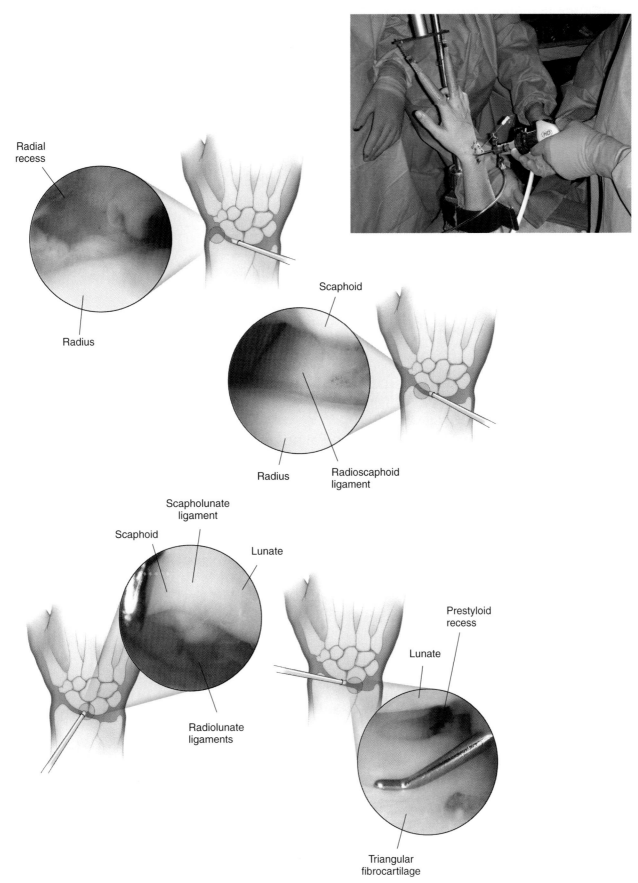

FIGURE HW-40 View from the 3-4 arthroscopic portal.

- Cannula is placed gently to avoid injury to carpal bones
  - Ulnar midcarpal portal is created under direct visualization with blunt trocar
  - Arthroscopic shaver and probe can be placed through these portals for diagnostic and therapeutic purposes
  - Capitohamate joint is identified and is an easily recognizable landmark **(Figure HW-41)**
  - Volar to capitohamate joint is lunotriquetral ligament
  - Radially, scapholunate ligament is identified **(see Figure HW-41)**
  - Probe is used to evaluate competency of these ligaments
  - Other portals (1,2 distal radioulnar joint, 6U, and STT) are for advanced arthroscopic techniques and should be used only by experienced surgeons

CLOSURE

- Skin is closed with sutures

HAZARDS

- Dorsal cutaneous ulnar nerve branch is at risk with placement of a 6U portal
- Radial artery and superficial sensory radial nerve are at risk with 1,2 portal placement
- Extensor tendons can be damaged if appropriate intervals are not used for each portal
- Cartilaginous injury to carpal bones or distal radius can occur with aggressive portal placement

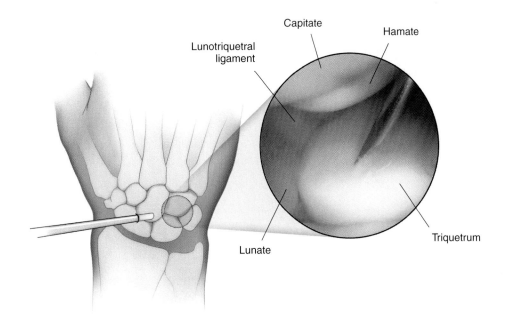

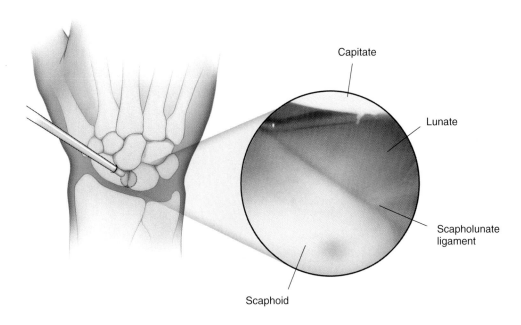

FIGURE HW-41   View from the radial midcarpal portal.

DORSAL APPROACH TO METACARPALS

Indications: ORIF of metacarpal fractures, repair of tendon lacerations, fasciotomy for compartment syndrome of the hand, extensor tenolysis

POSITIONING

● Supine, hand in pronation on hand table

INCISION (FIGURE HW-42)

● Longitudinal incision just ulnar or radial to metacarpal shaft

● To approach all 4 metacarpals or to release all interossei muscles for compartment syndrome, 2 longitudinal incisions can be used just off center to 2nd and 4th metacarpals

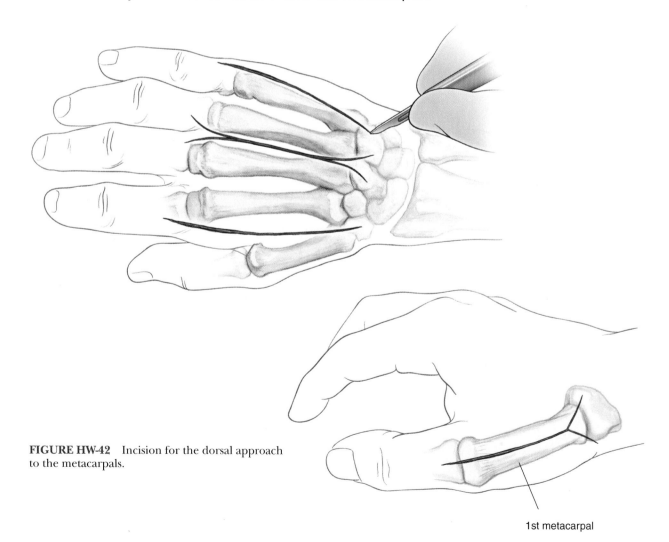

FIGURE HW-42   Incision for the dorsal approach to the metacarpals.

1st metacarpal

SUPERFICIAL DISSECTION (FIGURE HW-43)

- Skin and subcutaneous tissues are incised to expose extensor tendons and dorsal interossei muscles

  - Carefully identify and avoid any cutaneous nerve branches
  - Extensor tendon lacerations can be repaired at this point if identified

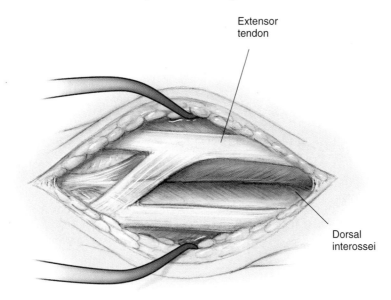

Extensor
tendon

Dorsal
interossei

FIGURE HW-43   Superficial dissection. Expose the extensor tendons.

DEEP DISSECTION

- Gently retract extensor tendon to expose metacarpal shaft (Figure HW-44)
- Subperiosteal dissection under extensor mechanism to expose metacarpal shaft

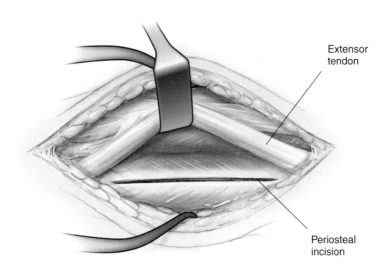

Extensor
tendon

Periosteal
incision

FIGURE HW-44   Deep dissection. Retract the extensor tendon to expose the metacarpal shaft.

- Place small Homan retractors to expose metacarpal shaft (Figure HW-45)
- For fasciotomies, divide fascia and intrinsic muscles
  - ▩ Hemostat is used to divide fascia over dorsal and volar intrinsic muscles through 2 dorsal incisions

CLOSURE

- Reapproximate periosteum over metacarpal if possible to limit adhesions to extensor tendon
  - ▩ Close skin with sutures

HAZARDS

- Extensor tendon injury
- Superficial cutaneous nerve injury

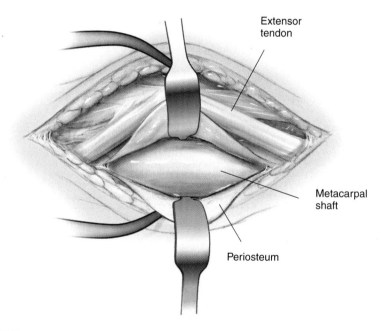

FIGURE HW-45 Deep dissection. Subperiosteally expose the metacarpal shaft.

DORSAL APPROACH TO FINGERS

Indications: Extensor tenolysis, extensor tendon repair, ORIF of phalanx fractures, excision of tumors and masses, capsulectomies of MCP and PIP joints, MCP and PIP arthroplasty and arthrodesis, intrinsic releases

POSITIONING

- Supine, hand in pronation on hand table

INCISION (FIGURE HW-46)

- Longitudinal or curvilinear incision just off center of MCP or PIP joints

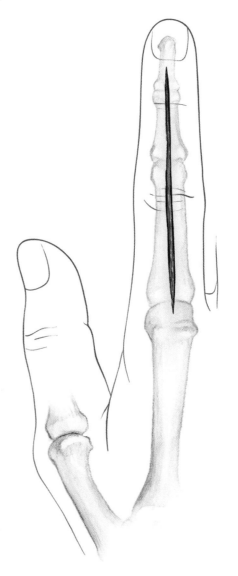

FIGURE HW-46   Incision for the dorsal approach to the fingers.

SUPERFICIAL DISSECTION (FIGURE HW-47)

- Skin and subcutaneous tissues are incised to expose extensor hood, avoiding superficial cutaneous nerves

- Extensor hood is incised longitudinally along radial side and elevated with extensor tendon to expose dorsal capsule of MCP joint

  - To expose proximal phalanx, divide interval between lateral band and central slip if area of interest is distal to MCP joint
  - Subperiosteal dissection is performed to expose proximal phalanx
  - Care should be taken to prevent injury to central slip insertion
  - Small Homan retractors are placed
  - Middle phalanx can be exposed in a similar manner by dissecting between central slip and lateral band. PIP joint can be exposed carefully by gently elevating extensor tendon to expose dorsal capsule. Insertion of central slip must be protected (**Figure HW-48**)

CLOSURE

- Repair interval between lateral band and central slip, or repair radial sagittal band with absorbable suture

- Close skin with suture

HAZARDS

- Cutaneous nerve branches
- Disruption of central slip insertion

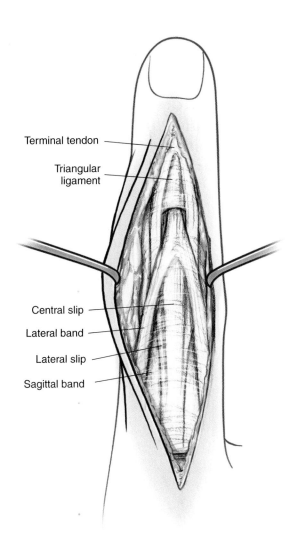

Terminal tendon

Triangular ligament

Central slip

Lateral band

Lateral slip

Sagittal band

FIGURE HW-47 Incision for the dorsal approach to the fingers—superficial dissection. Expose the extensor mechanism.

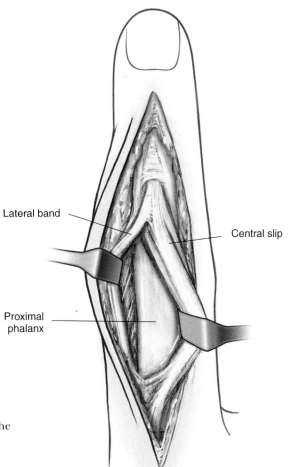

Lateral band

Central slip

Proximal phalanx

FIGURE HW-48 Exposure of the proximal phalanx between the lateral band and central slip.

VOLAR APPROACH TO THE FINGER

Indications: Flexor tendon repair, Dupuytren's contracture release, excision of tumors, volar plate arthroplasty, digital nerve repairs, flexor tendon tenolysis, flexor tendon staged reconstruction, PIP joint arthroplasty, drainage of flexor tendon sheath infections

POSITIONING

- Supine, hand in supination on hand table

INCISION (**FIGURE HW-49**)

- Bruner incisions with corners located at joint creases
  - Corner angles are not to be less than 60 degrees and incision should not pass too far dorsally to avoid injury to neurovascular bundle

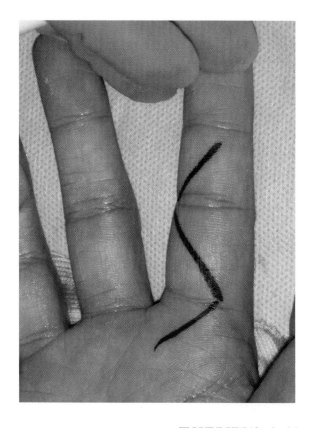

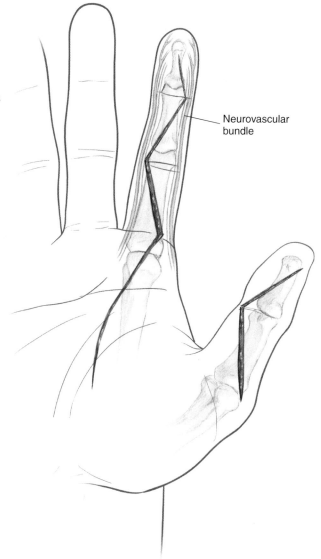

Neurovascular bundle

FIGURE HW-49   Incision for the volar approach to the finger.

SUPERFICIAL DISSECTION (FIGURE HW-50)

- Skin and subcutaneous tissues are incised to expose flexor tendon sheath
- Identify neurovascular bundles radially and ulnarly

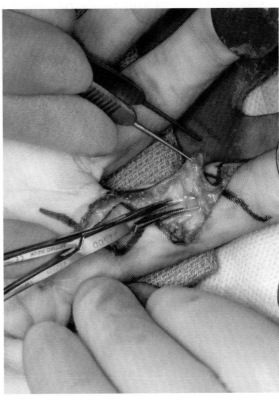

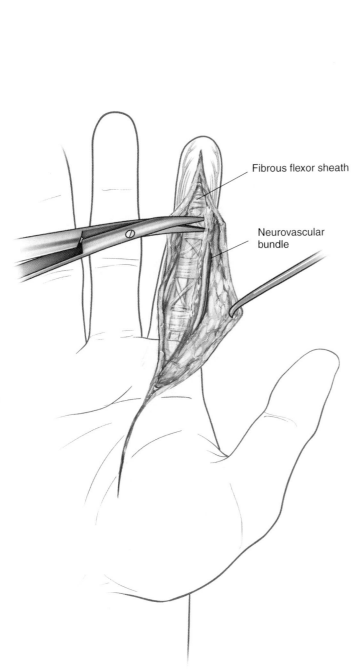

Fibrous flexor sheath

Neurovascular bundle

FIGURE HW-50   The skin and subcutaneous tissue are incised to expose the flexor tendon sheath, carefully protecting the radial and ulnar neurovascular bundles.

DEEP DISSECTION (FIGURE HW-51)

- Incise flexor tendon sheath as needed for tenolysis, exposure of PIP joint, or tendon repairs, but maintain A2 and A4 pulleys

CLOSURE

- Close skin with suture taking care to avoid strangulating tips of the skin flaps

HAZARDS

- Digital arteries, nerves

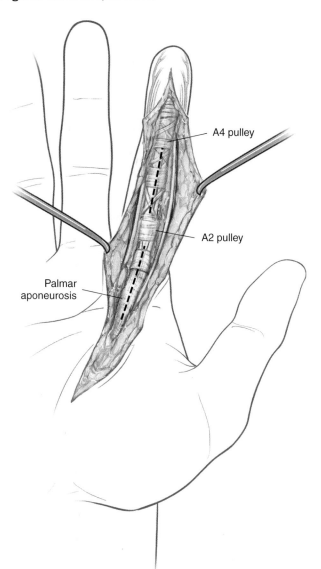

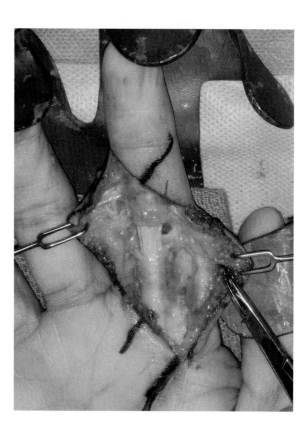

FIGURE HW-51 Exposure of the flexor tendon sheath and the neurovascular bundles.

MIDLATERAL APPROACH TO FINGERS

Indications: ORIF of phalanx fractures, extensor tendon or flexor tendon repairs, replantation of digits, excision of tumors or masses, digital nerve and artery repairs, drainage of flexor tendon sheath infections

POSITIONING

● Supine, hand in supination on hand table

INCISION (**FIGURE HW-52**)

● Longitudinal incision on lateral aspect of finger from lateral tip of proximal flexor crease, connecting to lateral tip of PIP flexor crease, and finally lateral crease of DIP flexor crease

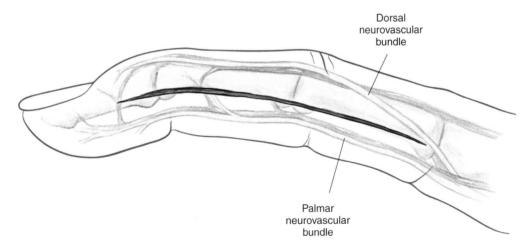

Dorsal neurovascular bundle

Palmar neurovascular bundle

FIGURE HW-52 Incision for the midlateral approach to the fingers.

SUPERFICIAL DISSECTION (**FIGURE HW-53**)

- Skin and subcutaneous tissues are carefully incised
- Bluntly dissect to identify neurovascular bundle on volar side of incision

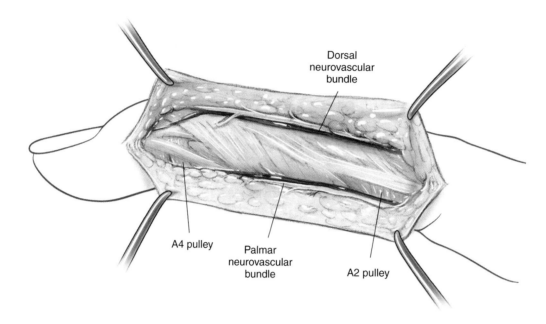

FIGURE HW-53   Superficial dissection. Identify the neurovascular bundles, and expose the extensor and flexor tendons.

DEEP DISSECTION

- Flexor tendon sheath may be incised with care taken to maintain A2 and A4 pulleys
- Skin and subcutaneous tissue can be elevated volarly to expose flexor tendon or elevated dorsally to expose extensor mechanism

CLOSURE

- Skin is closed with suture

HAZARDS

- Digital nerves, arteries, and veins

APPROACH FOR FINGER INFECTIONS

Paronychia

POSITIONING

- Supine, hand in pronation on hand table

INCISION (**FIGURE HW-54A AND B**)

- Two longitudinal incisions are made at nail eponychium, or one incision can be made if the infection is limited to one side

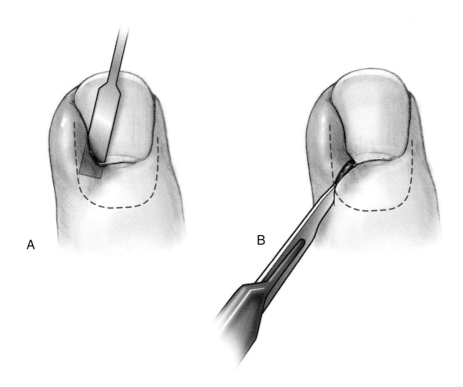

A B

FIGURE HW-54 Incision for treatment of paronychial infection.

SUPERFICIAL DISSECTION (FIGURE HW-54C AND D)

- Elevate nail fold to expose nail plate and drain infection

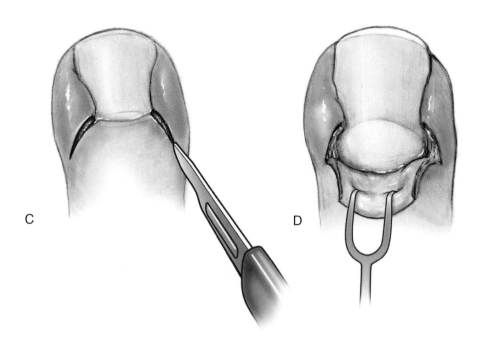

FIGURE HW-54, cont'd   Incision for treatment of paronychial infection.

CLOSURE

- Leave open to allow drainage of infection

HAZARDS

- Nail bed injury

Felon

POSITIONING

- Supine, hand in supination on hand table

INCISION (FIGURE HW-55A)

- Longitudinal incision on midlateral distal finger
- Place incision on ulnar side of index finger and radial side of thumb and small finger
- Incision can be made on either ulnar or radial sides for middle and ring fingers

SUPERFICIAL DISSECTION

Incise skin and subcutaneous tissue

DEEP DISSECTION (FIGURE HW-55B)

- Incise finger pulp taking care to open all septa with hemostat

CLOSURE

- Leave open to allow drainage of infection

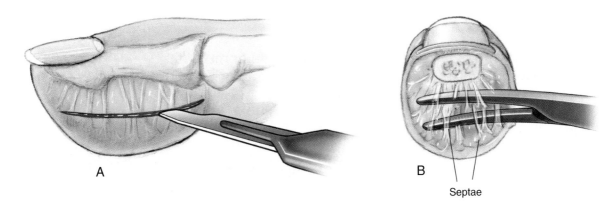

A

B

Septae

FIGURE HW-55 Incision for treatment of felon infection.

APPROACH FOR COMPARTMENT RELEASE IN THE HAND

Indications: Fasciotomies for compartment syndrome

POSITIONING

- Supine, hand in pronation on hand table

INCISION (FIGURE HW-56A AND B)

- Incision is made between 2nd and 3rd metacarpals and 4th and 5th metacarpals in a similar fashion as dorsal approach to metacarpals

  - Palmar and dorsal interossei are released through these incisions

- Two incisions are made along the volar palm, one over the thenars and the other over the hypothenar muscles
- See also approach for decompression of the median nerve in the palm and wrist

SUPERFICIAL DISSECTION

- Skin and subcutaneous tissue is incised including fascia overlying muscles of the intrinsics, thenars, and hypothenars

  - Thenar release also includes adductor pollicis muscle (Figure HW-56C)

DEEP DISSECTION

- Divide fascia of dorsal interossei muscles, and use hemostat to divide volar interossei fascia

CLOSURE

- Leave open, and return for wound closure versus skin grafting

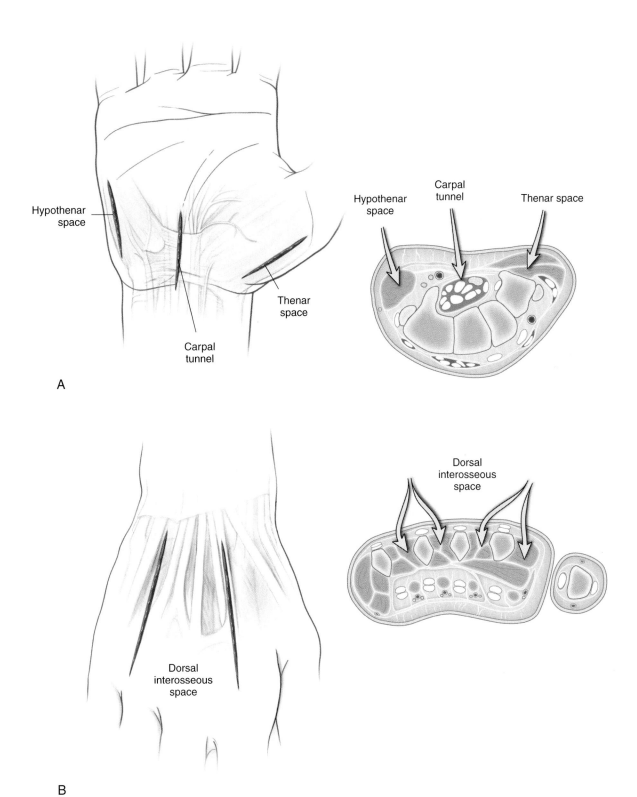

FIGURE HW-56   Approach for compartment releases for the hand, including incision for carpal tunnel release.

REFERENCES

Doyle JR, Botte MJ: Surgical Anatomy of the Hand and Upper Extremity. Philadelphia, Lippincott Williams & Wilkins, 2003.

Gelberman R: Master Techniques in Orthopedic Surgery: The Wrist, 2nd ed. Philadelphia, Lippincott Williams & Wilkins, 2002.

Hoppenfeld S, deBoer P: Surgical Exposures in Orthopedics, 3rd ed. Philadelphia, Williams & Wilkins, 2003.

Netter F: Atlas of Human Anatomy, 4th ed. Philadelphia, Saunders, 2006.

Standring S: Gray's Anatomy, 38th ed. Philadelphia, Churchill Livingstone, 1995.

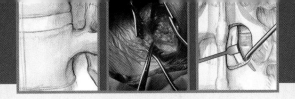

CHAPTER

5

SPINE

———

FRANCIS H. SHEN

REGIONAL ANATOMY

Osteology

- ● Occiput (Figure SP-1)
  - ▨ Foramen magnum
  - ▨ External occipital protuberance (inion)
    - ● Thickest portion of bone (4-18 mm)
  - ▨ Supreme, superior, and inferior nuchal lines
  - ▨ Transverse sinus

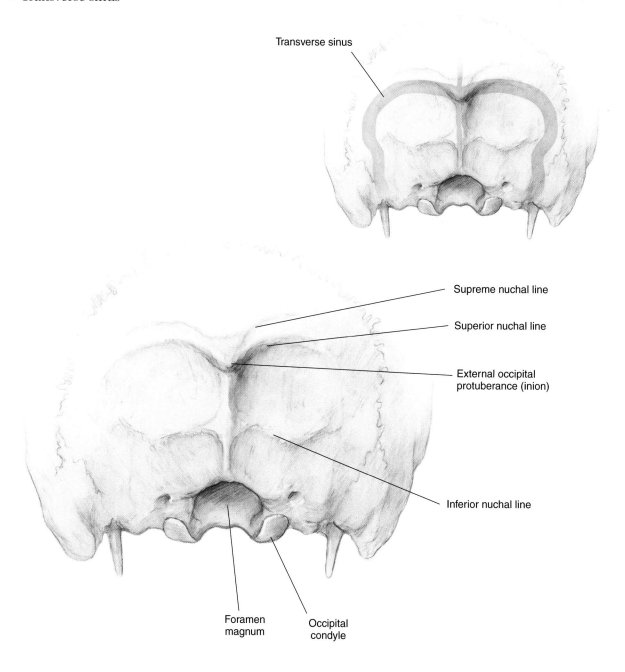

FIGURE SP-1   Posteroinferior view of occiput. Note the inion and the supreme, superior, and inferior nuchal lines.

- **Cervical Vertebrae (Figure SP-2)**
  - ▨ C1 (atlas)
    - ● Ring that lacks a centrum and spinous process
    - ● Groove for vertebral artery sits posterior and superiorly
  - ▨ C2 (dens)
    - ● Predental space
    - ● Prominent bifid spinous process
    - ● Superior articular facet lies anterior to inferior facets
  - ▨ Subaxial cervical spine C3-C7
    - ● Spinal canal triangular configuration
      - ○ Sagittal diameter varies from 17-18 mm (C3-C6) to 15 mm (C7)
    - ● Lateral masses thinnest at C6 and C7
    - ● Anterior and posterior tubercle
      - ○ Anterior tubercle C6
        - ❑ Carotid tubercle
        - ❑ Chassaignac's tubercle
    - ● Transverse foramen
    - ● C3-C6 bifid spinous process
    - ● C7 nonbifid spinous process (vertebra prominens)

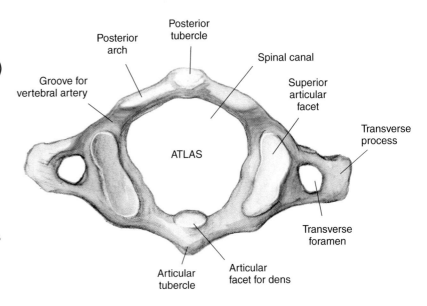

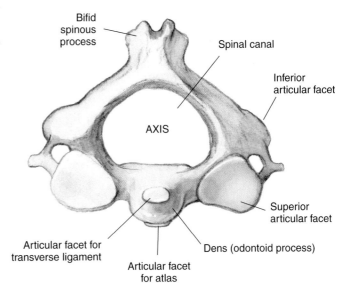

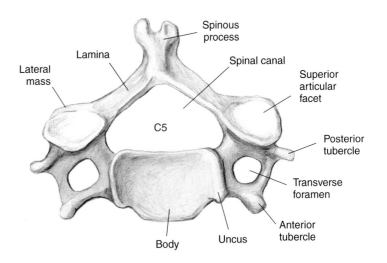

FIGURE SP-2 Superior view of atlas (C1), axis (C2), and C5 vertebrae.

- **Thoracic Vertebrae (Figure SP-3)**
  - Twelve heart-shaped vertebrae
  - Spinal canal circular in configuration
  - Canal diameter typically smaller than in cervical and lumbar regions
  - Ribs provide additional stability
    - Typically, ribs 1-10 articulate with the corresponding numbered vertebrae and the cephalad vertebra
    - Ribs 11 and 12 are floating vertebrae and attach to the corresponding vertebrae only

- **Lumbar Vertebrae (Figure SP-4)**
  - Five kidney-shaped vertebrae
  - Spinal canal triangular in configuration
  - Pedicles increase in width from L1 to L5
  - Pedicles increase in medial inclination from L1 to L5
  - Less motion at L5-S1 owing to iliolumbar ligament and transition zone to the sacrum

- **Sacrum**
  - Triangular shaped
  - Five fused vertebrae
  - Sacral ala
  - Sacral promontory

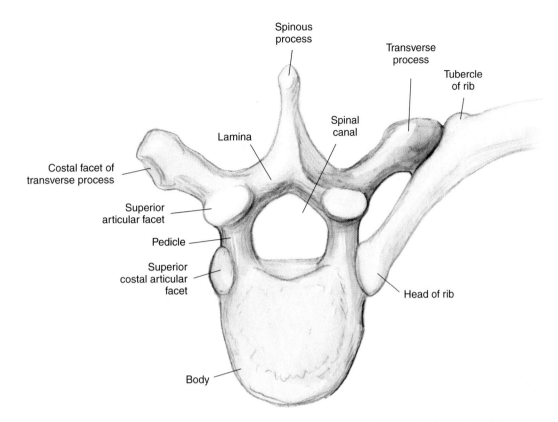

FIGURE SP-3 Superior view of thoracic vertebra and adjoining rib. Note the coronal orientation of thoracic facet joints.

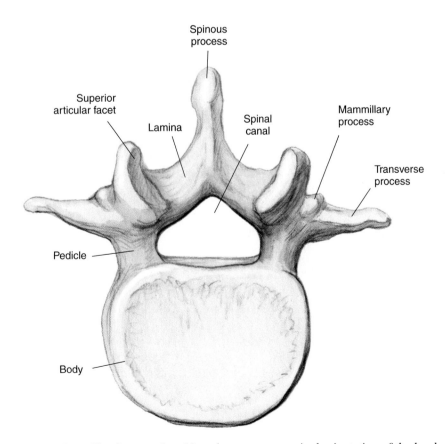

FIGURE SP-4 Superior view of lumbar vertebra. Note the more parasagittal orientation of the lumbar facet joints.

Arthrology

- Cervical
  - Occipitocervical (Figure SP-5)
    - 50% of cervical flexion-extension
    - Occipital condyles
    - Ligamentum nuchae
    - Tectorial membrane (following the foramen magnum becomes the posterior longitudinal ligament)

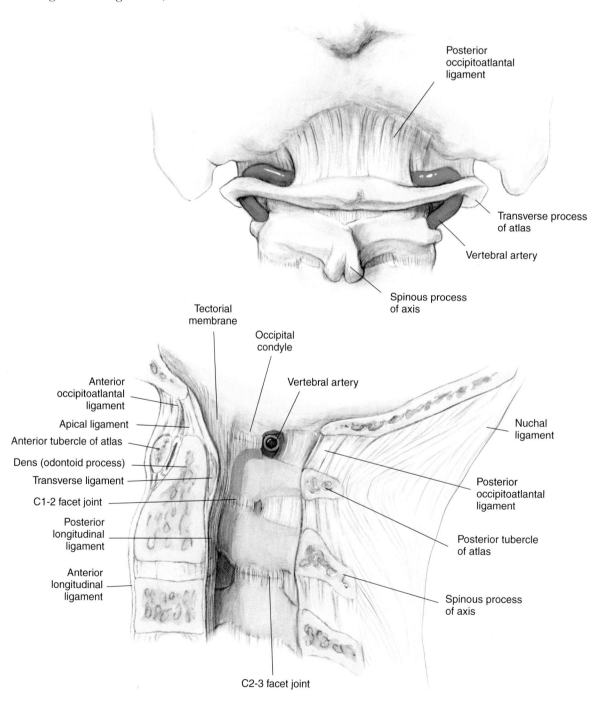

FIGURE SP-5 Occipitocervical junction. Note the location and course of the vertebral artery.

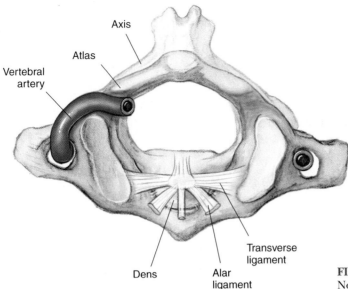

FIGURE SP-6   Superior view of atlantoaxial articulation. Note the relationship of the transverse ligament to C1-C2.

- Anterior longitudinal ligament (continues throughout the mobile spine)
- Posterior occipitoatlantal and anterior occipitoatlantal ligaments
- Apical and alar ligaments
- Atlantoaxial (Figure SP-6)
  - 50% of cervical rotation
  - Transverse ligament
  - Accessory ligament
  - No intervertebral disc
- Uncovertebral joint (Figure SP-7)
  - Not true diarthrodial joint
  - Forms anterior border of neuroforamen
- Facet joint
  - Coronal alignment
  - Shingled with superior articular facet anterior to inferior articular facet

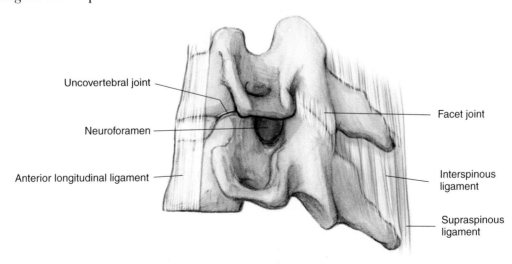

FIGURE SP-7   Lateral view of subaxial cervical spine. Note the anatomical location of the uncovertebral joints and neuroforamen.

- **Thoracic**
  - ■ Facet
    - Coronal alignment
    - Shingled with superior articular facet anterior to inferior articular facet
  - ■ Costovertebral (Figure SP-8)
    - Rib articulates vertebra at body and transverse process
    - Multiple ligamentous attachments

- **Lumbar and Sacrum (Figure SP-9)**
  - ■ Facet joint
    - Sagittal alignment
    - Superior articular facet lies lateral to inferior articular facet
  - ■ Sacroiliac joint

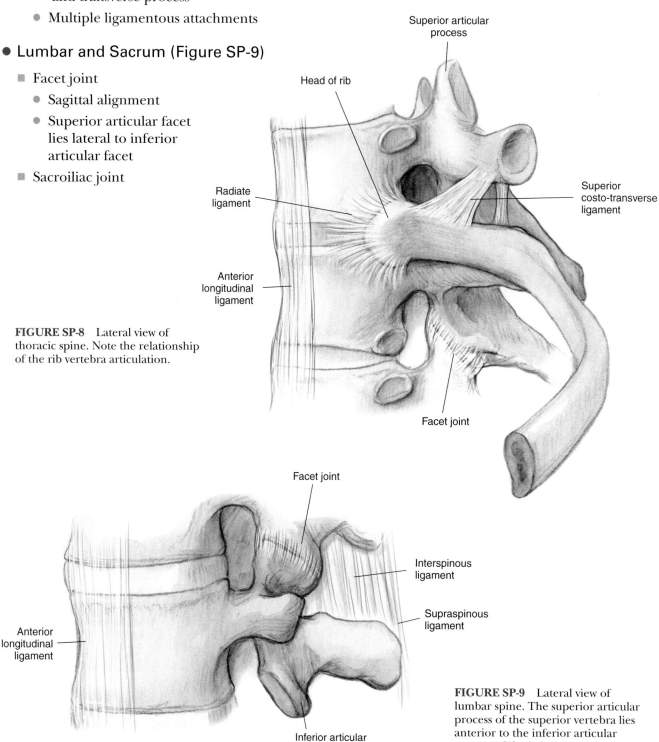

FIGURE SP-8   Lateral view of thoracic spine. Note the relationship of the rib vertebra articulation.

FIGURE SP-9   Lateral view of lumbar spine. The superior articular process of the superior vertebra lies anterior to the inferior articular process of the inferior vertebra.

Muscles

- ● Anterior
  - ▪ Best grouped by region
    - ● Cervical (Figure SP-10)
    - ● Thoracic (Figure SP-11)
    - ● Lumbar (Figure SP-12)

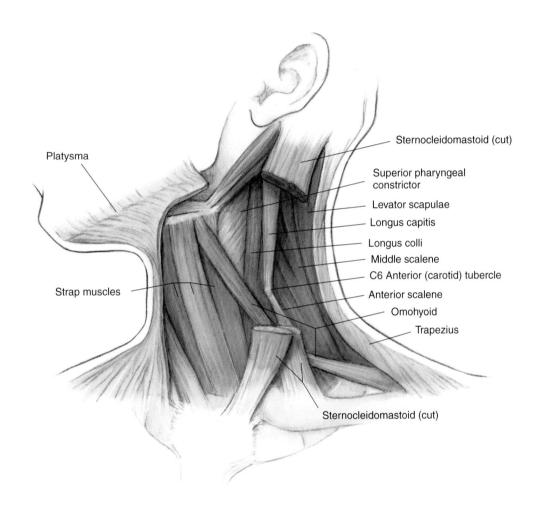

Platysma

Strap muscles

Sternocleidomastoid (cut)

Superior pharyngeal constrictor

Levator scapulae

Longus capitis

Longus colli

Middle scalene

C6 Anterior (carotid) tubercle

Anterior scalene

Omohyoid

Trapezius

Sternocleidomastoid (cut)

FIGURE SP-10   Muscles of the anterior cervical spine.

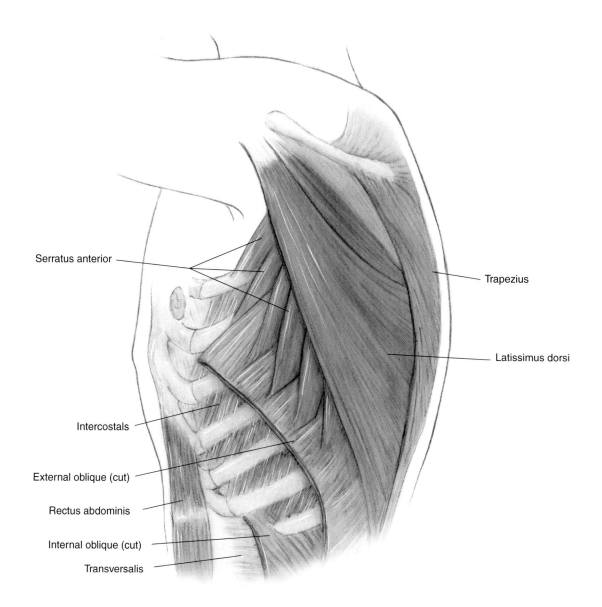

Serratus anterior

Trapezius

Latissimus dorsi

Intercostals

External oblique (cut)

Rectus abdominis

Internal oblique (cut)

Transversalis

FIGURE SP-11 Muscles of the anterior thoracic spine.

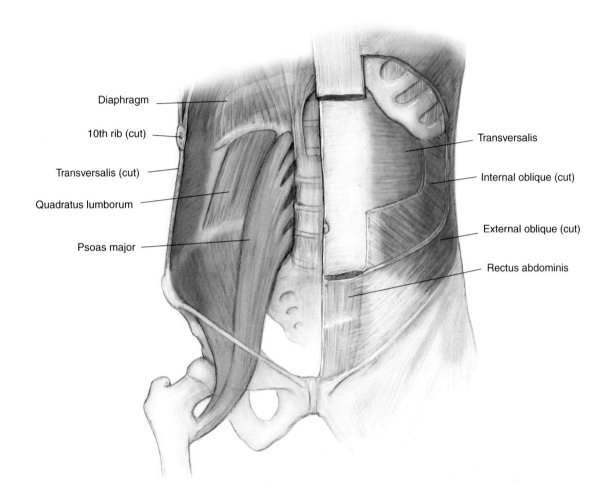

Diaphragm

10th rib (cut)

Transversalis (cut)

Quadratus lumborum

Psoas major

Transversalis

Internal oblique (cut)

External oblique (cut)

Rectus abdominis

FIGURE SP-12 Muscles of the anterior lumbar spine.

- ● **Posterior**
  - ▢ Best grouped by layers
    - ● Superficial (Figure SP-13, *left half*)
    - ● Intermediate (Figure SP-13, *right half*)
    - ● Deep (Figure SP-14)

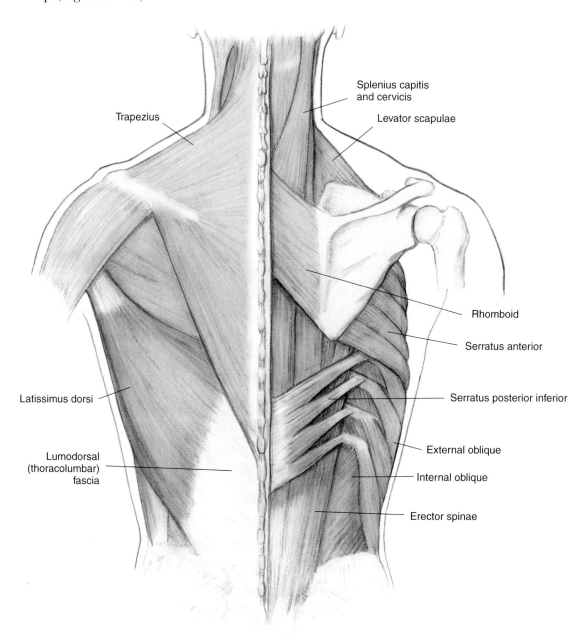

FIGURE SP-13 Superficial *(left half)* and intermediate *(right half)* musculature of the posterior spine.

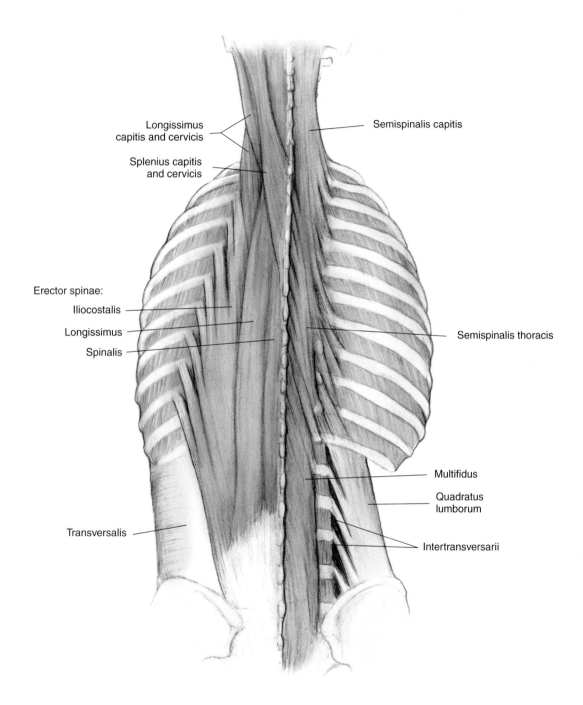

Longissimus
capitis and cervicis

Splenius capitis
and cervicis

Semispinalis capitis

Erector spinae:

Iliocostalis

Longissimus

Spinalis

Semispinalis thoracis

Multifidus

Quadratus
lumborum

Transversalis

Intertransversarii

FIGURE SP-14   Deep musculature of the posterior spine.

Nervous System

- **Spinal cord (Figure SP-15)**
  - Continuation of medulla as it exits foramen magnum
  - Terminates as conus medullaris at T12-L1 or L2-L3
  - Continues caudally as the cauda equina
  - Spinal cord diameter largest at C6 vertebra
  - Three meninges: dura (outermost covering), arachnoid, and pia mater (innermost covering)
  - Cerebrospinal fluid between arachnoid and pia mater
  - Dentate ligament (anchors spinal cord in position)

- **Gray matter**
  - Anterior/motor horn
    - Somatomotor neurons
  - Intermediolateral horn
    - Visceral center of gray matter
  - Posterior/sensory horn
    - Somatosensory neurons

- **White matter**
  - Anterior column
    - Anterior spinothalamic tract
      - Carries light/crude touch sensation
    - Anterior corticospinal tract
      - Delivers voluntary contraction
  - Posterior column
    - Fasciculus cuneatus laterally
    - Fasciculus gracilis medially
    - Carries deep touch, proprioception, vibratory sense
  - Lateral column
    - Lateral spinothalamic tract
      - Carries contralateral pain and temperature fibers
    - Descending motor lateral corticospinal tract
      - Delivers ipsilateral motor fibers

- **Nerve roots**
  - Spinal nerve
    - Formed by convergence of the dorsal and ventral roots
    - Exits foramen
      - Delivers dorsal primary rami
    - Supplies skin and muscle to neck and back
      - Delivers ventral primary rami

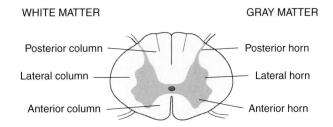

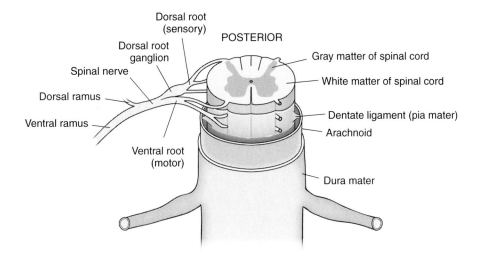

FIGURE SP-15 Cross-sectional spinal cord anatomy with surrounding pia, arachnoid, and dura mater.

- Supplies anteromedial trunk and limbs
  - Brachial plexus in the cervical spine
  - Lumbosacral plexus in the lumbar and sacral spine
- Thirty-one paired spinal nerves
  - Eight cervical
  - Twelve thoracic
  - Five lumbar
  - Five sacral
  - One coccygeal

- ● **Sympathetic chain**

  - Cervical
    - Posterior to carotid sheath
    - Lies anteriorly on longus colli bilaterally
    - Injury can result in Horner's syndrome
  - Lumbar
    - Typically, anterior to the psoas on the lateral aspect of the vertebral body
    - If divided, this results in a warm ipsilateral leg

Vascularity (Figure SP-16)

- **Cervical**
  - Carotid artery
  - Vertebral artery

- **Thoracic**
  - Aorta
  - Vena cava
  - Segmentals
  - Intercostal artery
  - Artery of Adamkiewicz (80% originating at T10)

- **Lumbar and Lumbosacral**
  - Aorta
  - Vena cava
  - Common iliac artery and vein
  - Iliolumbar vein
  - Middle sacral artery

- **Spinal Cord**
  - Segmentals/radicular arteries from the aorta
  - Single anterior spinal artery lying in anterior median fissure
  - Paired posterior spinal arteries running along posterolateral sulci

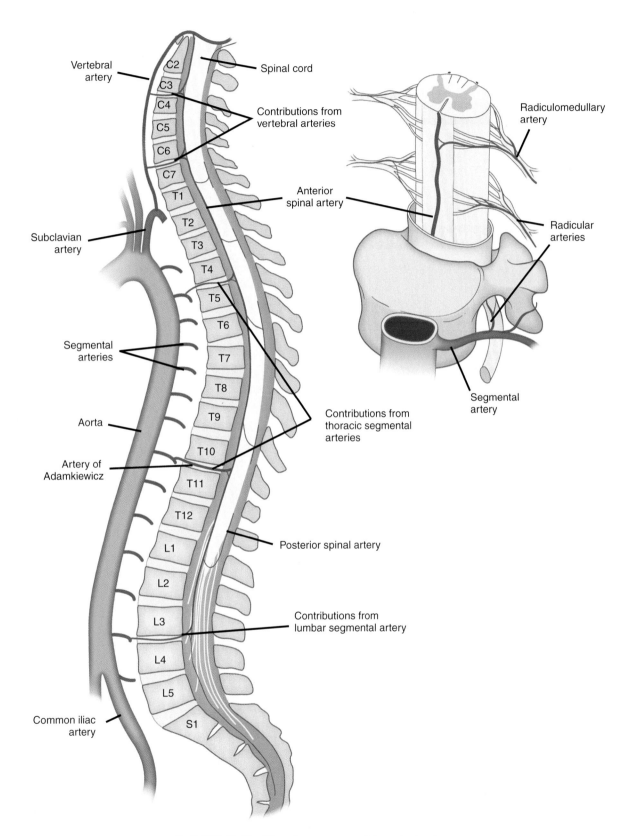

FIGURE SP-16   Vascular anatomy of the spinal column.

CROSS-SECTIONAL ANATOMY (Figure SP-17)

Cervical Spine Cross Section

Thoracic Spine Cross Section

Lumbar Spine Cross Section

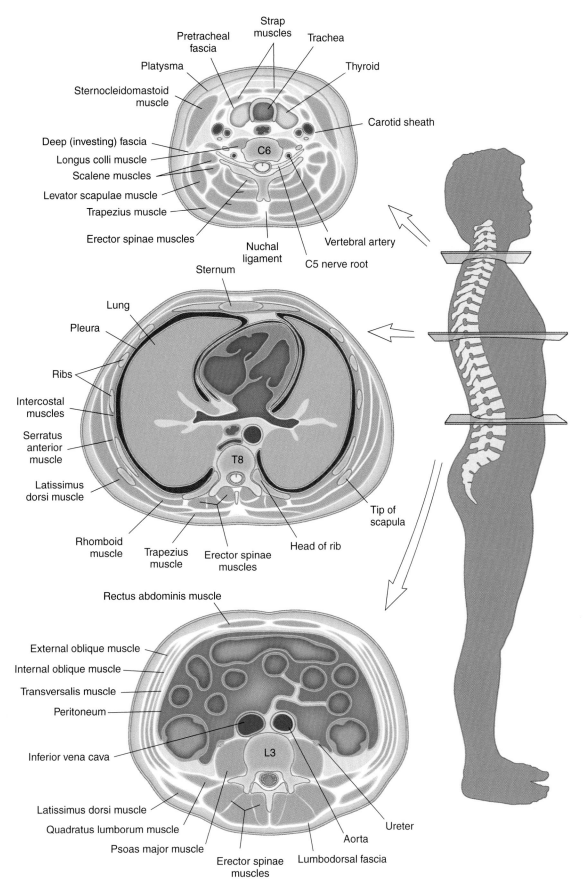

FIGURE SP-17   Cross-sectional anatomy of the cervical, thoracic, and lumbar spine.

LANDMARKS (Figure SP-18)

Cervical Spine

● Anterior

- Chin
- Angle of jaw
- Hyoid
- Thyroid cartilage
- Cricoid ring
- Carotid tubercle
- Sternal notch
- Sternocleidomastoid muscle
- Carotid pulse

● Posterior

- Inion
- C2 spinous process
- C7 spinous process

Thoracic Spine

● Anterior

- Ribs
- Sternal notch
- Tip of scapula

● Posterior

- Ribs
- Spinous processes

Lumbar and Lumbosacral Spine

● Anterior

- Pubic symphysis
- Pubic tubercle
- Anterior superior iliac spine (ASIS)
- Ribs

● Posterior

- Intercrestal line
- Posterior superior iliac spine (PSIS)
- Spinous processes

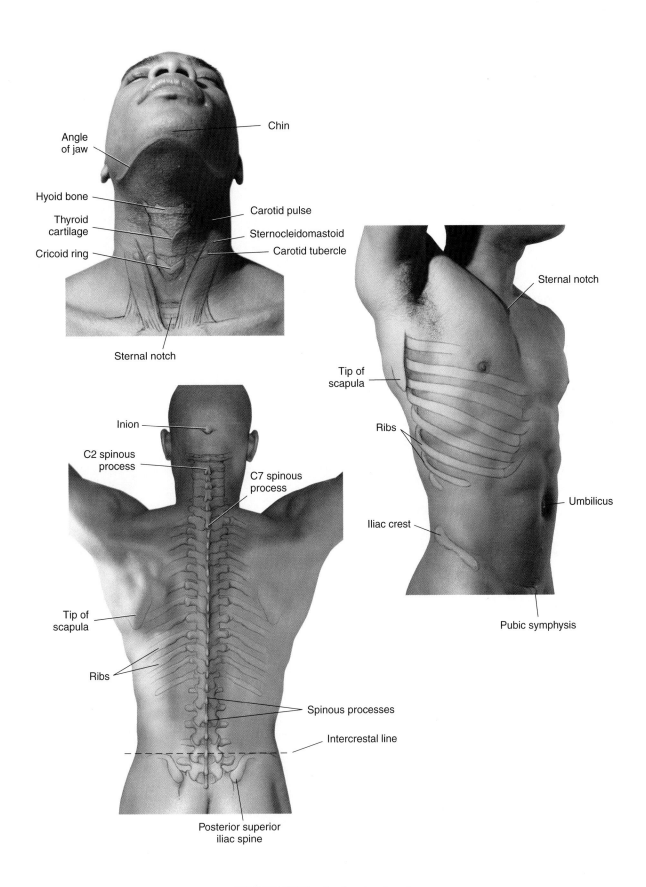

FIGURE SP-18 Surface landmarks.

ANTERIOR APPROACH TO THE CERVICAL SPINE

Indications

- **Anterior decompression of spinal canal**
  - Discectomy
  - Corpectomy
  - Epidural abscess
  - Ventral tumor

- **Anterior cervical fusion**
  - Fracture
  - Spinal malalignment
  - Tumor
  - Infection
  - Degenerative processes

- **Biopsy of vertebral body or disc space**
- **Placement of anterior cervical instrumentation**

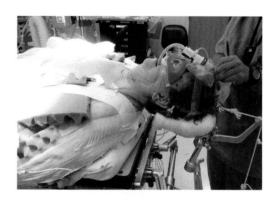

POSITIONING

- **Supine (Figure SP-19)**

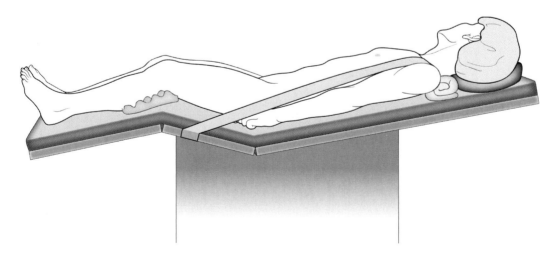

FIGURE SP-19   Supine positioning for surgery of the anterior cervical spine.

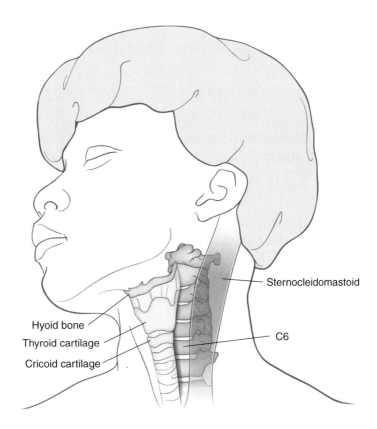

Hyoid bone

Thyroid cartilage

Cricoid cartilage

Sternocleidomastoid

C6

FIGURE SP-20   Relational anatomy of the anterior cervical spine.

- Head position (Figure SP-20)
  - Typically, the head is placed in a neutral alignment
  - Extension and contralateral head rotation can help improve surgical exposure if necessary
  - Care should be taken to ensure that the degree of extension necessary is possible before intubation
  - If there is any degree of myelopathy or neurologic changes with awake extension, an awake intubation should be considered
- Position of arms
  - At patient's side
  - Gentle taping of shoulders inferiorly can improve intraoperative radiographs
- Additional tricks
  - Neck extension can be facilitated by placement of a roll between the shoulder blades
  - Gardner-Wells or Halter traction can be used if distraction is required
  - Elevate operating table 30 degrees to reduce venous bleeding

HAZARDS

- Neural Structures
  - Spinal cord
  - Cervical nerve roots
  - Brachial plexus
    - Runs between anterior and middle scalene muscles
  - Recurrent laryngeal nerve
    - Branch of vagus nerve
    - Runs within tracheoesophageal groove
    - Left side crosses under arch of aorta
    - Right side crosses under subclavian artery and crosses surgical field at more variable level
  - Superior laryngeal nerve
  - Sympathetic chain
    - Sits anteriorly on the longus colli
    - Injury can lead to an ipsilateral Horner's syndrome
      - Ptosis
      - Miosis
      - Anhidrosis

- Vascular
  - Carotid artery
    - Runs in the medial aspect of the carotid sheath
  - Vertebral artery
    - Typically enters transverse foramen at level of C6
    - Ascends within the transverse foramen
    - Can be at risk during resection of the uncovertebral joint
  - Epidural veins

- Other
  - Trachea
  - Esophagus
  - Thoracic duct

INCISION

- **Transverse incision (Figure SP-21)**
  - In skin crease along Langer's lines
  - More cosmetic, but not extensile

- **Longitudinal incision**
  - Just anterior to sternocleidomastoid muscle
  - More extensile, but less cosmetically appealing

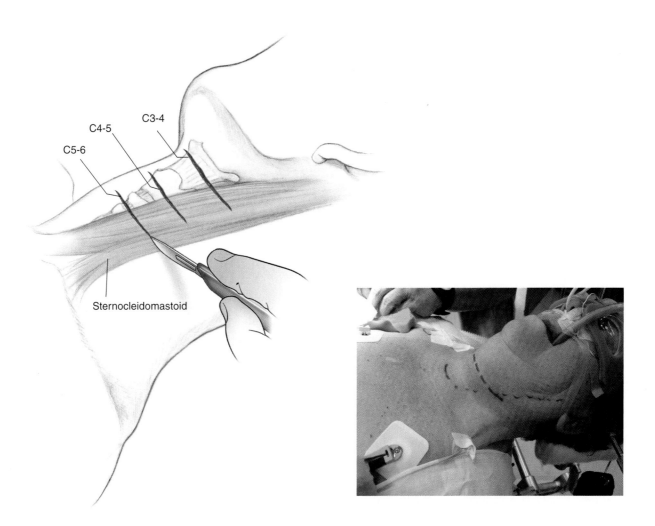

FIGURE SP-21 Relationship of hyoid bone, thyroid cartilage, and cricoid cartilage to level of the corresponding disc.

SUPERFICIAL DISSECTION

- ### Identify platysma (Figure SP-22)

  - Divide fibers of the platysma
  - Alternatively, split muscles of platysma in line with fibers
  - Elevate platysma superiorly and inferiorly

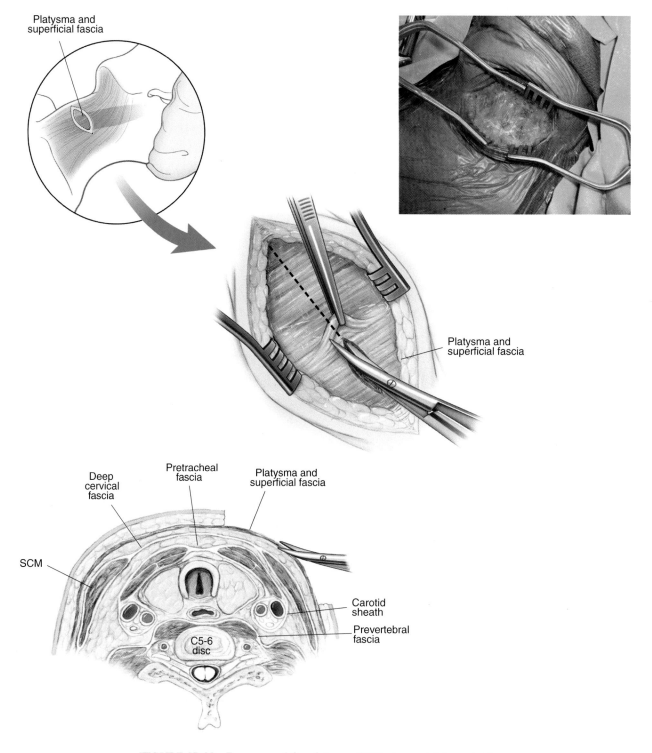

FIGURE SP-22 Exposure of the platysma. SCM, sternocleidomastoid.

● Identify anterior border of sternocleidomastoid muscle (Figure SP-23)

- ■ Divide fascia immediately anterior to sternocleidomastoid muscle (deep cervical fascia)

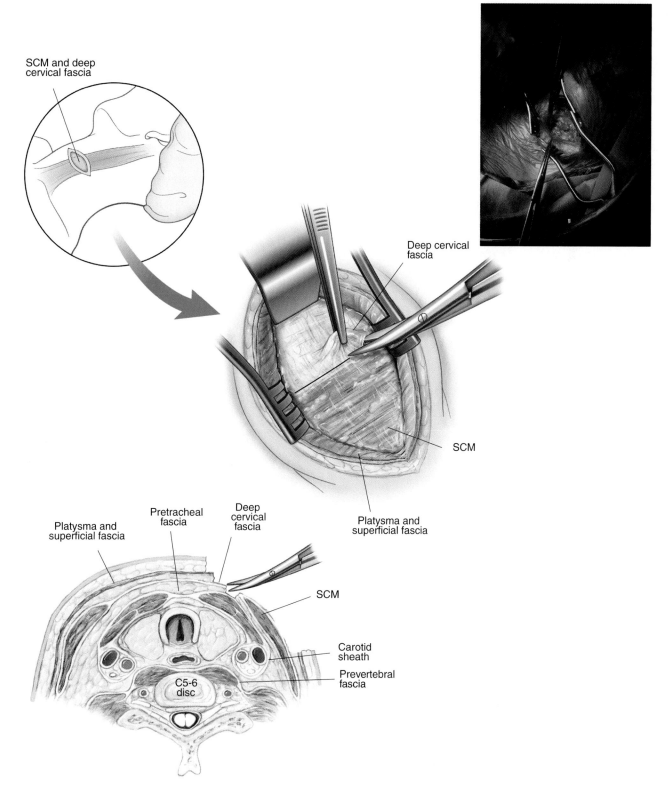

FIGURE SP-23   Identify anterior border of sternocleidomastoid (SCM), and divide deep cervical fascia.

● Palpate pulse of carotid artery (Figure SP-24)

 ▪ Divide fascia immediately anterior to carotid sheath (pretracheal fascia)

 ▪ Using blunt dissection, retract sternocleidomastoid and carotid sheath (common carotid artery, internal jugular vein, and vagus nerve) laterally

 ▪ Retract strap muscles (sternohyoid and sternothyroid) along with trachea and esophagus medially

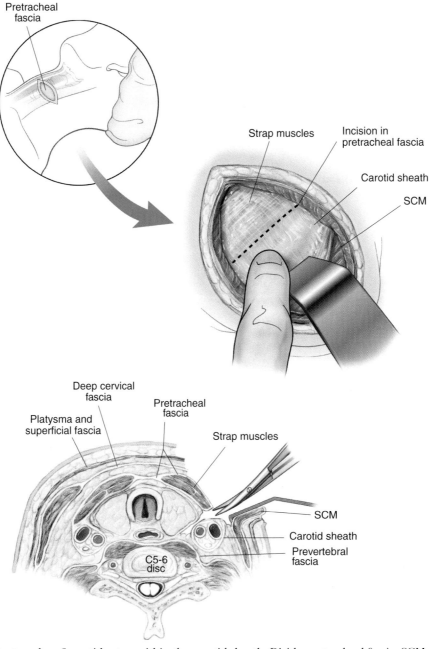

FIGURE SP-24 Palpate pulse of carotid artery within the carotid sheath. Divide pretracheal fascia. SCM, sternocleidomastoid.

- **Continue with blunt dissection to develop the plane down to the anterior surface of the cervical vertebra (Figure SP-25)**

  - Two arteries may be seen crossing the field from the carotid sheath toward the midline structures
    - Superior thyroid artery
    - Inferior thyroid artery
  - One or both may have to be divided to increase surgical exposure

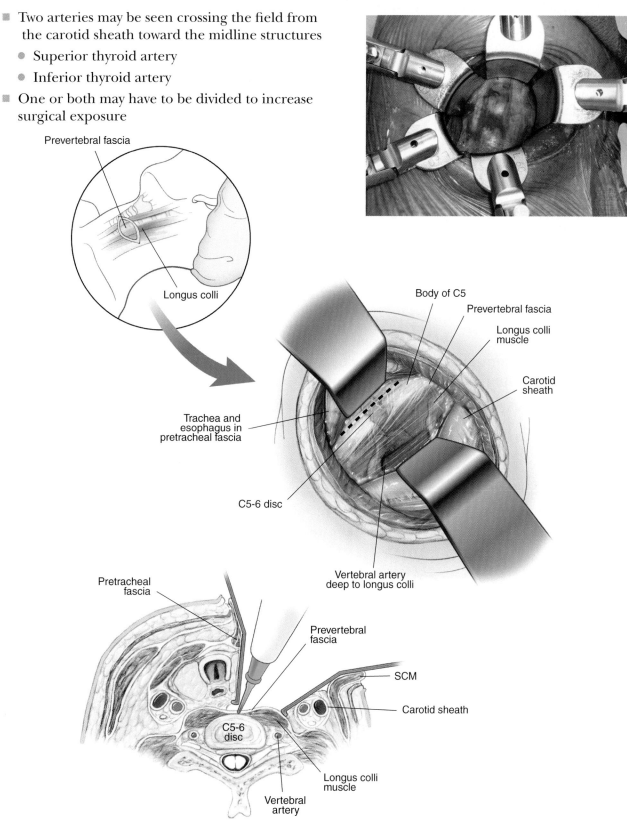

FIGURE SP-25   Identify anterior cervical spine and longus colli. SCM, sternocleidomastoid

DEEP DISSECTION

- This exposes the anterior cervical vertebra (Figure SP-26)
  - The longus colli muscles are now visible on either side
  - The prevertebral fascia also can be seen covering the cervical vertebra
  - The anterior longitudinal ligament can be seen as a gleaming white structure in the midline
  - Sympathetic chain lies on the longus colli lateral to the vertebral bodies

- Divide the prevertebral fascia
- Detach and elevate longus colli bilaterally for exposure
  - At the level of the vertebral body, the anterior tubercle of the transverse process can help protect the vertebral artery
  - Lateral dissection at the level of the disc should be performed carefully to reduce the risk of vertebral artery injury

- Careful placement of the retractors deep to the longus colli reduces the risk of inadvertent injury to surrounding structures

CLOSURE

- Hemostasis is achieved, and the deep structures are allowed to fall back into place
- A deep drain can be placed based on the surgeon's preference
- The platysma, subcutaneous layer, and skin are closed in layers

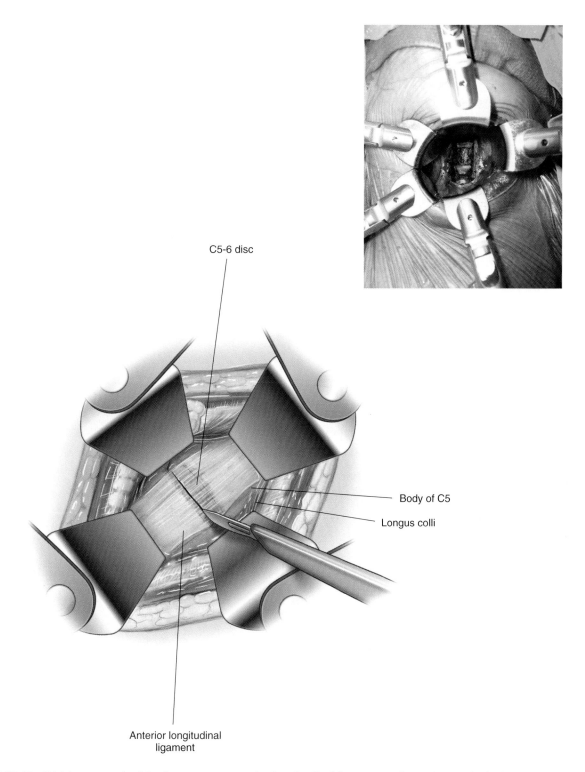

C5-6 disc

Body of C5

Longus colli

Anterior longitudinal
ligament

FIGURE SP-26   Divide prevertebral fascia to expose anterior longitudinal ligament and anterior cervical spine.
Photo courtesy of Vincent Arlet, MD.

ANTERIOR TRANSTHORACIC APPROACH TO THORACIC SPINE

Indications

- **Anterior spinal cord decompression**
  - Fracture
  - Tumor
  - Herniated disc
  - Infection

- **Correction of deformity**
  - Anterior release for scoliosis or kyphosis

- **Fusion for instability or deformity**

- **Biopsy**

POSITIONING

- **Lateral decubitus position with the side to be approached oriented up (Figure SP-27)**
  - For deformity, the convexity of the curve is typically oriented up
  - For decompressions, the side with the greatest stenosis to be addressed is typically oriented up

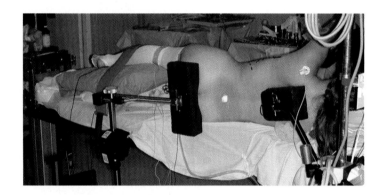

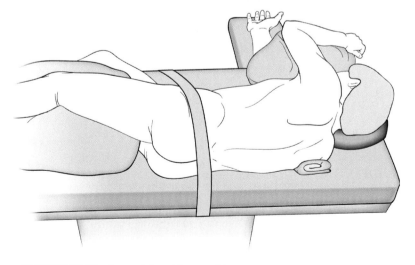

FIGURE SP-27 Lateral decubitus position. *Photo courtesy of Vincent Arlet, MD.*

- Secure the patient firmly to the operating table
  - Stabilize the patient with either beanbags or hip positioners
  - Carefully note the orientation of the spine before draping
    - This reduces the risk of disorientation and inadvertent entry into the spinal canal
    - This is particularly important if rotation of the table is required intraoperatively
  - Place a well-padded small roll in the axilla of the dependent side to avoid prolonged axillary artery, vein, and brachial plexus compression
  - Place the hand and arm on the side to be approached above the head

HAZARDS

- Neural Structures
  - Spinal cord
  - Segmental thoracic nerve roots

- Vascular
  - Aorta
  - Vena cava
  - Segmental artery and vein
    - Crosses at the level of the midvertebral body
  - Intercostal segmental feeders
    - Lies on the undersurface of the rib
  - Artery of Adamkiewicz
    - Variable course
    - Traditionally left-sided from T9-T11
  - Epidural veins

- Other
  - Esophagus
  - Thoracic duct

INCISION

- **It is easier to extend the dissection distally than proximally**
  - ■ It is best to center the incision on the rib associated with the vertebra of interest or of the one more superior (Figure SP-28)
    - Rib articulates with the corresponding vertebra and the one more cranial
      - ○ The 8th rib typically articulates with the T7 vertebra and the T8 vertebra
  - ■ Correlate the number of ribs from preoperative imaging with the number of ribs palpated on the patient after positioning
    - Typically, the 12th rib cannot be felt, and the most inferior rib palpated is the 11th rib
    - The tip of the scapula is mobile and varies in location; however, an incision centered approximately 1-2 finger breadths below the tip usually overlies the 7th or 8th rib

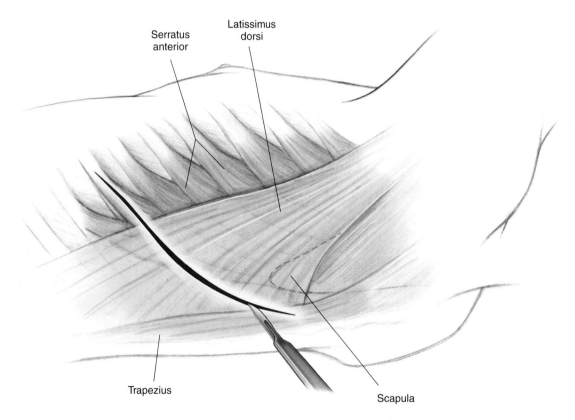

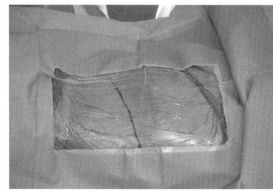

FIGURE SP-28 Thoracotomy incision following path of underlying rib.

SUPERFICIAL DISSECTION

- Identify the latissimus dorsi and trapezius muscles
  (Figure SP-29)
  - Divide the latissimus dorsi in line with the skin incision
    - Because this is not performed in the intramuscular plane, bleeding can be an issue
  - The scapula can now be elevated
    - Although unnecessary, the surgeon can carefully develop the plane between the scapula and ribs to obtain confirmation of the appropriate rib level
      - The most proximally palpated rib is typically the 2nd rib
  - If necessary, the rhomboids can be detached to improve the posterior exposure

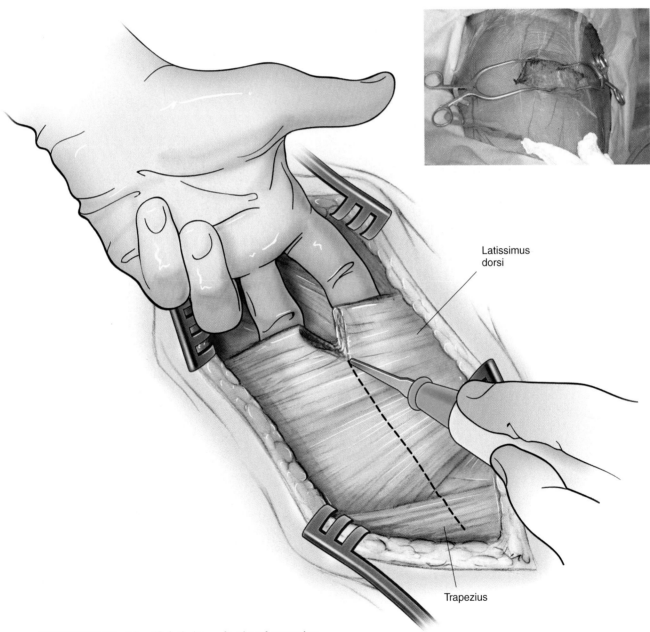

Latissimus dorsi

Trapezius

FIGURE SP-29 Identify latissimus dorsi and trapezius.

- ● The serratus anterior can now be identified better (Figure SP-30)

  - ▨ Divide the serratus anterior in line with the incision to expose the rib

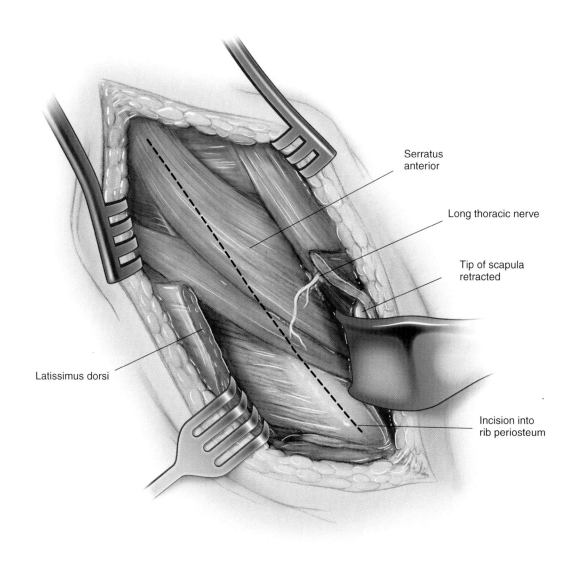

FIGURE SP-30 Identify underlying rib and serratus anterior.

● Subperiosteally elevate the musculature from the ribs
  (Figure SP-31)

   ▪ Detachment of the muscular attachments

      ● Above the rib, proceed posterior to anterior (Figure SP-32)

      ● Below the rib, proceed anterior to posterior

   ▪ If possible, preserve the intercostal neurovascular bundle, which runs along the
     inferior border of the rib

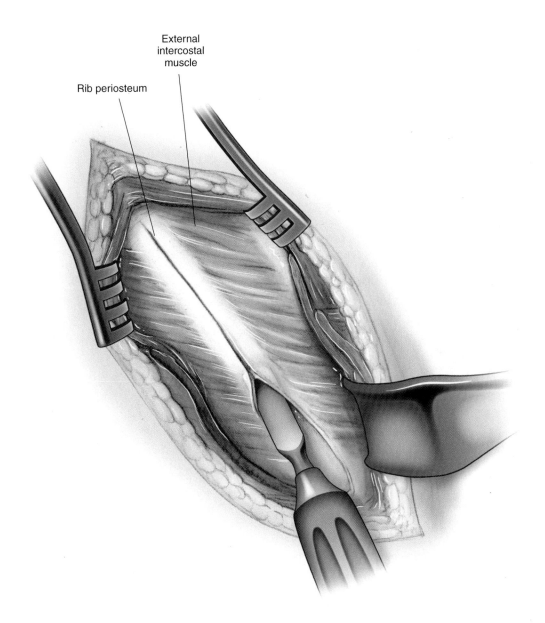

FIGURE SP-31   Subperiosteal exposure of the rib.

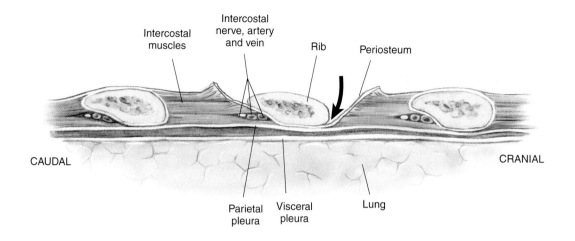

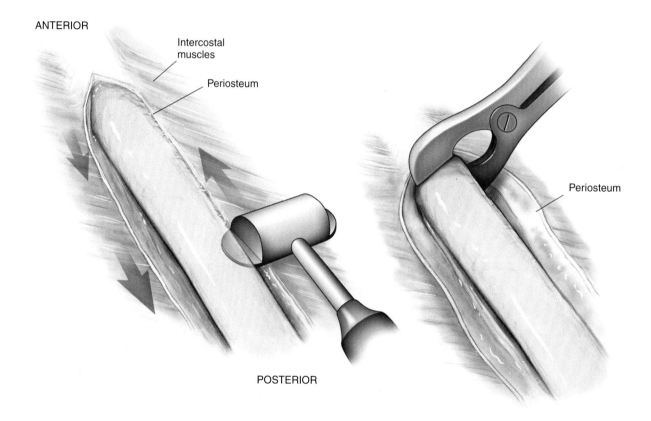

FIGURE SP-32 Detach the intercostal muscles from posterior to anterior on the superior edge of the rib and from anterior to posterior on the inferior edge.

■ Continue the subperiosteal dissection as far posteriorly as necessary

　● Using a rib cutter, resect as much rib as necessary to obtain the needed exposure

　● Bleeding at the posterior angle of the rib after it is resected can be controlled with bone wax

　● Save the rib as bone graft if needed

- The thoracic cavity can be entered now by cutting the periosteum and pleura above the rib (Figure SP-33)
  - Notify the anesthesia team at this point that you are entering the chest

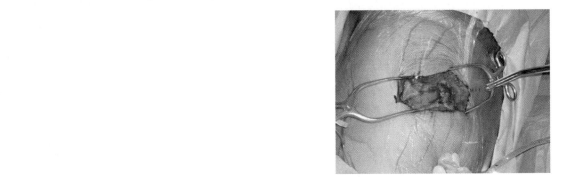

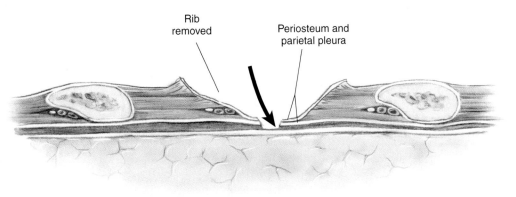

Rib removed

Periosteum and parietal pleura

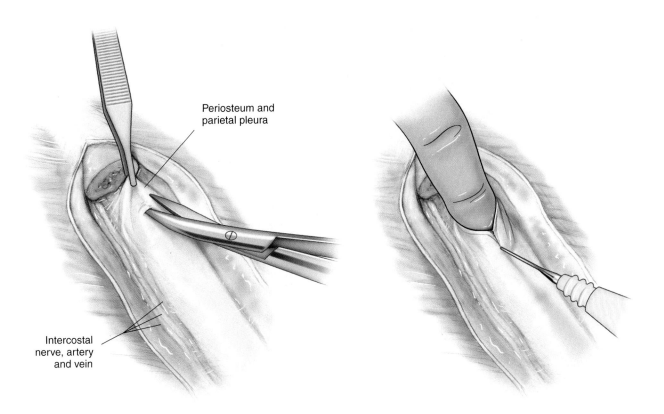

Periosteum and parietal pleura

Intercostal nerve, artery and vein

FIGURE SP-33 Enter chest cavity by dividing the periosteum and parietal pleura.

DEEP DISSECTION

- Insert a rib spreader (Figure SP-34)
- The lung can be readily identified
  - Typically, a double-lumen tube is unnecessary
  - Pack moist laporotomy sponges to assist in the exposure

- Identify the posterior mediastinum and associated structures
  - The lateral aspect of the spine can be readily identified
    - The "hills" are the intervertebral discs
    - The "valley" is the vertebral body

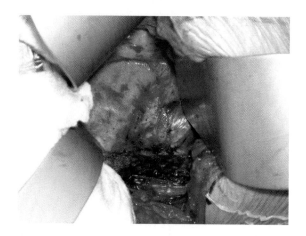

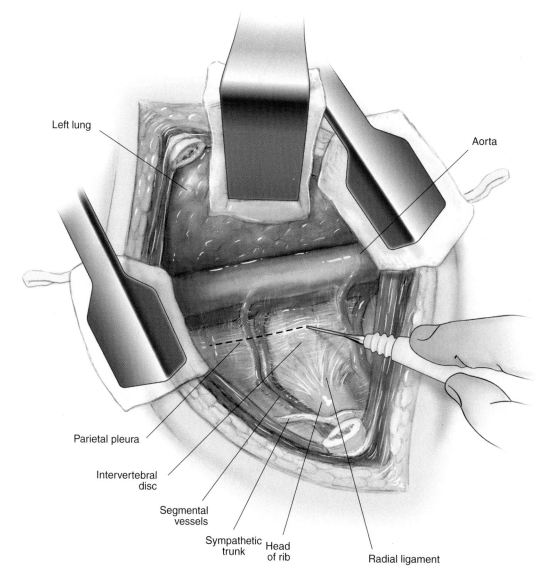

FIGURE SP-34   Thoracic spine exposed. The intervertebral discs are the "hills," whereas the vertebral bodies are the "valleys."

● Incise the pleura (Figure SP-35)

■ This allows for mobilization of the posterior mediastinal structures off the anterior aspect of the vertebra

■ The intercostal vessels can be seen crossing the operative field at the level of the midvertebral body

● Preserve the intercostal vessels if possible

● Tying off more intercostal vessels than necessary should be avoided

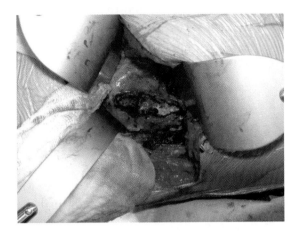

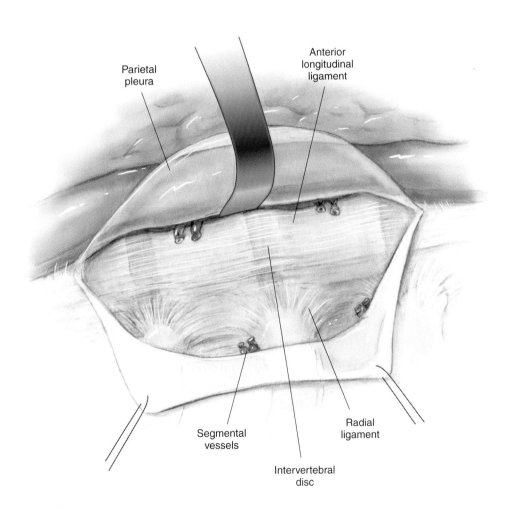

FIGURE SP-35   Parietal pleura divided. The segmental vessels (divided and ligated) cross at the level of the midvertebral body.

CLOSURE

- A careful complete instrument and sponge count should be performed before final closure
- Before final closure, have the anesthesiologist re-expand the lung to reduce the risk of postoperative atelectasis
- Placement of chest tube
  - Make the skin incision for the chest tube 1-2 ribs inferior to the level of the thoracotomy
  - Tunnel subcutaneously to the thoracotomy, and place the chest tube above the rib
  - Secure the chest tube at the skin with a heavy stitch
- Approximate the ribs with heavy suture
- Close the remaining muscles in layers

ANTERIOR THORACOABDOMINAL APPROACH TO THE THORACIC AND LUMBAR SPINE

Indications

- Anterior spinal cord decompression
  - Fracture
  - Tumor
  - Herniated disc
  - Infection

- Correction of deformity
  - Anterior release for scoliosis or kyphosis

- Fusion for instability or deformity
- Biopsy

POSITIONING

- Lateral decubitus position
  - See anterior thoracic approach

HAZARDS

- See anterior transthoracic and retroperitoneal/transperitoneal lumbar approaches

INCISION (FIGURE SP-36)

- It is easier to extend the dissection distally than proximally
  - A curvilinear incision is used centered on the rib of interest proximally, typically either the 9th or 10th rib
  - Anteriorly, the incision is carried inferiorly along the lateral border of the rectus abdominis
  - Posteriorly, the incision follows the rib

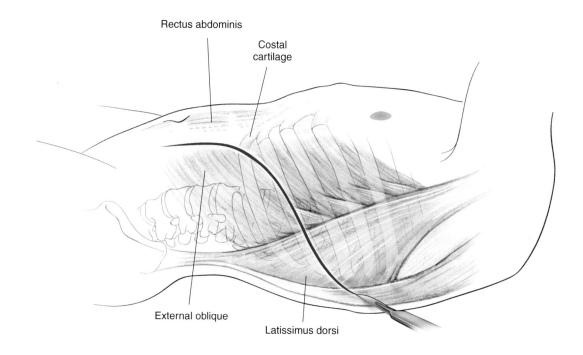

Rectus abdominis

Costal cartilage

External oblique

Latissimus dorsi

FIGURE SP-36 Incision for thoracoabdominal approach.

SUPERFICIAL DISSECTION

- Identify the latissimus dorsi (Figure SP-37)
  - Divide the latissimus dorsi in line with the skin incision
    - Because this is not performed in the intramuscular plane, bleeding can be an issue

- The serratus anterior can be better identified now
  - Divide the serratus anterior in line with the incision to expose the rib

- Subperiosteally elevate the musculature from the ribs
  - Detachment of the muscular attachments
    - See thoracic approach

- The thoracic cavity can be entered now by cutting the periosteum and pleura above the rib
  - Notify the anesthesia team at this point that you are entering the chest

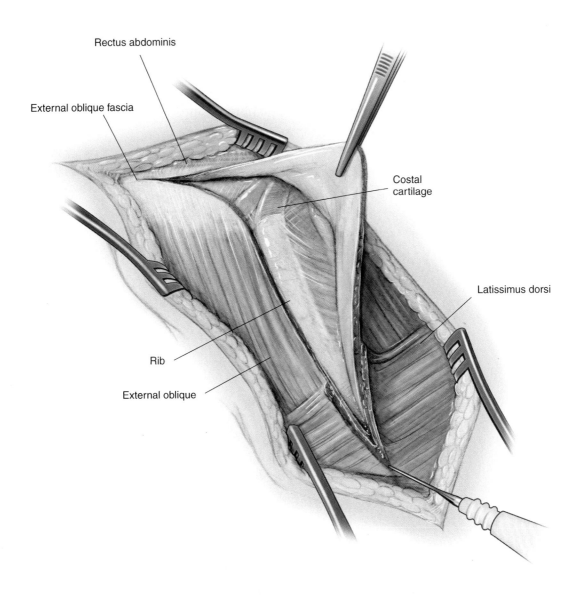

Rectus abdominis

External oblique fascia

Costal
cartilage

Latissimus dorsi

Rib

External oblique

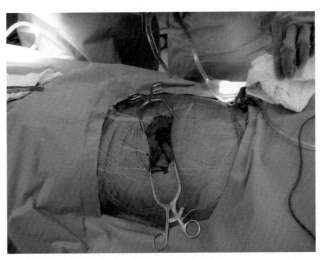

FIGURE SP-37   Exposure of the rib and costal cartilage.

- ● Split the costal cartilage with a knife along its length (Figure SP-38)

  - ▣ The preperitoneal fat can be visualized at this time
  - ▣ Bluntly dissect the peritoneum off the inferior surface of the diaphragm
  - ▣ Sweep peritoneum from the undersurface of the diaphragm and the transversalis fascia and abdominal wall

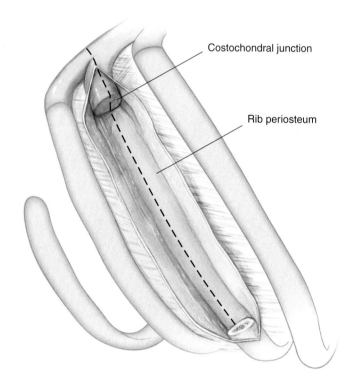

Costochondral junction

Rib periosteum

FIGURE SP-38   Split and tag costochondral cartilage. This helps with reapproximation during closure.

- ● Next, the three abdominal muscles are sequentially encountered: external oblique, internal oblique, and transversus abdominis (Figure SP-39)

  - ▣ Open abdominal musculature—aponeurosis of external oblique, internal oblique, transversus abdominis, and transversalis fascia
  - ▣ See anterior retroperitoneal approach to lumbar spine

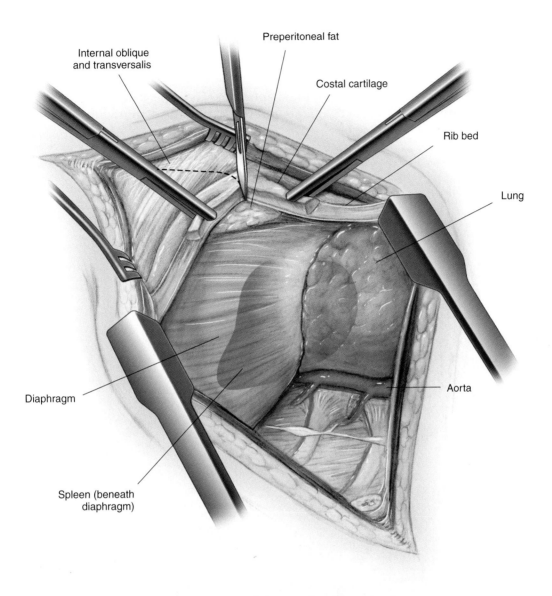

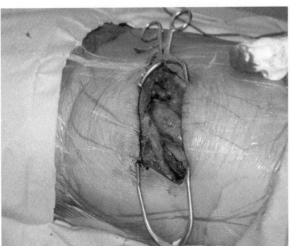

FIGURE SP-39 Split costal cartilage. This assists in identifying the preperitoneal fat.

● Incise the diaphragm (Figure SP-40)

■ Detach the diaphragm approximately 2 cm from its peripheral attachment to the chest wall

■ Mark the diaphragm with suture or ligature clips to allow for accurate reapproximation

■ For added exposure, complete separation of the diaphragm can be performed by dividing the medial and lateral arcuate ligaments and the crus of the diaphragm

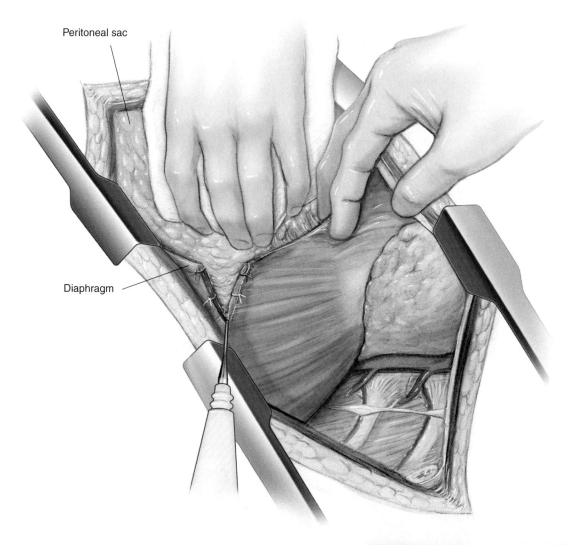

Peritoneal sac

Diaphragm

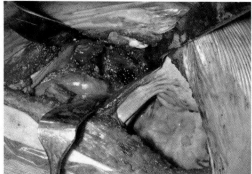

FIGURE SP-40 Detach diaphragm approximately 2 cm from chest wall. Colored suture tags help with reapproximation. *Photo courtesy of Vincent Arlet, MD.*

DEEP DISSECTION

- Insert a rib spreader and abdominal retractor into the respective cavities (Figure SP-41)
- Thoracic cavity (see thoracic approach)
  - ▪ The lung can be readily identified
  - ▪ Identify the posterior mediastinum and associated structures
    - • The lateral aspect of the spine can be readily identified
  - ▪ Incise the pleura
    - • The intercostal vessels can be seen crossing the operative field at the level of the midvertebral body

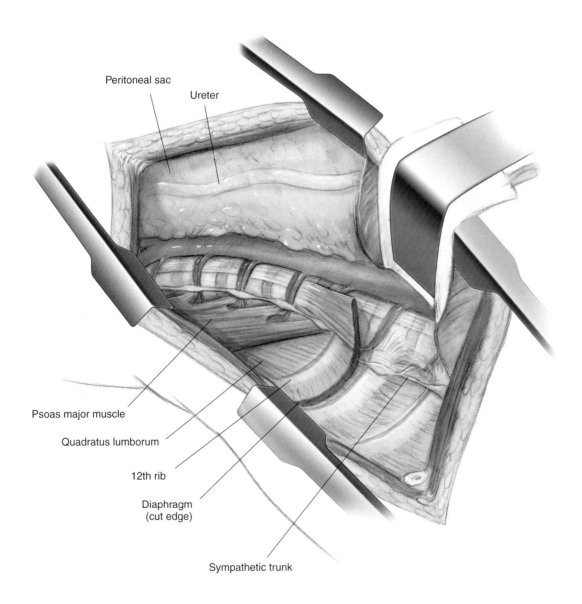

Peritoneal sac

Ureter

Psoas major muscle

Quadratus lumborum

12th rib

Diaphragm
(cut edge)

Sympathetic trunk

FIGURE SP-41 Diaphragm detached providing extensile exposure of the thoracic and lumbar spine.

- Abdominal cavity (see anterior retroperitoneal approach)
  - Identify the psoas fascia, but do not enter the muscle
  - Identify and preserve the genitofemoral nerve
  - Identify and, if possible, preserve the sympathetic chain
  - Identify the segmental vessels as they cross the field at the level of the midvertebral body

CLOSURE

- Key to closure is reapproximation of the costal cartilage
  - The diaphragm attaches to the superior aspect of the costal cartilage
  - The transverse abdominal fascia and abdominal musculature insert into the distal split cartilage

- Diaphragm
  - Carefully repair the diaphragm with interrupted suture based on the predivision markings

- Insert a chest tube, and close the chest cavity in the standard fashion
- The abdominal musculature is closed in layers in the standard fashion

ANTERIOR RETROPERITONEAL APPROACH TO THE LUMBAR SPINE

Indications

- ● Anterior spinal cord decompression
  - ▪ Fracture
  - ▪ Tumor
  - ▪ Herniated disc
  - ▪ Infection

- ● Drainage of psoas infection
- ● Correction of deformity
  - ▪ Anterior release for scoliosis or kyphosis

- ● Fusion for instability or deformity
- ● Biopsy
- ● Total disc replacement

POSITIONING

- ● Semilateral or lateral decubitus position (Figure SP-42)
  - ▪ For deformity, the convexity of the curve is typically oriented up
  - ▪ For decompressions, the side with the greatest stenosis to be addressed typically is oriented up

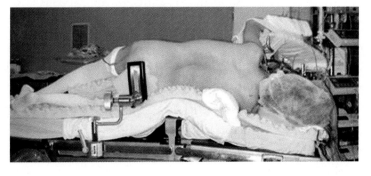

FIGURE SP-42 Lateral decubitus position. Note the flexion in the table to assist in opening up the interspace. *Photo courtesy of Vincent Arlet, MD.*

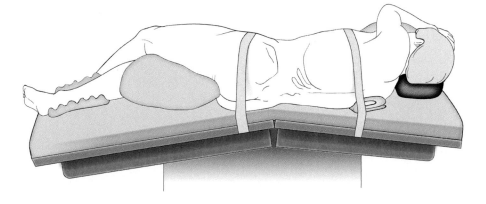

- If both sides are equivalent, the left-sided exposure is typically preferred
  - Left-sided approach places the more durable descending aorta into the surgical field, in contrast to a right-sided approach, which exposes the thin-walled inferior vena cava
- Secure the patient firmly to the operating table
  - See description for the anterior transthoracic approach
- Flexion of the down leg may help reduce the amount of rolling experienced by the patient intraoperatively
  - Pad the bony prominences well—particularly the lateral malleolus and the fibular head
- Flexion of the leg on the side of the approach may help reduce psoas tension

- **Supine on the operating table**
  - Table hyperextension assists in the exposure
  - Insert a urinary catheter to decompress the bladder
  - Additional tricks
    - Place the patient into Trendelenburg position
    - This helps move the abdominal contents superiorly to improve visibility
    - It also provides improved access to the L5-S1 disc by bringing it into better view

HAZARDS

- **Neural structures**
  - Cauda equina
  - Segmental lumbar nerve roots
  - Lumbosacral plexus
    - May be at risk if the substance of the psoas is entered
  - Superior hypogastric plexus
    - Particularly during approaches to the L4-L5 and L5-S1 disc space
    - Use of bipolar electrocautery can reduce the risk of injury
    - Injury can lead to retrograde ejaculation in men
  - Sympathetic chain
    - Lies on the anterior border of the psoas muscle
    - Injury can result in increase in warmth to the ipsilateral lower extremity
  - Hypogastric nerve

- **Vascular**
  - Aorta
  - Vena cava
  - Common iliac artery and vein
  - Iliolumbar vein
    - Frequently must be identified and ligated for mobilization of the great vessels, particularly during exposure of L4-L5
    - Middle sacral artery

- Other
  - Ureter
    - Typically rests against the posterior aspect of the peritoneal cavity during the retroperitoneal exposure
    - Crosses the brim of the pelvis over the common iliac vessels
  - Bladder

INCISION

- Identify the pubic symphysis, ASIS, and inferiormost rib (Figure SP-43)
  - Correlate the number of ribs from preoperative imaging with the number of ribs palpated on the patient after positioning
    - Typically, the 12th rib cannot be felt, and the most inferior rib palpated is the 11th rib

- Identify the umbilicus, and palpate the lateral border of the rectus abdominis muscle

- Design the skin incision based on the bony landmarks and the corresponding spinal level to be addressed

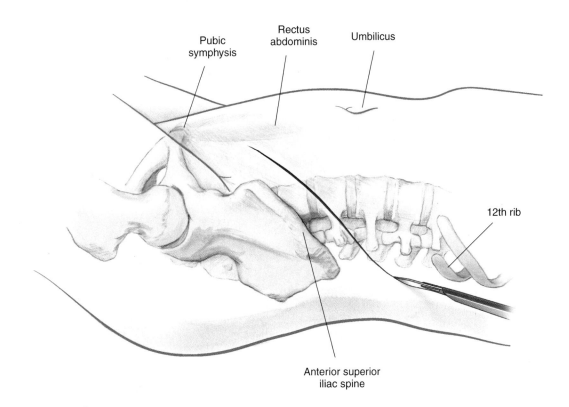

FIGURE SP-43 Oblique incision for extensile retroperitoneal approach to the lumbar spine.

SUPERFICIAL DISSECTION (FIGURE SP-44)

- ● Deepen the skin incision through the subcutaneous fat

- ● Next, the three abdominal muscles are sequentially encountered: external oblique, internal oblique, and transverse abdominis

  - ■ Depending on the surgeon's preference, the muscles can be divided in line with the skin incision or separated in line with the fibers

  - ■ Because these muscles are innervated segmentally, division of the fibers partially denervates the muscle

  - ■ This may result in a postoperative hernia.

- ● The aponeurosis of the external oblique enters into view

  - ■ Muscle fiber orientation is from superolateral to inferomedial

  - ■ Muscle fibers of the external oblique may not be present below the level of the umbilicus

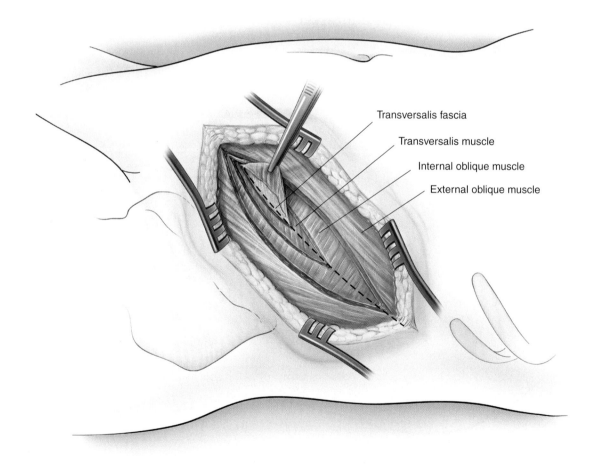

FIGURE SP-44   External oblique, internal oblique, and transversalis muscle and fascia exposed. Note fiber orientation of each layer.

- The internal oblique muscles are identified next
  - Muscle fiber orientation is perpendicular to the external oblique and is oriented from superomedial to inferolateral

- The transversus abdominis is the next muscle to be identified
- The transversalis fascia is encountered
  - Careful division of the transversalis fascia provides access to the retroperitoneal space

- Using blunt dissection, develop the plane between the peritoneum and the retroperitoneal space
  - Avoid entering into the peritoneal cavity
    - If this occurs, the peritoneum can be repaired with 4-0 polyglactin 910 (Vicryl)

- Mobilize the peritoneal cavity and its contents anteromedially until the fascia of the psoas is identified
  - Do not mistake the quadratus lumborum for the psoas muscle
  - The ureter typically is carried forward with the peritoneal cavity
    - If there is any doubt, the ureter can be gently stroked with a DeBakey forcep to induce peristalsis

DEEP DISSECTION

- Identify the psoas fascia, but do not enter the muscle (Figure SP-45)
  - If a psoas abscess is present, this can be palpated easily at this point and entered with gentle finger dissection
  - If a trans-psoas approach is planned, neuromonitoring should be considered to reduce the risk of lumbosacral plexus injury because the lumbosacral plexus typically runs in the posterior aspect of the psoas

- Identify the genitofemoral nerve
  - Typically, the genitofemoral nerve is lying on the anteromedial aspect of the psoas within the psoas fascia
  - This should be preserved

- Identify the sympathetic chain
  - The sympathetic chain lies even more anterior and medial to the genitofemoral nerve
  - Typically, this lies anterior to the psoas on the lateral aspect of the vertebral body
  - Preserve the sympathetic chain if possible
    - If divided, this results in a warm leg on the ipsilateral side of the surgical approach
    - Postoperatively, the more commonly identified complaint is a cool contralateral lower extremity

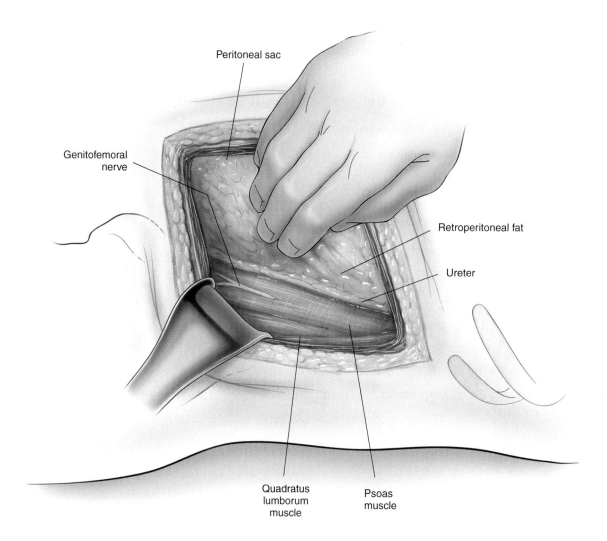

Peritoneal sac

Genitofemoral nerve

Retroperitoneal fat

Ureter

Quadratus lumborum muscle

Psoas muscle

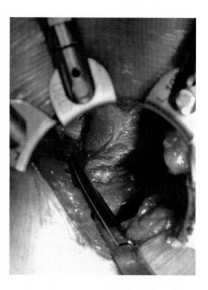

FIGURE SP-45   Psoas muscle exposed. Do not mistake the quadratus lumborum for the psoas muscle. Note location of the genitofemoral nerve.

- Identify the segmental vessels as they cross the field at the level of the midvertebral body (Figure SP-46)

  - Depending on the procedure to be performed, these vessels can be either spared or tied and cut
  - Access to the anterior portion of the vertebral bodies requires mobilization of the great vessels by ligating the segmental vessels
    - Do not cut the lumbar segmental vessels flush with the great vessels
  - For the L5-S1 disc, and occasionally the L4-5 disc, a transperitoneal lumbar approach also can be used (see transperitoneal approach)

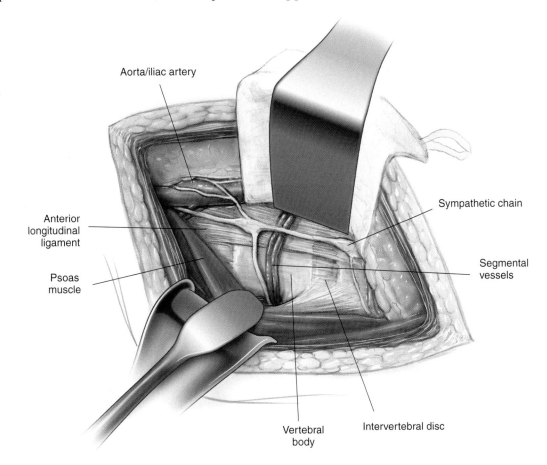

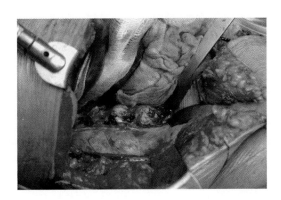

FIGURE SP-46 Retract psoas muscle. Note location of segmental vessels at the level of the midvertebral body. *Photo courtesy of Vincent Arlet, MD.*

CLOSURE

- A careful complete instrument and sponge count should be performed before final closure
- Peritoneal contents are allowed to fall back into place
- Closure of the abdominal muscles can be either in layers or as a single layer
  - The muscle fascia provides the strength of closure
- Skin and subcutaneous tissues are closed in the standard fashion

ANTERIOR TRANSPERITONEAL APPROACH TO THE LUMBOSACRAL SPINE

Indications

- Decompression
  - L5-S1 intervertebral disc
  - Occasionally L4-5 discectomy

- Fusion
  - L5-S1 intervertebral disc

- Biopsy

- Total disc replacement

POSITIONING

- Supine on the operating table (Figure SP-47)
  - Table hyperflexion assists in the exposure
  - Insert a urinary catheter to decompress the bladder

- Additional tricks
  - Place the patient into Trendelenburg position
  - This helps move the abdominal contents superiorly to improve visibility
  - It also provides improved access to the L5-S1 disc by bringing it into better view

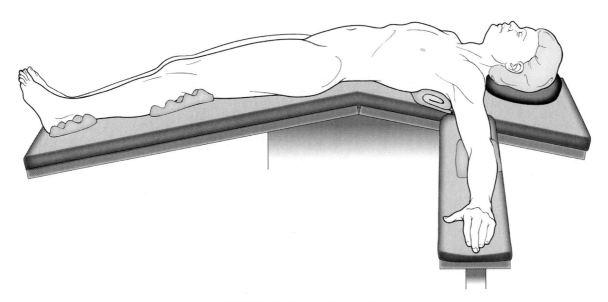

FIGURE SP-47   Supine positioning.

LANDMARKS

- Identify the umbilicus, which is variable in level, but approximates the L3-4 disc in a typical patient
- Identify the pubic symphysis
  - If this is difficult to palpate, the pubic tubercle lies just lateral to the midline on the upper border of the pubis and may serve as another bony landmark

HAZARDS

- See retroperitoneal lumbar approach

INCISION (FIGURE SP-48)

- Longitudinal midline from umbilicus to pubic symphysis
  - Curve the incision just lateral to the umbilicus to allow for appropriate closure
- Transverse (Pfannenstiel's) incision
  - Typically, a more cosmetic, but less extensile exposure
  - Gentle curved incision approximately 4-8 cm above pubis

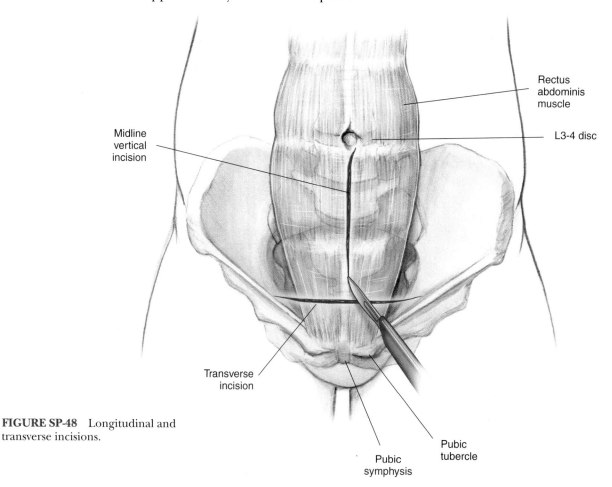

Rectus abdominis muscle

L3-4 disc

Midline vertical incision

Transverse incision

Pubic symphysis

Pubic tubercle

FIGURE SP-48 Longitudinal and transverse incisions.

SUPERFICIAL DISSECTION

- Deepen in line with skin incision down to rectus sheath
- Identify the rectus sheath (Figure SP-49)
  - Incise the sheath in the midline in line with skin incision
  - The linea alba marks the midline of the rectus abdominis muscles
    - This is typically more apparent above the umbilicus and less distinct below

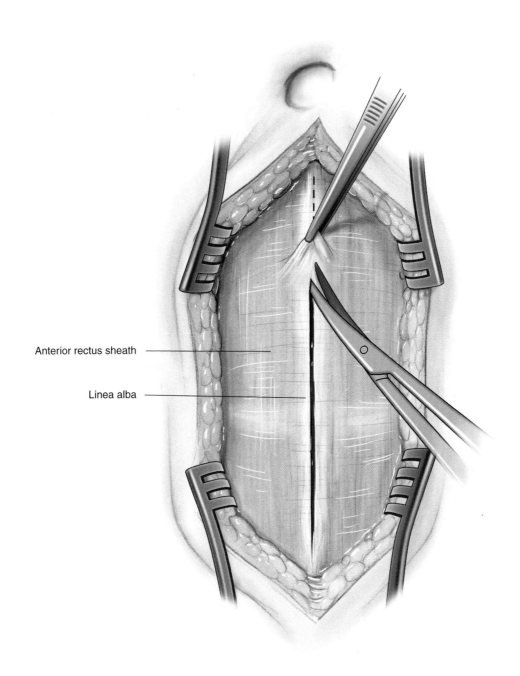

Anterior rectus sheath

Linea alba

FIGURE SP-49   Identify rectus sheath.

- Entering the peritoneal cavity (Figure SP-50)

  - ▪ The linea alba may be divided in the midline

    - ● Next, bluntly dissect between the rectus muscles with your fingertips

    - ● Alternatively, the rectus fascia may be divided longitudinally over its lateral margin

- Mobilize the rectus medially to expose the posterior rectus fascia

- Entering lateral to the rectus allows the surgeon to proceed with either a transperitoneal or a retroperitoneal approach to the lumbar spine

  - ▪ Identify and carefully incise the peritoneum

    - ● Avoid injury to the underlying visceral structures

    - ● The dome of the bladder is at risk if the incision is distal and deep

    - ● Placing one hand or a moist laparotomy sponge within the abdominal cavity helps protect the viscera

DEEP DISSECTION

- Insert an abdominal self-retainer

  - ▪ This assists in retracting the rectus abdominis and the bladder

  - ▪ Additional blades may be inserted as needed to provide access to the deep structures

    - ● Place moist laparotomy sponges between the blades and the abdominal contents to reduce the risk of iatrogenic visceral injury

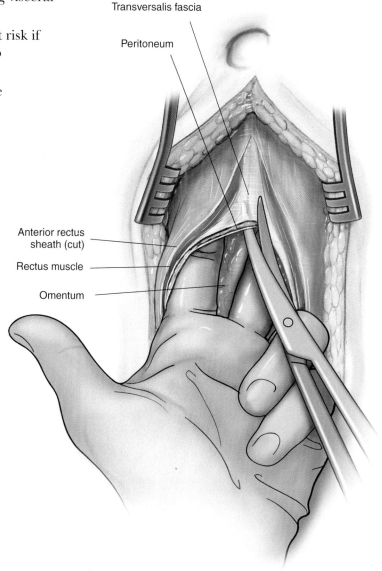

FIGURE SP-50   Divide linea alba in the midline to enter peritoneal cavity.

● The posterior peritoneum can be seen overlying the retroperitoneal structures (Figure SP-51)

  ■ Identify the common iliac vein and artery underneath the peritoneum

    ● Typically, the bifurcation lies at the level of the L4-5 intervertebral disc or the L5 body

  ■ Identify the ureter passing over the pelvic brim bilaterally

    ● This structure can be confirmed by gently pinching it with a pair of nontoothed forceps to induce peristalsis

  ■ Palpate the sacral promontory through the posterior peritoneum

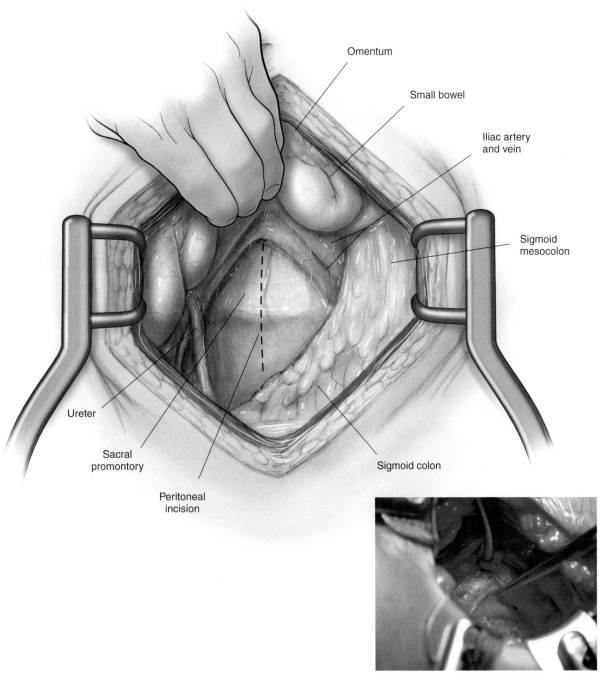

FIGURE SP-51 Transperitoneal exposure of L5-S1 disc space between the bifurcation of the great vessels.

- **Open the posterior peritoneum by incising it over the sacral promontory (Figure SP-52)**

  - Ligate the middle sacral artery, which runs down the anterior sacrum
  - Presacral sympathetic nerves (superior hypogastric plexus) also run in this area
    - Although variable, most of the fibers overlie the left iliac vessels
    - Injury to these nerves may result in retrograde ejaculation and impotence in men
    - Expose the presacral space using blunt dissection as much as possible
    - Limit the use of monopolar electrocautery if possible

- **Identify the L5-S1 disc and the sacral promontory**

  - Confirm the level with an intraoperative radiograph if necessary

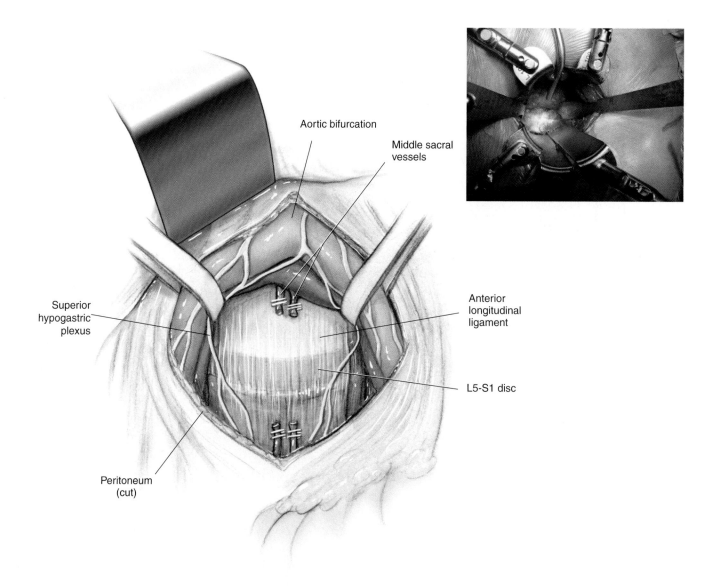

FIGURE SP-52 Ligate middle sacral artery and vein. Injury to the superior hypogastric plexus may lead to retrograde ejaculation in men. *Photo courtesy of Vincent Arlet, MD.*

CLOSURE

- A careful complete instrument and sponge count should be performed before final closure
- Close the peritoneum as a separate layer
- Close the fascia as a separate layer
- Skin and subcutaneous tissues are closed in a standard fashion

POSTERIOR APPROACH TO THE OCCIPITOCERVICAL JUNCTION (O-C2)

Indications

- **Posterior decompression**
  - Skull base
  - Foramen magnum
  - Spinal canal
  - Nerve root

- **Posterior occipitocervical fusions and C1-C2 fusions**
  - Atlanto-occipital dissociation
  - C1 and C2 fractures
  - Transverse cervical ligament disruption
  - Tumors
  - Infections

POSITIONING

- **Prone (Figure SP-53)**
  - Head position
    - Halo or Mayfield tongs are applied for stabilization
    - Head and neck flexion separates the occiput and ring of C1
    - If a fusion and instrumentation are to be performed, the head and neck should be returned to neutral position after the decompression
  - Position of arms
    - At patient's side
    - Gentle taping of shoulders inferiorly can improve intraoperative radiographs
  - Additional tricks
    - Elevate operating table 30 degrees to reduce venous bleeding
    - Knee flexion prevents patient from sliding inferiorly during reverse Trendelenburg position

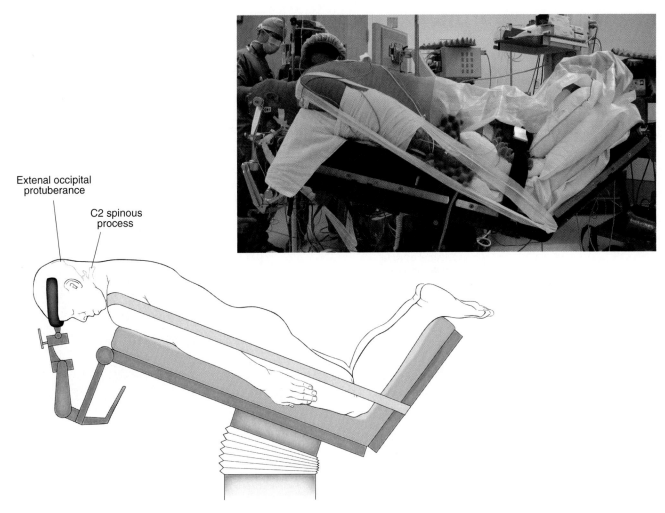

Extenal occipital
protuberance

C2 spinous
process

FIGURE SP-53 Prone positioning.

HAZARDS

- **Neural structures**
  - Spinal cord
  - Cervical nerve roots
    - Greater occipital nerve (C2)
      - Lies posterior to the C1-C2 joint
      - Injury may result in numbness to the posterior aspect of the skull

- **Vascular**
  - Vertebral artery
    - Lies anterior to the lateral mass in the subaxial region
    - Lies on the posterior cranial portion of the C1 ring within the vertebral sulcus
    - Dissection of the ring of C1 should be within 1.5 cm of the midline to reduce the risk of injury to the vertebral artery
  - Transverse sinus
    - Lies anterior to the superior nuchal line
  - Epidural veins

INCISION

- ### Longitudinal midline incision (Figure SP-54)
  - External occipital protuberance and spinous process of C2 and C7 help assist in identifying the midline
  - Typically, exposure should be extended from the external occipital protuberance distally to at least C3 (approximately 6-7 cm)

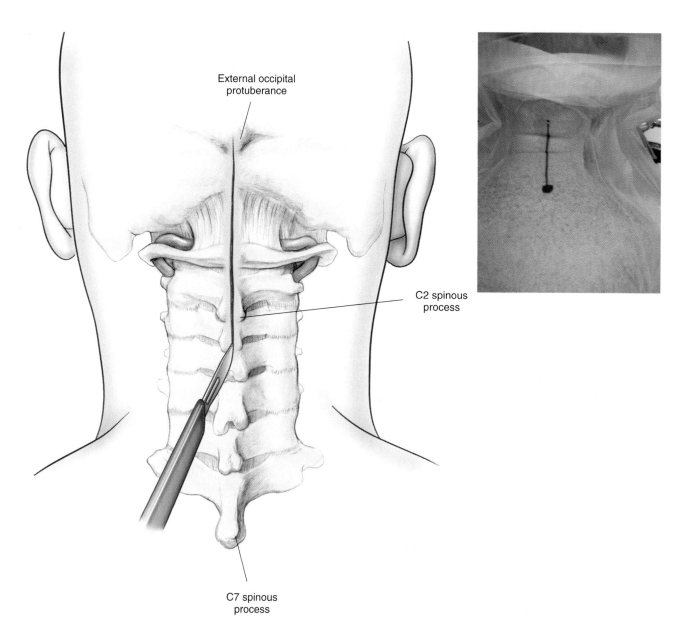

FIGURE SP-54   Midline longitudinal posterior cervical incision.

SUPERFICIAL DISSECTION

- Divide subcutaneous fat and deep cervical fascia in line with skin incision (Figure SP-55)

- Identify the nuchal ligament

  - This is a relatively avascular plane, typically seen as a thin white line in the midline
  - Because the posterior cervical musculature is extremely vascular, the dissection should remain in midline to reduce bleeding

- Deepen incision to external occipital protuberance and down to posterior tubercle of C1 and bifid spinous process of C2 and C3

  - Ring of C1 has no spinous process
  - The dissection should be done carefully to prevent inadvertently entering the spinal canal

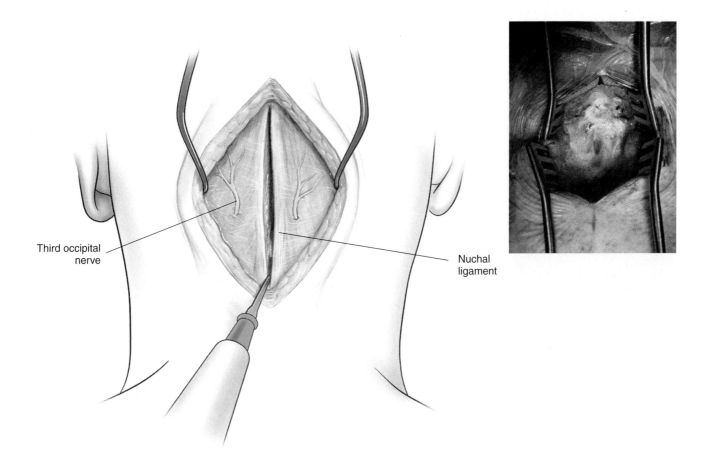

Third occipital nerve

Nuchal ligament

FIGURE SP-55   Remain in the midline by dividing the nuchal ligament to minimize bleeding.

DEEP DISSECTION

● **Expose the occiput**

  ■ A leash of veins is frequently present at the base of the skull near the foramen magnum

● **Expose the ring of C1 (Figure SP-56)**

  ■ Subperiosteal elevation and judicious use of electrocautery as the dissection progresses laterally reduce the risk of inadvertent vertebral artery injury

  ■ Preoperative planning should include assessment of vertebral artery location

  ■ The vertebral artery runs in a sulcus on the superior aspect of the posterior ring of C1

    ● Approximately 10 mm from midline on the superior aspect of C1 and 15 mm from the midline on the posterior aspect of C1

  ■ The ligamentum flavum and the tectorial membrane can be detached from the ring of C1 using a fine curette and subperiosteal dissection

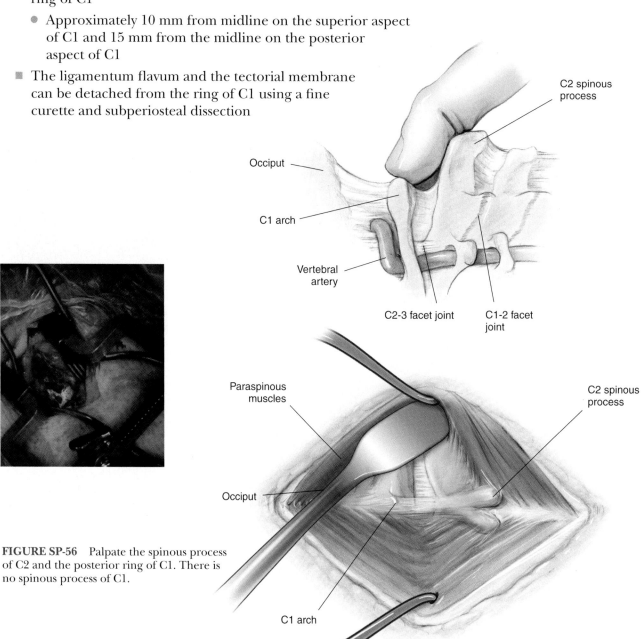

FIGURE SP-56 Palpate the spinous process of C2 and the posterior ring of C1. There is no spinous process of C1.

- **Expose C2**
  - Spinous process of C2 is bifid and typically palpable
  - Identify C1-C2 joint (Figure SP-57)
    - Follow the spinous process to the lamina and then superiorly to the C1-C2 joint
      - The C1-C2 joint lies approximately 2-3 cm anterior to the facet joint of C2-C3
      - The greater occipital nerve (C2) traverses the field just superficial to the C1-C2 joint and is at risk during this exposure
      - A plexus of veins typically overlies the greater occipital nerve

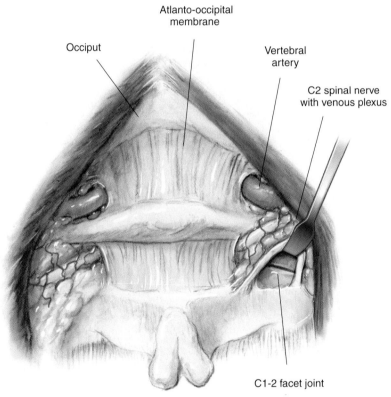

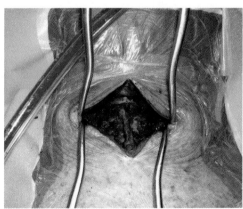

FIGURE SP-57   Identify the C1-C2 facet joint. The C2 nerve lies posterior to the C1-C2 joint.

- Enter the C1-C2 joint (Figure SP-58)
  - Allows for visualization of the C1 lateral mass and placement of C1 screw
  - Allows for identification of the medial border of the C2 pedicle for placement of C2 pedicle screw
  - Alternatively, allows for direct visualization for the placement of the C1-C2 transarticular screw or posterior wire or bone graft fixation or both

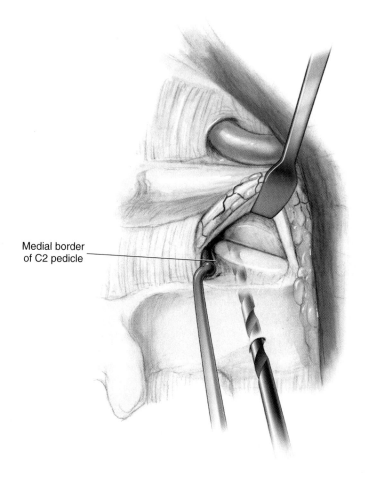

Medial border
of C2 pedicle

FIGURE SP-58   Exposure of the C1-C2 joint allows for palpation of the medial border of the C2 pedicle and visualization of the undersurface of the C1 lateral mass.

CLOSURE

- Deep drain is placed based on the surgeon's preference
- Careful reattachment of the fascia of the posterior cervical musculature to each side and a layered closure can help reduce the risk of a wide unsightly scar, which is common after posterior cervical procedures

POSTERIOR APPROACH TO THE SUBAXIAL CERVICAL SPINE AND CERVICOTHORACIC JUNCTION

Indications

- Posterior decompression of spinal canal and nerve root
  - Laminectomy
  - Laminoplasty
  - Keyhole laminoforaminotomy

- Posterior spinal fusion
  - Fracture
  - Tumor
  - Infection

POSITIONING

- Prone (see posterior approach to occipitocervical junction)

HAZARDS

- See posterior approach to occipitocervical junction

INCISION

- Longitudinal midline (see posterior approach to occipitocervical junction) (Figure SP-59)

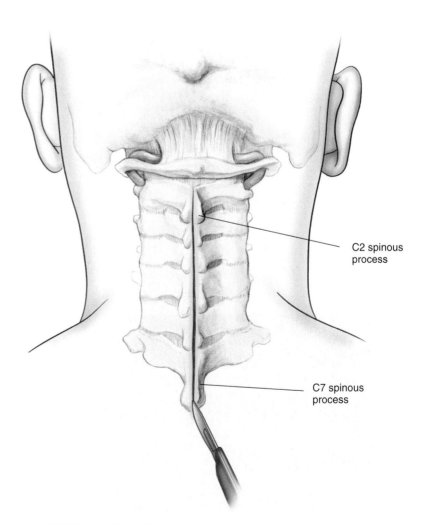

C2 spinous process

C7 spinous process

FIGURE SP-59 Midline longitudinal posterior cervical incision.

SUPERFICIAL DISSECTION

- Divide subcutaneous fat and deep cervical fascia in line with the skin incision (Figure SP-60)
- Identify the nuchal ligament (see previous description)
- The supraspinous and interspinous ligaments should be protected during the initial dissection

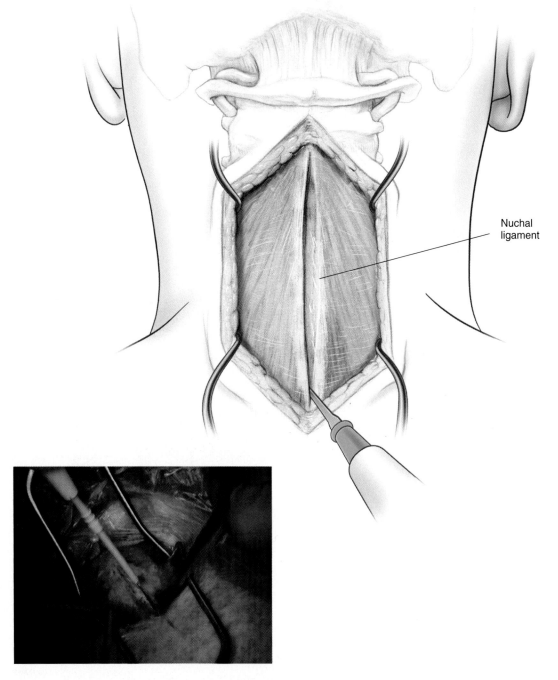

Nuchal
ligament

FIGURE SP-60   Remain in the midline by dividing the nuchal ligament to minimize bleeding.

- Subperiosteally, follow the spinous process out laterally first onto the lamina and then to the lateral mass (Figure SP-61)
  - If possible, protect the facet capsule unless a fusion is to be performed at that level
  - The lateral mass is the rectangular mass of bone that lies between the superior articular and inferior articular facet of the same vertebra
    - Starting point of lateral mass screws is 1 mm medial of the center of the lateral mass angulated superiorly (approximately 15 degrees) and laterally (approximately 30 degrees)
- Exposure of the cervicothoracic junction
  - Posterior cervicothoracic junction typically can be identified by the characteristic bony landmarks
    - Because the transverse process of the cervical vertebra lies more anteriorly, it is typically not seen during the exposure of the C7 lateral mass
    - This is in contradistinction to the T1 transverse process, which is readily identified and travels in a lateral superior direction and is partially overlapped by the C7 lateral mass, giving it a distinct anatomical appearance

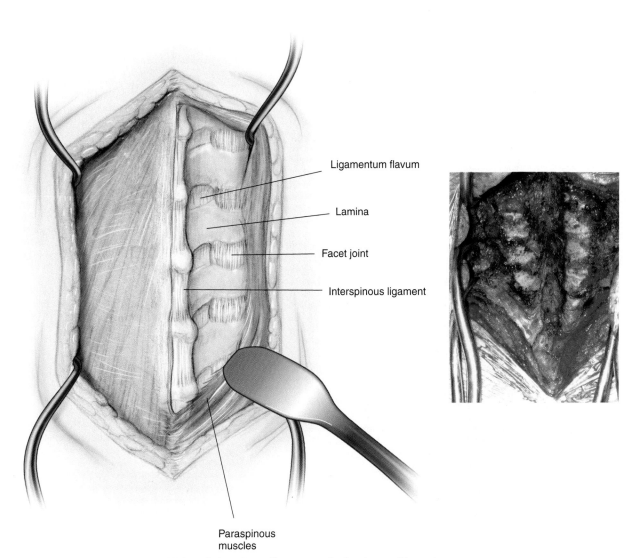

Ligamentum flavum

Lamina

Facet joint

Interspinous ligament

Paraspinous muscles

FIGURE SP-61   Subperiosteally, expose the lamina and lateral masses.

DEEP DISSECTION

- ● Identify the ligamentum flavum running between the lamina
  - ▪ Using a fine curette, carefully detach the ligamentum flavum from the lamina

- ● Laminectomy or laminotomy (Figure SP-62)
  - ▪ Typically, this can be performed using a no. 1 or 2 Kerrison, depending on the space available and the thickness of the lamina

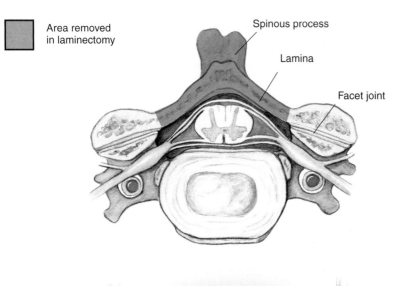

Area removed in laminectomy

Spinous process

Lamina

Facet joint

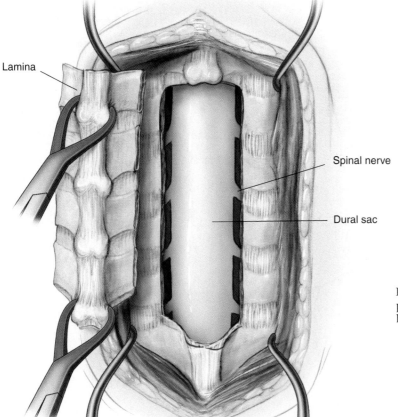

Lamina

Spinal nerve

Dural sac

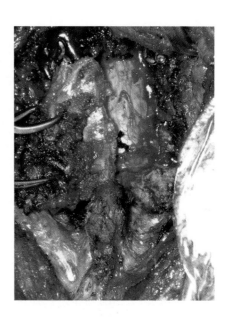

FIGURE SP-62 En bloc removal of spinous process and lamina during a cervical laminectomy.

- If the lamina is too thick, it can be carefully thinned using a rongeur or power burr
- The epidural fat overlying the translucent blue-white dura is visible after the ligamentum flavum and lamina are removed

Multilevel laminectomies

- Thin the lamina at the laminofacet junction at each level of interest using a power burr, creating a trough bilaterally
- Complete the trough using a 1 mm or 2 mm Kerrison
- Carefully remove the ligamentum flavum at the superior and inferior edges of the decompression
- Carefully remove the lamina en bloc using multiple towel clips secured into the spinous processes
- Depending on the level, consideration should be given to placement of either lateral mass or pedicle screws (Figure SP-63)

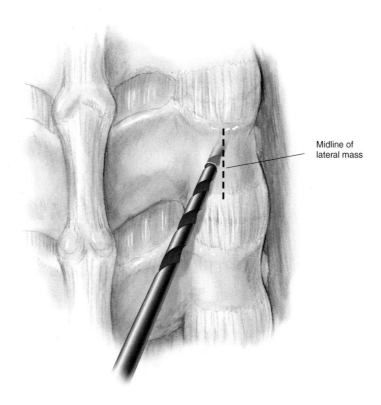

Midline of
lateral mass

FIGURE SP-63   Starting point and trajectory of lateral mass screw.

● Keyhole laminoforaminotomy

▪ Create a laminotomy at the level of interest (as described previously) (Figure SP-64)

● Center half of the laminotomy in the inferior lamina of the vertebra above and the other half in the superior lamina of the vertebra below

● This forms the circular portion of the "keyhole"

▪ Trace the path of the exiting nerve root with a Woodson

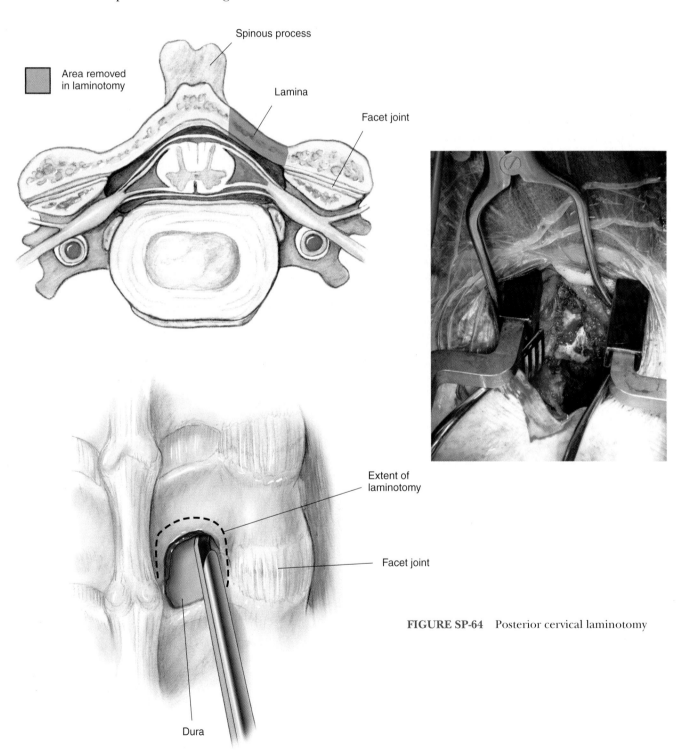

Spinous process

Area removed in laminotomy

Lamina

Facet joint

Extent of laminotomy

Facet joint

Dura

FIGURE SP-64 Posterior cervical laminotomy

■ Using a power burr, thin the medial 50% of the facet joint (Figure SP-65)

- ● Perform this from a medial-to-lateral direction
- ● Remove the remaining thinned bone with a Kerrison
- ● Do not remove greater than 50% of the facet
    - ○ If greater than 50% is removed, a fusion should be included

● **Pedicle screw fixation is not routinely placed in the cervical spine**

■ In selected cases, pedicle screws can be placed at levels from C2 to C7

■ Lateral mass screws are typically used from C3 to C6

● **Epidural bleeding can be brisk and hard to control during any portion of the deep dissection**

■ Use of thrombostatic agents and neuropaddies typically can control most bleeding

CLOSURE

● **Close in layers (as previously described)**

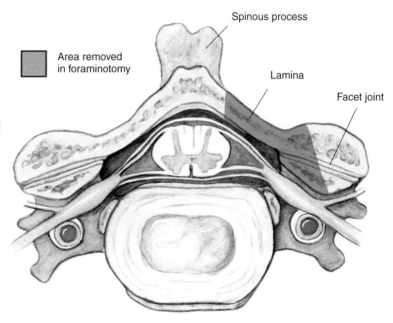

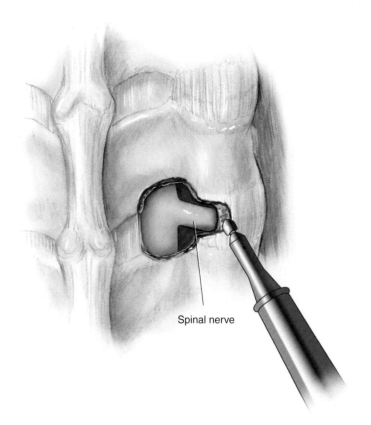

FIGURE SP-65   Posterior cervical keyhole laminoforaminotomy.

POSTERIOR MIDLINE APPROACH TO THE THORACIC SPINE

Indications

- Posterior decompression of spinal canal and nerve root
  - Laminectomy

- Posterior spinal fusion
  - Deformity
  - Fracture
  - Tumor
  - Infection

- Biopsy

- Tumor resection

POSITIONING

- Prone (Figure SP-66)
  - Use well-padded, longitudinally placed bolsters
    - Make sure that the chest wall is free to allow for chest expansion
    - Make sure the abdominal wall is free to allow for emptying of the epidural veins and abdominal vasculature to reduce intraoperative bleeding
  - Alternatively, numerous standard radiolucent spine frames exist that allow for chest and abdominal cavity decompression

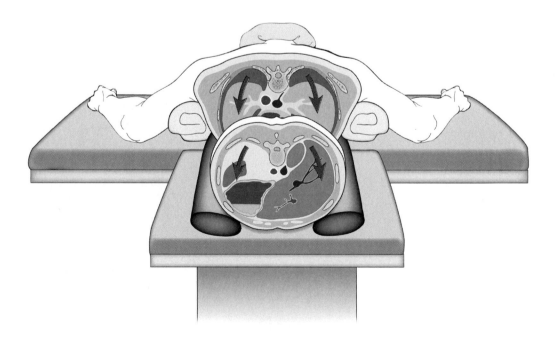

FIGURE SP-66   Prone positioning. Note the use of pads to decompress the chest and abdominal cavities.

HAZARDS

- **Neural Structures**
  - Spinal cord
  - Segmental thoracic nerve roots

- **Vascular**
  - Aorta
  - Vena cava
  - Segmental artery and vein
  - Epidural veins

- **Other**
  - Lung

INCISION

- **Longitudinal midline incision (Figure SP-67)**
  - The spinous processes of C7 and T1 are typically palpable proximally, and the gluteal cleft helps identify the midline distally

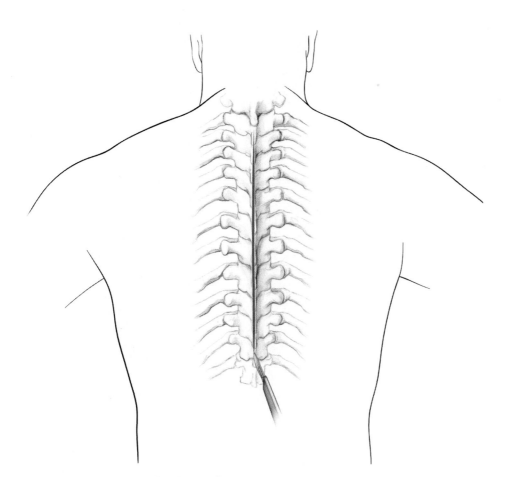

FIGURE SP-67   Midline longitudinal posterior thoracic incision.

SUPERFICIAL DISSECTION

- ● Identify individual spinous processes (Figure SP-68)

  - ▪ They may be rotated off the midline, or a palpable step-off or widening may be present in patients with scoliosis or spinal fractures

- ● Subperiosteally dissect off the paraspinous musculature bilaterally

  - ▪ In adults, identify and preserve the supraspinous and interspinous ligaments whenever possible

  - ▪ In children, the apophyses of the spinous process can be split longitudinally and dissected to each side with a Cobb elevator

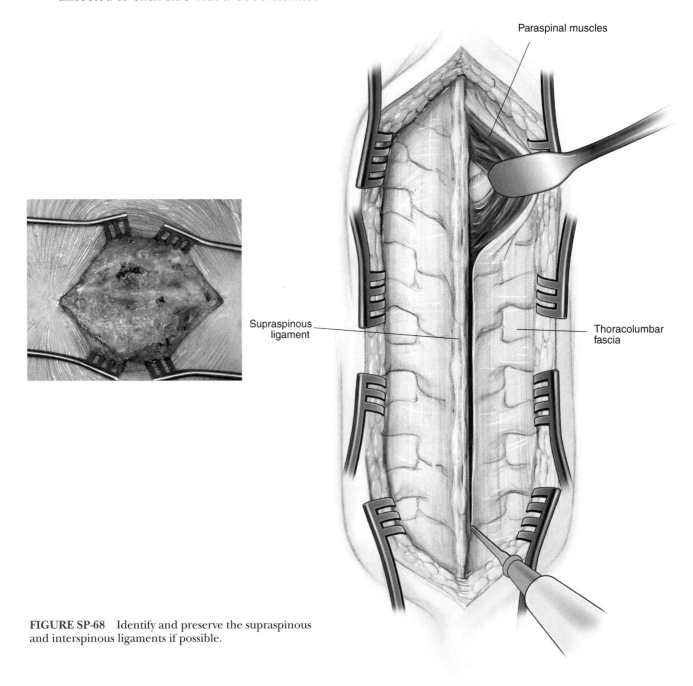

FIGURE SP-68 Identify and preserve the supraspinous and interspinous ligaments if possible.

● Expose the lamina and transverse processes bilaterally (Figure SP-69)

▪ Depending on the procedure to be performed, follow the spinous process subperiosteally out to the tips of the transverse processes

▪ The transverse processes of the thoracic spine are oriented laterally and superiorly

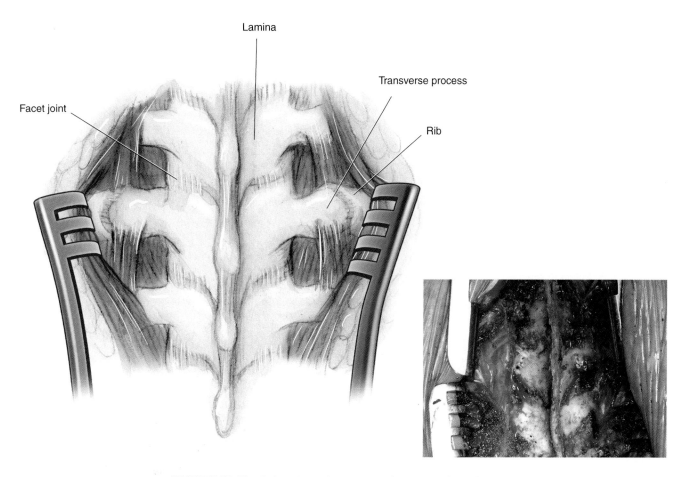

FIGURE SP-69 Subperiosteal exposure of posterior thoracic spine.

DEEP DISSECTION

● Laminotomy/laminectomy

▪ Using a combination of the Woodson and curettes, carefully develop the plane between the ligamentum and the inferior aspect of the superior lamina

● Next, a laminectomy or laminotomy can be performed using a no. 2 or 3 Kerrison, depending on the space available and the thickness of the lamina

● If the lamina is too thick, it can be carefully thinned using a rongeur or power burr

▪ The epidural fat overlying the translucent blue-white dura is visible after the ligamentum flavum and lamina are removed

- ## Multiple posterior wedge (modified Smith-Peterson) osteotomies (Figure SP-70)

  - Number of levels should be based on magnitude of kyphosis to correct
  - Each osteotomy is a wedge-shaped "V"
    - Begin medially, and carefully enter into the spinal canal as described previously

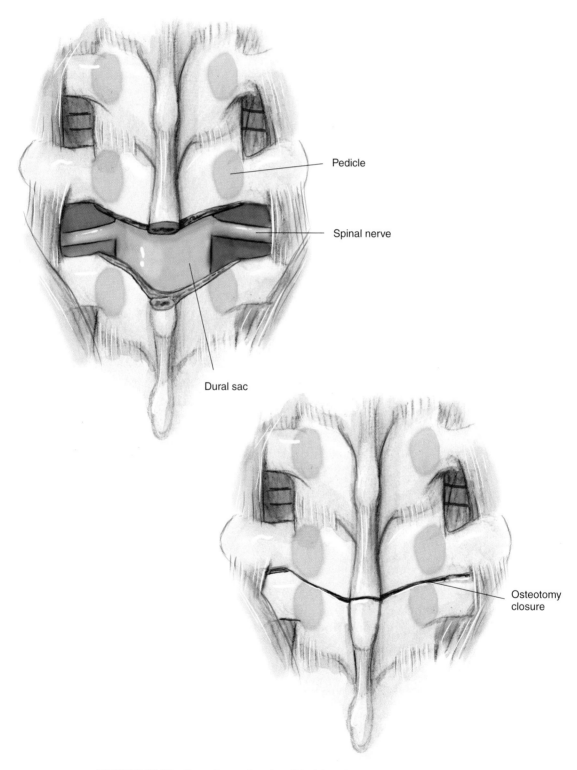

FIGURE SP-70 Posterior wedge (modified Smith-Peterson) osteotomies.

- Typically, the spinous process and supraspinous and interspinous ligaments must be removed
- Using a Woodson, carefully palpate the medial wall of the pedicle
- Each osteotomy is performed superior to the corresponding pedicle through the neuroforamen of the level above
  - First, using either an osteotome or a power burr, remove the inferior articular facet of the vertebra above
  - This exposes the superior articular facet of the vertebra below
  - Next, remove the superior articular facet using a Kerrison
  - This is done bilaterally at as many levels as planned

- **Identification of the thoracic pedicle**
  - Use of fluoroscopic guidance can help assist in pedicle localization
  - Anatomical landmarks for pedicle entry site
    - The line bisecting the transverse process intersecting the vertical line at the lateral edge of the superior articular facet
    - Alternatively, the corner of the superior border of the transverse process and lateral edge of the superior articular facet defines the lateral superior edge of the pedicle

CLOSURE

- **Skin and subcutaneous tissue is closed in layers (as previously described)**

POSTERIOR EXTRACAVITARY/ COSTOTRANSVERSECTOMY/ POSTEROLATERAL APPROACH TO THE THORACIC SPINE

Indications

- Decompression
  - Discectomy
  - Corpectomy
  - Anterior column resection

- Spinal fusion
  - Anterior interbody fusion
  - Strut grafting

- Irrigation and débridement for infections
- Drainage of abscess
- Biopsy
- Resection of tumors

POSITIONING

- Prone (Figure SP-71)
  - See description under posterior thoracic approach
  - Drape wide over the rib cage to allow for lateral exposure as necessary

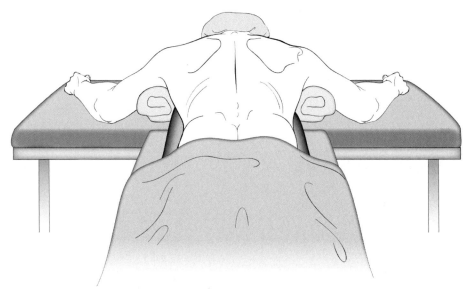

FIGURE SP-71 Prone positioning. Note the use of pads to decompress the chest and abdominal cavities.

HAZARDS

- See posterior midline approach to the thoracic spine

INCISION

- Palpate the spinous processes in the midline (Figure SP-72)
- Confirm the level with intraoperative radiographs to help plan the surgical incision
- Several skin incisions have been described
  - Midline longitudinal over the spinous process
    - This approach is completely extensile and utilitarian for revisions, but may need to be extended in length to achieve adequate lateral exposure
  - Paramedian longitudinal
    - Approximately 2.5 cm lateral to the spinous process
  - Curvilinear
    - Approximately 10-12 cm in length with the apex 6-8 cm lateral to the midline centered at the level of the pathology
  - "T" incisions also have been described, but are typically not required

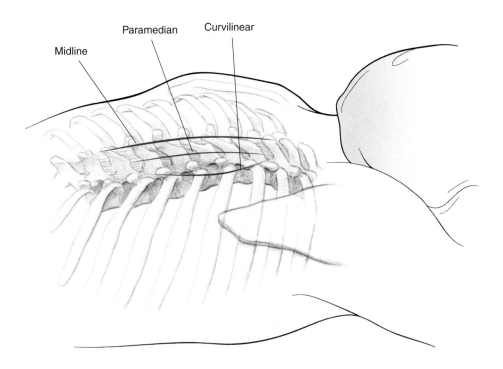

FIGURE SP-72   Various incisions used for extracavitary exposures of the thoracic spine.

SUPERFICIAL DISSECTION

- Divide subcutaneous tissue in line with skin incision

- Identify the trapezius as the next muscle layer, and split this in line with the incision (Figure SP-73)

  - The trapezius is innervated by the spinal accessory nerve proximally and is not denervated

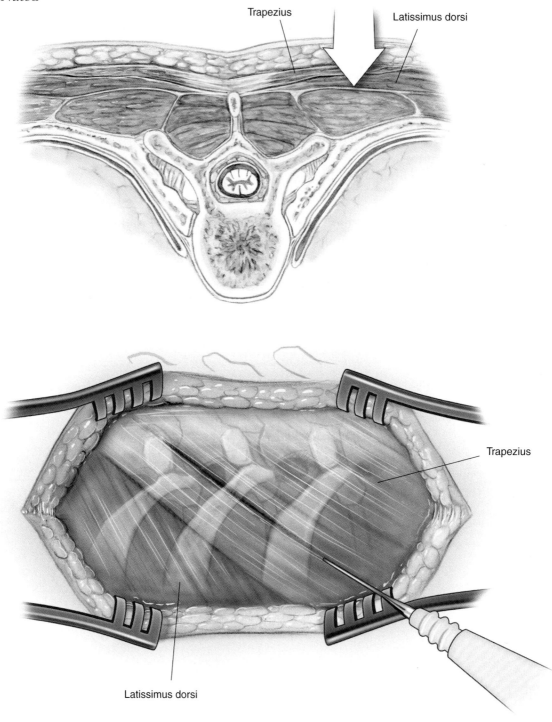

FIGURE SP-73 Identify the trapezius and latissimus dorsi muscles.

- Next, identify the erector spinae and transversospinales muscles (deep paraspinal muscles), and divide these in line with the incision (Figure SP-74)

  ▪ These muscles are segmentally innervated and are not significantly denervated by this approach

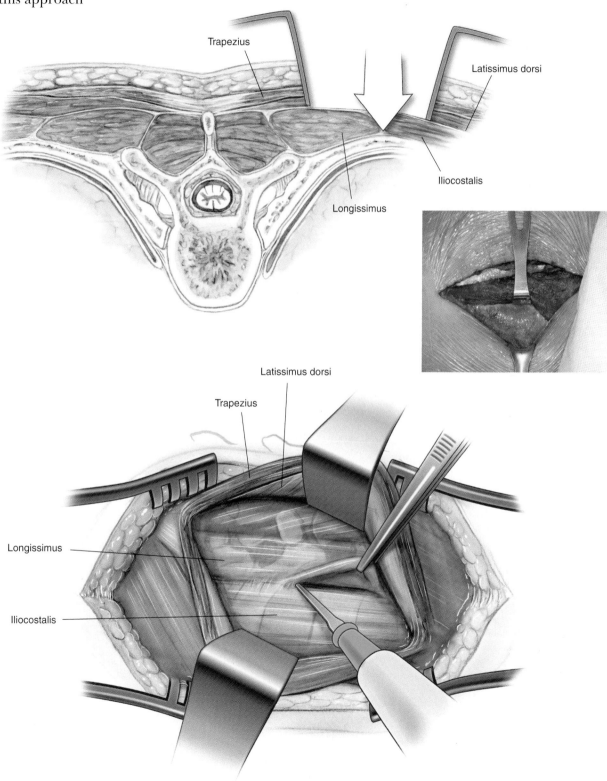

FIGURE SP-74 Divide the trapezius, and expose the deep paraspinal (longissimus and iliocostalis) muscles.

- ## Identify the junction of the rib–transverse process articulation (Figure SP-75)

  - Subperiosteally dissect the fascia, muscle attachments, and periosteum circumferentially around the rib

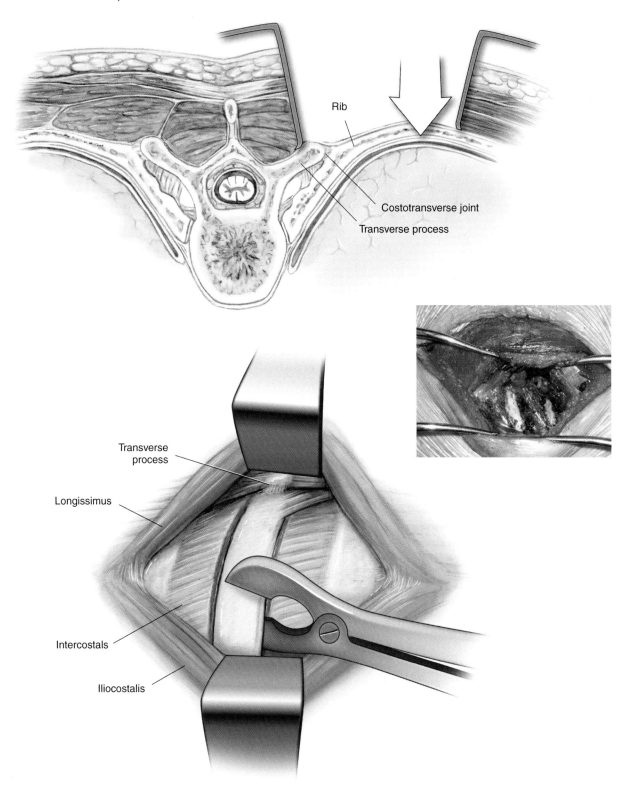

FIGURE SP-75 Expose the rib, the tip of the transverse process, and the costotransverse joint.

DEEP DISSECTION

- The amount of rib resection varies based on exposure required (2-8 cm of rib from the midline) (Figure SP-76)
  - Because of the numerous ligamentous attachments between the rib and transverse process and rib head and spine, removal of the rib can be difficult

- If wider exposure is required, detach the muscular attachments to the transverse process, and remove the process at the base

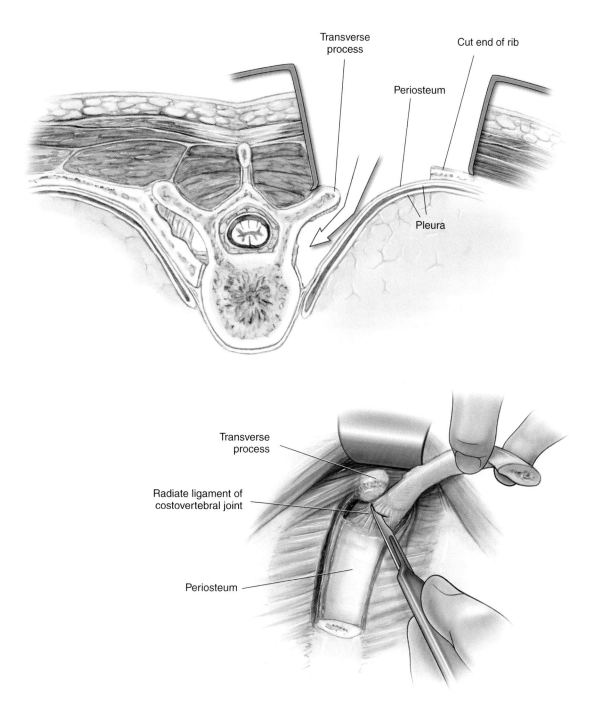

FIGURE SP-76 Disarticulate and resect the rib from the transverse process. Subperiosteal rib dissection allows for an extrapleural exposure.

- Enter the retropleural space, and identify the lateral vertebral body and corresponding disc space (Figure SP-77)

  - This can be done by careful subperiosteal dissection along the lateral pedicle wall onto the lateral vertebral body wall

  - Avoid entering the pleural cavity if possible

  - Rotating the patient away from the side of the surgical exposure can improve visualization of the lateral aspect of the vertebral body

    - This can be performed at several levels as necessary

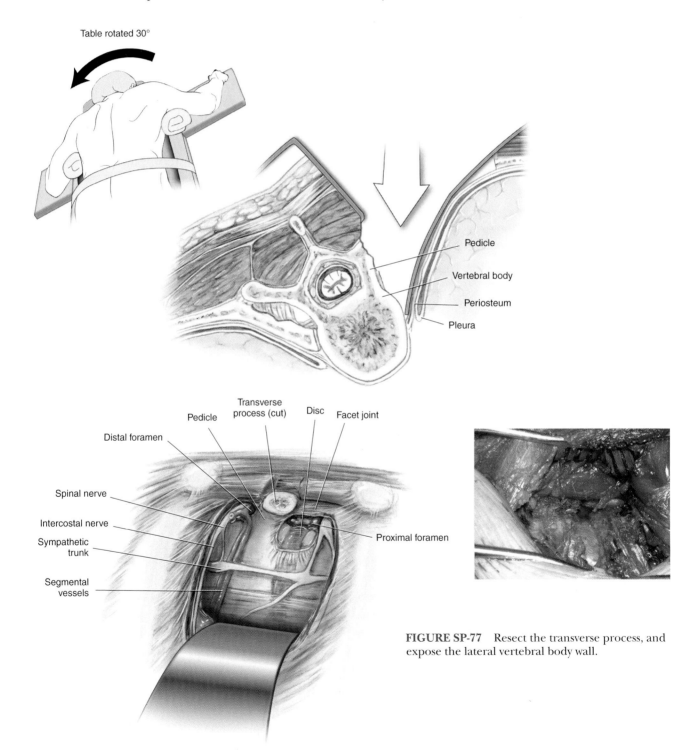

FIGURE SP-77 Resect the transverse process, and expose the lateral vertebral body wall.

CLOSURE

- If the pleural cavity has not been entered, a chest tube is unnecessary

  - If the chest cavity has been entered, a chest tube should be placed

    - Make a skin incision for the chest tube 1-2 ribs inferior to the level of the rib resection

    - Subcutaneously, tunnel superiorly up to the level, and place the chest tube above the rib

    - Place the chest tube posteriorly and superiorly toward the apex of the chest

    - Secure the chest tube at the skin with a heavy stitch

- Skin and subcutaneous tissues are closed in a standard fashion

POSTERIOR MIDLINE APPROACH TO LUMBAR SPINE

Indications

- Decompression
  - ▨ Discectomy
  - ▨ Laminotomy
  - ▨ Laminectomy
  - ▨ Facetectomy

- Posterior spinal fusion
  - ▨ Fracture
  - ▨ Instability
  - ▨ Deformity

- Osteotomy
  - ▨ Pedicle subtraction osteotomy
  - ▨ Smith-Peterson osteotomy

- Biopsy

- Tumor resection

POSITIONING

- Prone
  - ▨ Use well-padded, longitudinally placed bolsters
    - Make sure the chest wall is free to allow for chest expansion
    - Make sure the abdominal wall is free to allow for emptying of the epidural veins and abdominal vasculature to reduce intraoperative bleeding
  - ▨ Alternatively, numerous standard radiolucent spine frames exist that allow for chest and abdominal cavity decompression

- Kneeling (Figure SP-78)
  - ▨ Use a well-padded specialized kneeling table
    - Make sure chest and abdomen are free as in the prone position
    - Because the kneeling position reverses normal lumbar lordosis, it can make access into the spinal canal easier by splaying the spinous process and opening up the interlaminar space
    - Cases that require a fusion with instrumentation should not be performed in the kneeling position to avoid iatrogenic flatback syndrome

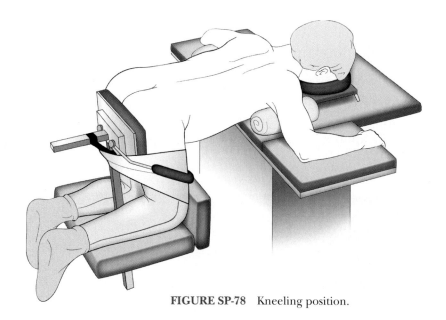

FIGURE SP-78   Kneeling position.

● Lateral (Figure SP-79)

■ Occasionally used

● Simultaneous anterior and posterior approaches

■ See description under anterior thoracic spine approach

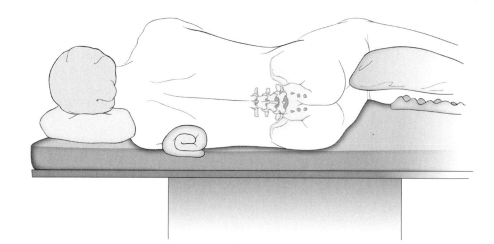

HAZARDS

● Neural structures

■ Cauda equina

■ Lumbar nerve roots

■ Lumbosacral plexus

■ Dorsal root ganglion

● Is at particular risk during transforaminal approaches

FIGURE SP-79   Lateral position.

● Vascular

■ Aorta

● Can be at risk during aggressive discectomies

■ Vena cava

● Can be at risk during aggressive discectomies

■ Epidural veins

INCISION

● **Longitudinal midline incision (Figure SP-80)**

- ■ The spinous processes are easily palpable
- ■ Gluteal cleft helps identify the midline distally
- ■ Superior aspects of the iliac crest help identify the approximate level of the L4-5 interspace (Figure SP-81)

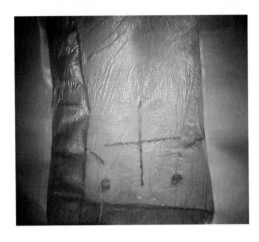

FIGURE SP-80   Intercrestal line approximates the L4-5 intervertebral disc space.

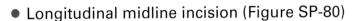

L3 spinous process

L4-5 interspace

Iliac crest

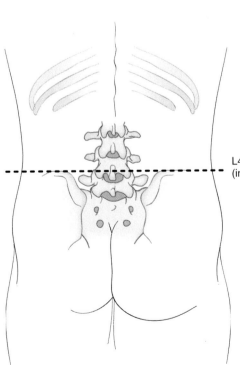

L4-5 level (intercrestal line)

FIGURE SP-81   Midline longitudinal posterior lumbar incision.

SUPERFICIAL DISSECTION

● Divide the fat and fascia in line with skin incision
  (Figure SP-82)

● Palpate for the spinous process intermittently to help identify
  the midline

  ▪ This is particularly important in larger patients and patients with scoliotic
    deformity

● Using a Cobb elevator, dissect down to the spinous process

● Detach the paraspinous muscles subperiosteally from the
  midline (Figure SP-83)

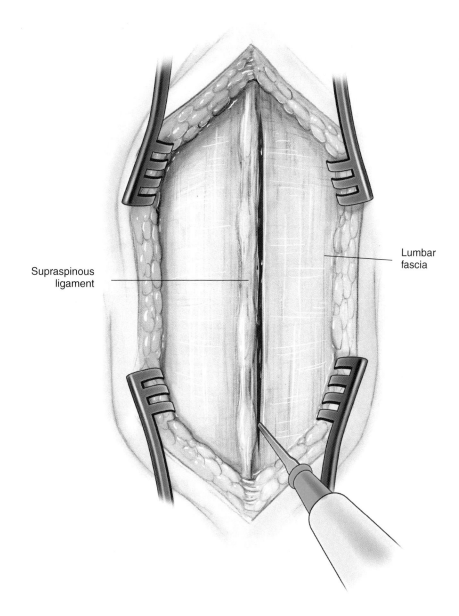

Supraspinous
ligament

Lumbar
fascia

FIGURE SP-82   Divide the fascia.

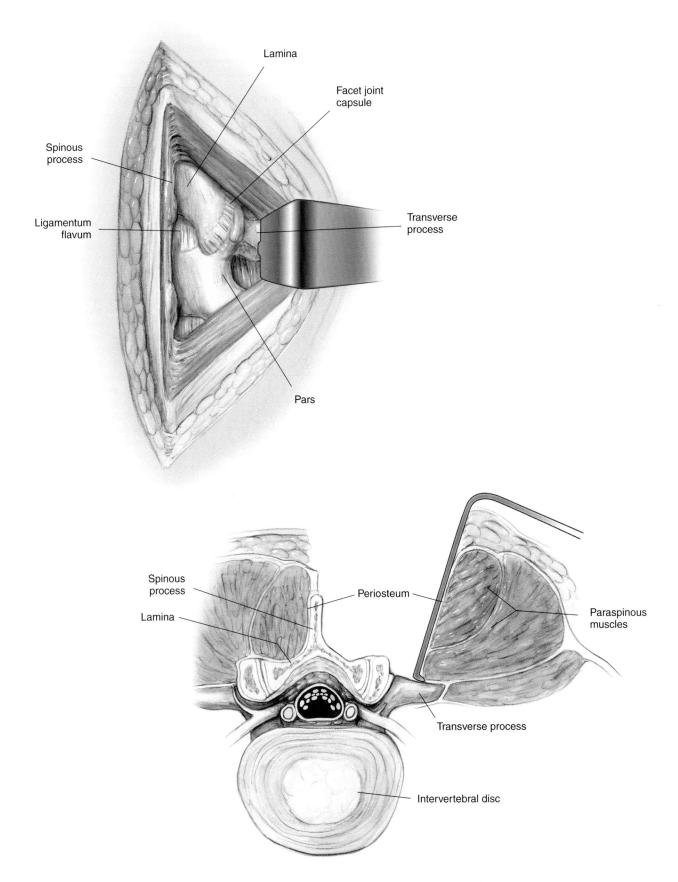

FIGURE SP-83 Subperiosteal dissection of the lumbar spine. Note the location of the pars.

■ Subperiosteal dissection helps reduce bleeding

■ In young patients, the tips of the spinous process are cartilaginous apophyses

● These can be split or detached to assist in the subperiosteal muscle dissection

■ In adults, the supraspinous and interspinous ligaments should be preserved if possible to reduce the risk of junctional kyphosis

● **Follow the spinous process laterally to the lamina and out to the facet joint capsule (Figure SP-84)**

■ If a fusion is not planned, preserve the facet joint and overlying capsule

■ Facet joints in the lumbar spine are oriented in a parasagittal plane

■ The inferior articular facet of the superior vertebra lies medial and posterior to the superior articular facet of the inferior vertebra

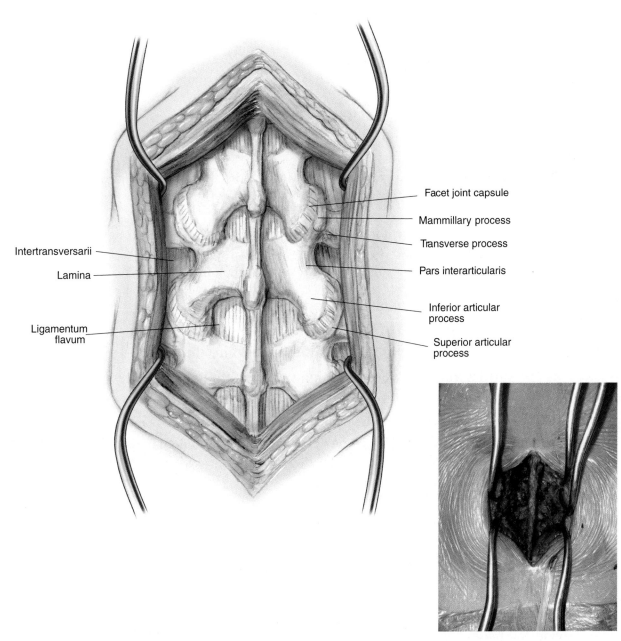

FIGURE SP-84 Preserve the facet capsule, and the supraspinous and interspinous ligaments if possible. Note the natural widening of each subsequent vertebra from superior to inferior.

- Identify the pars interarticularis

  - This lies between the superior and inferior articular facet of the same vertebra

- If necessary, the dissection can be continued laterally to the mammillary process, then onto the transverse process

  - Care should be taken to stay on the transverse process. Straying inadvertently deep to the intertransverse ligament can result in injury to the exiting nerve root
    - Occasionally, excision of a far lateral disc requires that the intertransverse ligament be divided
  - Dissection lateral to the facet joint may result in injury to the articular branches of the segmental vessels
    - This would not cause a problem; however, these vessels can bleed vigorously and should be controlled with careful cauterization or packing

DEEP DISSECTION

- Identify the ligamentum flavum (Figure SP-85)

  - The superior attachment is on the superior lamina halfway up its anterior/undersurface.
    - The canal can be entered superiorly by removing the distal end of the superior lamina with a Kerrison until the attachment of the ligamentum flavum is reached.
  - The inferior attachment on the inferior lamina is at its superior (leading) edge.
    - The canal can be entered inferiorly by cutting the attachment of the ligamentum flavum directly from the leading edge of the inferior lamina

- Variable amounts of epidural fat are seen on entering the spinal canal

- Immediately beneath the epidural fat is the blue-white dura

- Success for almost all procedures in the lumbar spine lies in identifying the location of the pedicle (Figure SP-86)

  - The disc space lies just superior to the pedicle
  - The exiting nerve root first travels just medial to the pedicle and then exits the foramen just inferior to the pedicle

- Identify the pars interarticularis

  - This should be exposed and defined during the superficial dissection
    - If no fusion is to be performed, care should be taken not to remove too much of the pars interarticularis during the laminotomy and foraminotomy
    - Complete resection of the pars interarticularis results in an iatrogenic spondylolysis and possible spondylolisthesis
    - Bilateral pars defects result in segmental instability and an iatrogenic spondylolisthesis

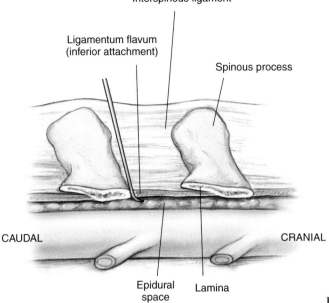

Interspinous ligament

Ligamentum flavum
(inferior attachment)

Spinous process

CAUDAL

CRANIAL

Epidural
space

Lamina

FIGURE SP-85 Note the superior attachment of the ligamentum flavum midway up the anterior surface of the superior lamina and the inferior attachment on the superior aspect of the inferior lamina.

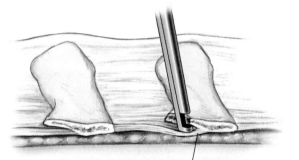

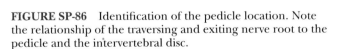

Ligamentum flavum
(superior attachment)

FIGURE SP-86 Identification of the pedicle location. Note the relationship of the traversing and exiting nerve root to the pedicle and the intervertebral disc.

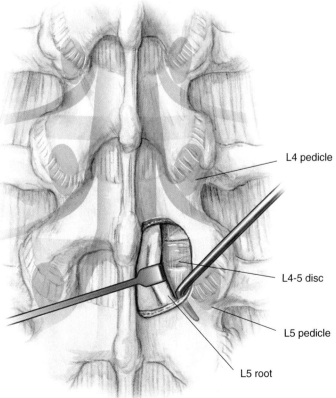

L4 pedicle

L4-5 disc

L5 pedicle

L5 root

- Laminotomy/laminectomy (Figure SP-87)

  - Depending on the etiology and location of the spinal compression, a laminotomy (windowing), a laminectomy, or a variation of the two can be used to gain access to the spinal canal (Figure SP-88)

- Discectomy

  - Before surgery, preoperative imaging should be studied carefully to understand fully the location of the herniated disc

  - The most common location for disc herniations remains posterolateral

    - There is a natural weakening just lateral to where the posterior longitudinal ligament begins to thin

    - Posterolateral herniations typically impinge on the shoulder of the nerve root traversing that level to the more inferior vertebra

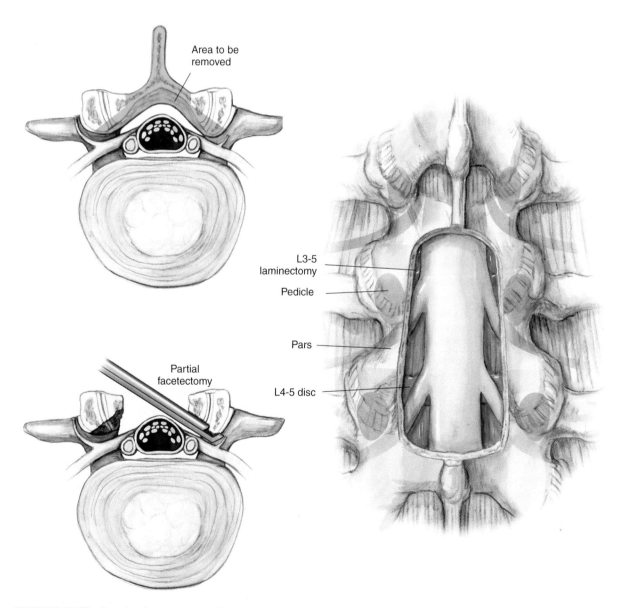

FIGURE SP-87 Lumbar laminectomy. Note the importance of undercutting the facet joint to provide room for the nerve root while preserving segmental stability.

- **Foraminotomy**
  - In the case of neuroforaminal stenosis, direct nerve impingement from facet capsule hypertrophy or bony osteophytes can result
    - This typically results in impingement of the nerve root exiting at that level

- **Identification of the lumbar pedicle**
  - Use of fluoroscopic guidance can help assist in pedicle localization
  - Anatomical landmarks for pedicle entry site
    - Variations exist, but typically the entry site can be identified by the confluence of several lines
      - The line bisecting the midpoint of the transverse process
      - The lateral edge of the superior articular facet
      - The superomedial edge of the mammillary process
      - A curvilinear line following the pars proximally to the crossing point of the other lines

CLOSURE

- **Skin and subcutaneous tissues are closed in the standard fashion**

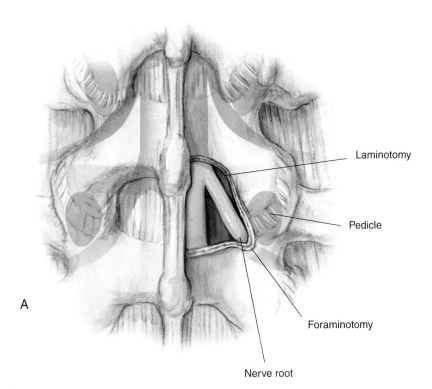
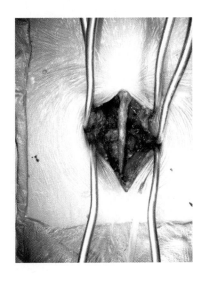

A

Laminotomy

Pedicle

Foraminotomy

Nerve root

FIGURE SP-88 **A,** Hemilaminotomy and foraminotomy. **B,** Hemilaminectomy. **C,** Fenestrations (bilateral hemilaminotomy and laminectomy).

(figure continues)

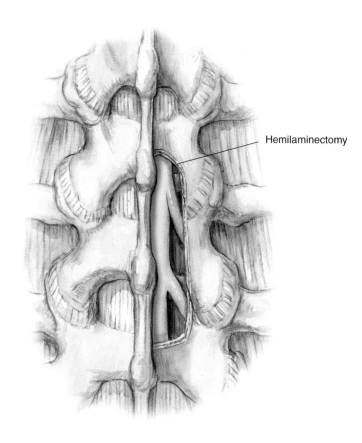

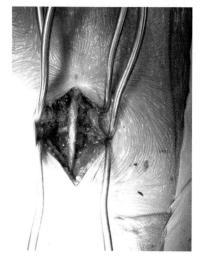

Hemilaminectomy

B

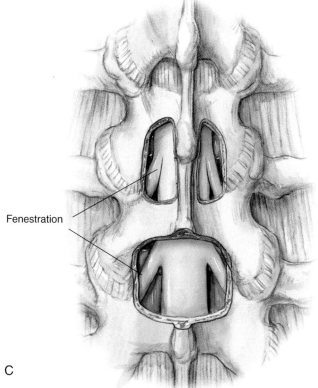

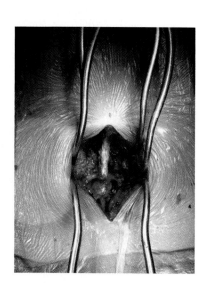

Fenestration

C

FIGURE SP-88 *(continued)*

POSTERIOR MUSCLE SPLITTING APPROACH TO THE LUMBAR SPINE

Indications

- Decompression
  - Far lateral disc herniations
  - Foraminal decompression

- Fusion
  - Posterior intertransverse fusion

- Placement of pedicle screws
- Biopsy

POSITIONING

- Prone
  - See description under posterior lumbar approach

- Kneeling
  - See description under posterior lumbar approach

HAZARDS

- See posterior midline lumbar approach

LANDMARKS

- Before making the surgical incision, identification of the appropriate landmarks is vital
  - Identify the midline
    - The spinous processes are easily palpable
    - Gluteal cleft helps identify the midline distally
  - Identify the cephalad and caudal levels
    - Superior aspects of the iliac crest help identify the approximate level of the L4-5 interspace
  - The use of fluoroscopy before the surgical incision can be useful, especially for percutaneous and limited-open techniques
    - Identify the middle of the pedicle on the anteroposterior view
    - Identify the level of the intervertebral disc space on the anteroposterior view
    - Identify the direction of the intervertebral disc on the lateral fluoroscopic view

INCISION

- Longitudinal incision approximately 2 finger breadths (3 cm) lateral to the midline centered evenly over the site of the pathology (Figure SP-89)

  - ▪ A spinal needle and intraoperative radiographs should be used as necessary

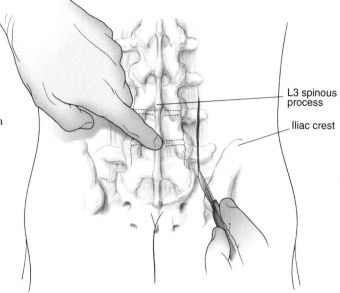

L3 spinous process

Iliac crest

FIGURE SP-89 Posterior muscle splitting approach to lumbar spine. Note incision is approximately 2 finger breadths (3 cm) lateral to the midline.

SUPERFICIAL DISSECTION

- Divide the skin and subcutaneous tissue down to the lumbodorsal fascia (Figure SP-90)

- Gently feel for the natural interval between the multifidus and longissimus with the fingertip

  - ▪ Sharply divide the fascia longitudinally with either electrocautery or scalpel blade

- Using blunt dissection, this plane can be gently developed down to the lumbar spine

  - ▪ Depending on the specific procedure, this plane can be developed down to the transverse process, facet joint, pars interarticularis, or lamina
  - ▪ This can be done with finger dissection or over sequential dilators
  - ▪ If the proper plane is identified and developed, this is a relatively bloodless approach

- When the appropriate location is identified, retractors are placed

  - ▪ Currently, dozens of commercially available retractors are available
  - ▪ Alternatively, for limited-open procedures, a traditional Taylor retractor can be used

    - • Place the spike tip just lateral to either the facet joint or the pars interarticularis
    - • Care should be taken not to place the spike tip inadvertently within the neuroforamen

- Clear off the overlying soft tissue, and carefully identify the bony anatomy with a combination of electrocautery, pituitaries, and curettes

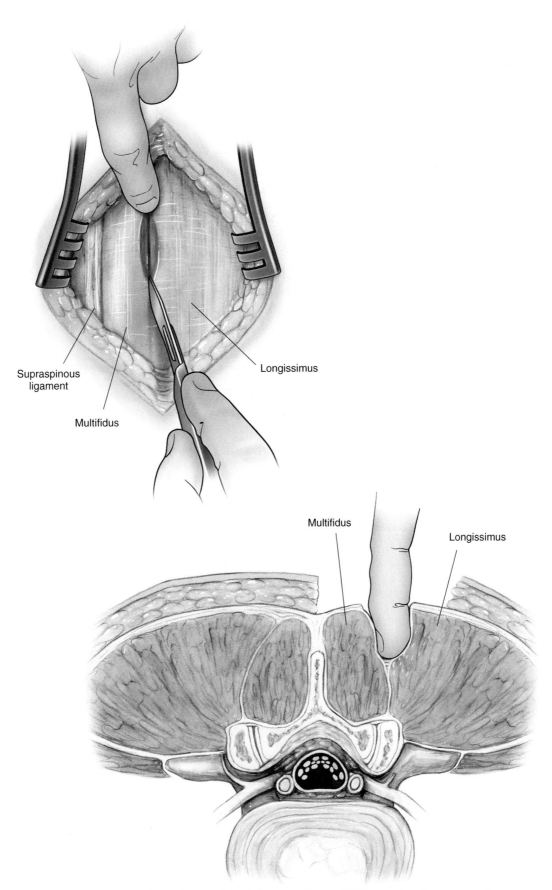

FIGURE SP-90   Divide lumbodorsal fascia between the multifidus and longissimus muscles.

DEEP DISSECTION

● **Far lateral disc**

  ▪ Identify the transverse processes superior and inferior to the herniated disc
  ▪ Identify the pars interarticularis
  ▪ Retract the muscle off the intertransverse ligament (Figure SP-91)
  ▪ Detach the intertransverse ligament (Figure SP-92)
    ● This can be done with a combination of a straight and curved curette
    ● Detach the ligament from the superior transverse process and pars
    ● Hook the ligament with a nerve hook or fine Kerrison, and gently retract it laterally
  ▪ Identify the exiting nerve root traversing just below the pedicle
    ● Using a Penfield no. 4, gently trace the nerve from the inferomedial aspect of the pedicle laterally
  ▪ Identify the intervertebral disc just inferior to the exiting nerve
    ● The location of the nerve may be more superficial or inferior than expected, depending on the location of the disc herniation

● **Transforaminal approach**

  ▪ Identify the inferior articular facet of the superior vertebra
    ● Remove a portion of the inferior articular facet using a combination of osteotome, Kerrison, and pituitaries
  ▪ This now exposes the superior articular facet of the inferior vertebra

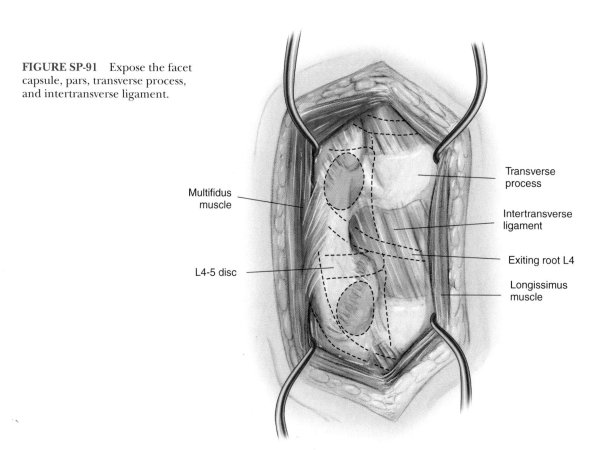

FIGURE SP-91 Expose the facet capsule, pars, transverse process, and intertransverse ligament.

Multifidus muscle

L4-5 disc

Transverse process

Intertransverse ligament

Exiting root L4

Longissimus muscle

- Remove the superior articular facet down to the pedicle
- Care should be taken to identify and protect the common dural sac
  - The intervertebral disc is clearly exposed just above the inferior pedicle
    - Depending on the amount of exposure required, the exiting nerve root may or may not be identified
  - The transforaminal approach is particularly destabilizing and in most cases results in segmental instability and should be performed in conjunction with a fusion procedure

Laminotomy/laminectomy

  - This is performed analogous to the midline lumbar approach

Identification of the lumbar pedicle

  - This is performed analogous to the midline lumbar approach
  - Access to the pedicle is typically easier from this approach than from the standard midline approach
    - This is because the direction of this approach is from a more lateral-to-medial position, mimicking the normal pedicle trajectory
    - There is less force against the paraspinous muscles as there is in the midline approach

CLOSURE

- Skin and subcutaneous tissues are closed in the standard fashion

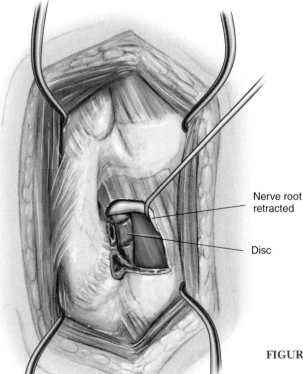

Nerve root retracted

Disc

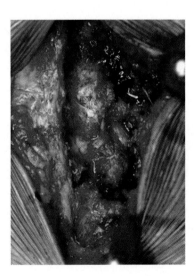

FIGURE SP-92   Carefully detach the intertransverse ligament.

ANTERIOR ILIAC CREST BONE GRAFT

Indications

- Bone graft harvest
  - Tricortical autograft
  - Cancellous autograft
  - Corticocancellous autograft

POSITIONING

- Supine on the operating table
- A bump under ipsilateral buttocks can help the exposure and accessibility of the iliac crest

HAZARDS

- Neural structures
  - Lateral femoral cutaneous nerve
    - Lies approximately 1 cm distal to the ASIS
    - In a small percentage of patients may cross over the iliac wing

- Vascular
  - Femoral artery and vein
    - Rarely at risk, but may be injured if exposure strays anteriorly into the femoral triangle

- Other
  - Avulsion fracture of ASIS
    - Risk may be reduced by performing osteotomy at least 1 cm proximal to ASIS
  - Inguinal ligament
    - Takes origin off of ASIS
    - Do not inadvertently cut or detach the inguinal ligament, which can result in an inguinal hernia

LANDMARKS

- Identify the ASIS
- Identify the iliac tubercle

INCISION (FIGURE SP-93)

- Parallel the incision in line with the iliac crest
- Center incision based on type of graft required
  - Tricortical (Smith-Robinson) graft
    - Focus incision at least 2 cm posterior to ASIS
  - Corticocancellous/cancellous bone graft
    - Focus incision over iliac tubercle

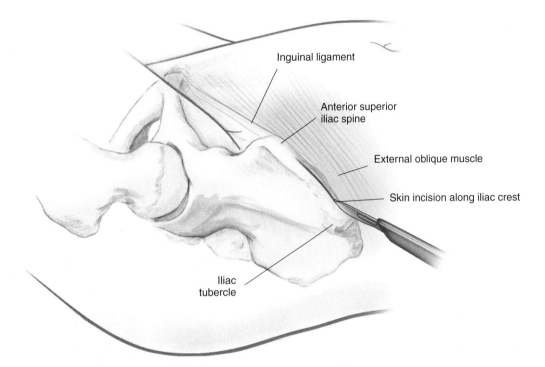

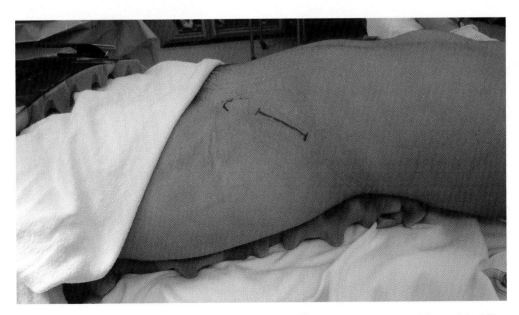

FIGURE SP-93 Incision for exposure of the anterior iliac crest. *Photo courtesy of Vincent Arlet, MD.*

SUPERFICIAL DISSECTION

- Deepen in line with skin incision down to iliac wing
  - Do not stray anterior to the ASIS
    - Lateral femoral cutaneous nerve
      - Course varies
      - Typically, it runs 1 cm anterior to the ASIS underneath the inguinal ligament
    - Inguinal ligament
      - Takes origin off of ASIS
      - Do not inadvertently cut or detach the inguinal ligament, which can result in an inguinal hernia

- Identify the natural raphe between the fascia overlying iliac wing (Figure SP-94)
  - Fascia of external oblique anteriorly
  - Fascia of gluteus medius posteriorly

- Incise directly on the iliac wing

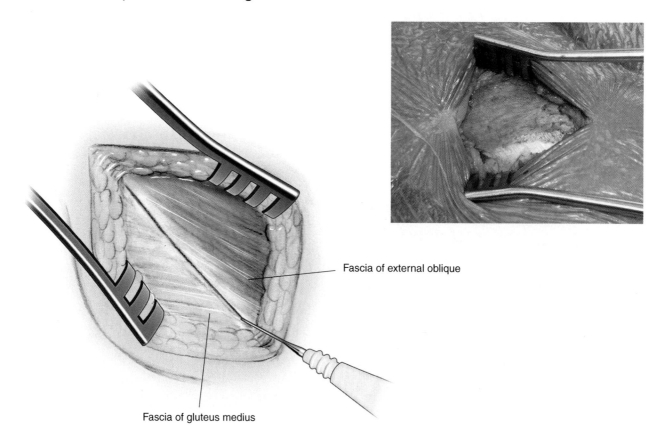

Fascia of external oblique

Fascia of gluteus medius

FIGURE SP-94 Identify the fascia over the external oblique and gluteus medius.

DEEP DISSECTION

- ## Subperiosteal dissection (Figure SP-95)
  - Using a Cobb elevator, subperiosteally dissect the abdominal musculature and the psoas off the inner table of the iliac wing
  - Using a Cobb elevator, subperiosteally dissect the gluteus medius and tensor fasciae latae off the outer table of the iliac wing

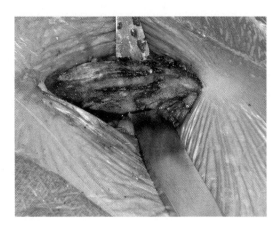

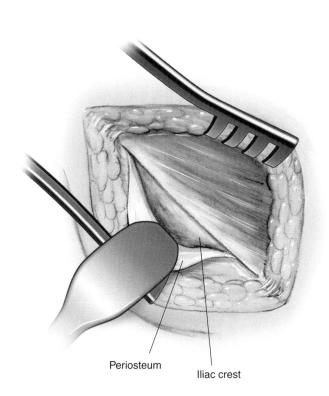

Periosteum   Iliac crest

FIGURE SP-95   Subperiosteally dissect the outer and inner table of the anterior iliac crest. *Photo courtesy of Vincent Arlet, MD.*

- Place Taylor retractors to protect the surrounding structures
- Osteotomies (Figure SP-96)
  - Tricortical graft
    - Make osteotomy at least 2 cm from the ASIS
      - This reduces risk of iatrogenic ASIS avulsion
    - Make parallel osteotomies to ensure that the graft has parallel end plates
      - Measure the length and depth of graft required
    - One-level and two-level grafts are typically obtained without difficulty
    - There may be insufficient crest available for longer strut grafts
    - Natural curvature of the iliac wing also may prohibit long strut grafts
  - Corticocancellous graft
    - Strips can be harvested using an osteotome
  - Cancellous bone
    - The iliac tubercle provides the largest supply of cancellous bone and can be accessed via a variety of methods

CLOSURE

- Close in layers in the standard fashion
- A drain is typically not required

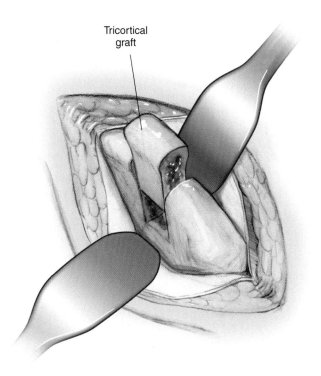

Tricortical graft

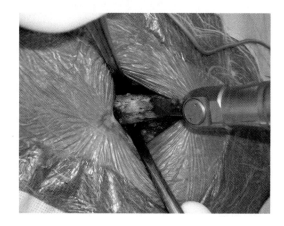

FIGURE SP-96 Tricortical iliac crest harvest. The osteotomies are made at least 2 cm proximal to the ASIS to reduce the risk of fracture. *Photo courtesy of Vincent Arlet, MD.*

POSTERIOR ILIAC CREST BONE GRAFT

Indications

- Bone graft harvest
  - Cancellous autograft
  - Corticocancellous autograft

POSITIONING

- Prone or lateral decubitus
  - Based on primary procedure being performed

HAZARDS

- Neural structures
  - Superior cluneal nerve
    - Lies approximately 8 cm lateral to PSIS
    - Injury can result in variable degree of numbness to the buttock region
  - Sciatic nerve
    - Exits pelvis through greater sciatic notch
    - At risk during the osteotomy

- Vascular
  - Superior gluteal artery
    - Branch of internal iliac
    - Exits through sciatic notch
    - If cut, the vessel may retract into the pelvis and result in vigorous bleeding

- Other
  - Sciatic notch fracture
    - Inadvertent osteotomy through the sciatic notch results in the equivalent of a pelvic fracture
  - Sacroiliac joint
    - Can occur during bone graft harvest by violating the inner table

LANDMARKS

- Identify the PSIS

INCISION

● Variety of incisions described (Figure SP-97)

   ■ All separate surgical incisions are centered on PSIS

   ■ Alternatively, can be obtained from same midline incision as primary procedure

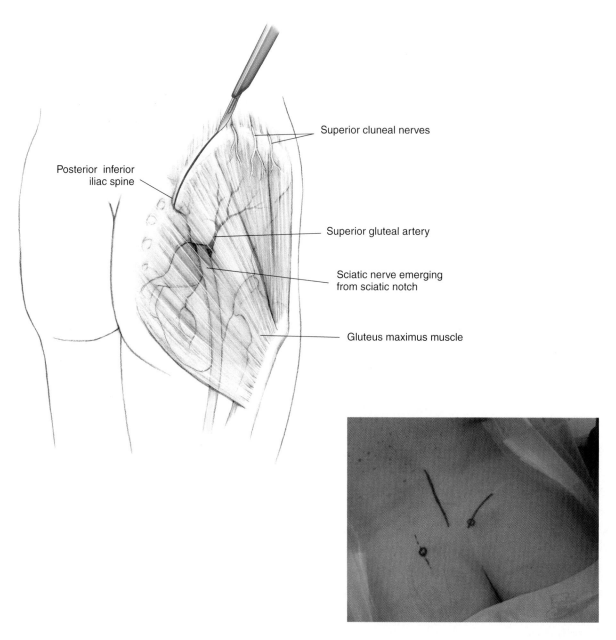

Posterior inferior iliac spine

Superior cluneal nerves

Superior gluteal artery

Sciatic nerve emerging from sciatic notch

Gluteus maximus muscle

FIGURE SP-97 Incision for exposure of the posterior iliac crest.

SUPERFICIAL DISSECTION

- **Separate incision**
  - Dissect directly down onto the PSIS
  - Do not stray greater than 8 cm lateral to the PSIS to reduce risk of injury to cluneal nerves

- **Midline incision**
  - Divide skin and subcutaneous tissue down to the lumbodorsal fascia
  - Remain subfascial and dissect laterally to PSIS

DEEP DISSECTION

- **Exposure of outer table (Figure SP-98)**
  - Using a Cobb elevator, subperiosteally dissect the musculature of the outer table
  - Place a Taylor retractor after dissection

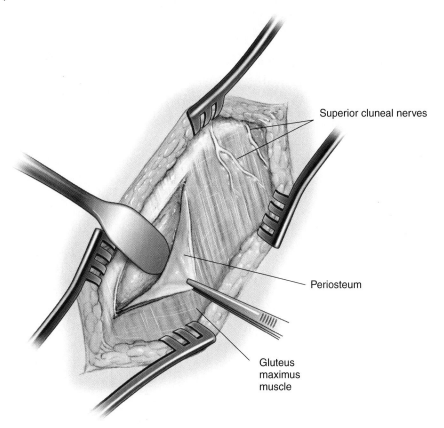

FIGURE SP-98 Subperiosteally dissect the outer table of the posterior iliac crest. Lateral dissection greater than 8 cm from the PSIS places the superior cluneal nerve at risk.

- Bone graft harvest (Figure SP-99)

  - Variety of methods described
    - The iliac tubercle provides the largest supply of cancellous bone

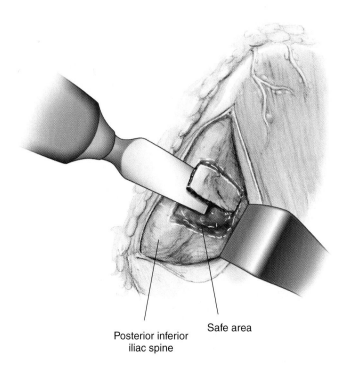

Posterior inferior
iliac spine

Safe area

FIGURE SP-99   Harvest of corticocancellous strips from the posterior iliac crest.

- Dangers

  - Greater sciatic notch
    - Identification of this anatomical structure remains one of the keys to this procedure

- Sciatic nerve

  - Exits pelvis through greater sciatic notch
  - At risk during the osteotomy

- Superior gluteal artery

  - Branch of internal iliac
  - Exits through sciatic notch
  - If cut, the vessel may retract into the pelvis and result in vigorous bleeding

- Sciatic notch
  - Inadvertent osteotomy through the sciatic notch results in the equivalent of a pelvic fracture
  - Sacroiliac joint
    - During harvest of the corticocancellous or cancellous autograft, do not violate the inner table
    - This may result in injury to the sacroiliac joint and be one source of persisent postoperative pain

CLOSURE

- Close in layers in the standard fashion
- The use of a closed suction drain is based on surgeon preference

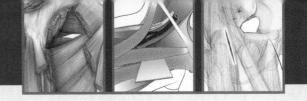

CHAPTER

6

HIP AND PELVIS

———

WILLIAM M. MIHALKO

MARK J. ANDERS

QUANJUN CUI

THOMAS BROWN

KHALED SALEH

REGIONAL ANATOMY

Osteology

- Pelvis (Figures HP-1 and HP-2)
  - Iliac crest (palpable throughout its entire length)
    - Internal lip
    - External lip
    - Tubercle (outer surface of iliac crest about 5 cm posterior to the anterior superior iliac spine [ASIS])
  - Wing of the ilium (broad surface for muscle attachments)
    - Gluteal lines
      - Anterior
      - Inferior
      - Posterior
  - Posterior superior iliac spine (PSIS) (at level of second sacral spine and may have a dimple in the skin at its level)
  - Posterior inferior iliac spine
  - Greater sciatic notch
  - Body of ilium

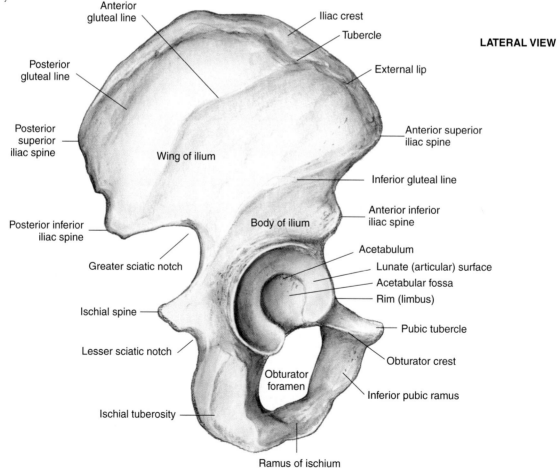

LATERAL VIEW

Anterior gluteal line — Iliac crest — Tubercle — External lip — Posterior gluteal line — Anterior superior iliac spine — Posterior superior iliac spine — Wing of ilium — Inferior gluteal line — Anterior inferior iliac spine — Posterior inferior iliac spine — Body of ilium — Acetabulum — Lunate (articular) surface — Acetabular fossa — Rim (limbus) — Greater sciatic notch — Ischial spine — Pubic tubercle — Lesser sciatic notch — Obturator crest — Obturator foramen — Inferior pubic ramus — Ischial tuberosity — Ramus of ischium

FIGURE HP-1 Osseous anatomy of the outer portion of the hemipelvis and the acetabulum.

- Ischial spine (sacrospinous ligament attachment and separates lesser and greater sciatic notches)
- Lesser sciatic notch
- Ischial tuberosity (palpated at the lower aspect of the buttocks and in the sitting position covered only by skin and bursa)
- Ramus of ischium
- Wing of ilium
- ASIS (attachment of inguinal ligament)
- Anterior inferior iliac spine (origin of the long head of the rectus femoris)
- Acetabulum
  - Lunate (articular) surface
  - Acetabular fossa
  - Rim (limbus)
- Pubic tubercle (attachment of the inguinal ligament)
- Obturator foramen
- Obturator crest
- Inferior pubic ramus
- Arcuate line
- Pectineal line
- Obturator groove

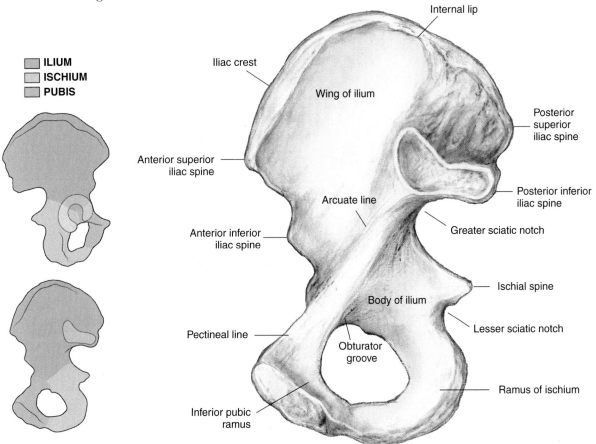

FIGURE HP-2 Osseous anatomy of the inner portion of the hemipelvis from the sacroiliac joint to the pubic symphysis.

- Proximal femur
  (Figures HP-3 and HP-4)

  - Head
  - Fovea (ligament of the femoral head attachment)
  - Greater trochanter (abductor attachment for increased moment arm and mechanical advantage)
  - Piriformis fossa
  - Intertrochanteric line
  - Lesser trochanter (insertions of the iliacus and the psoas muscles)
  - Intertrochanteric crest
  - Calcar
  - Pectineal line
  - Gluteal tuberosity
  - Linea aspera

ANTERIOR VIEW

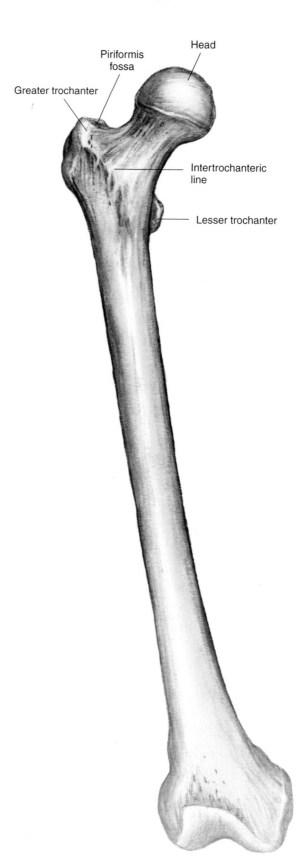

FIGURE HP-3 Osseous anatomy of the anterior portion of the proximal femur.

POSTERIOR VIEW

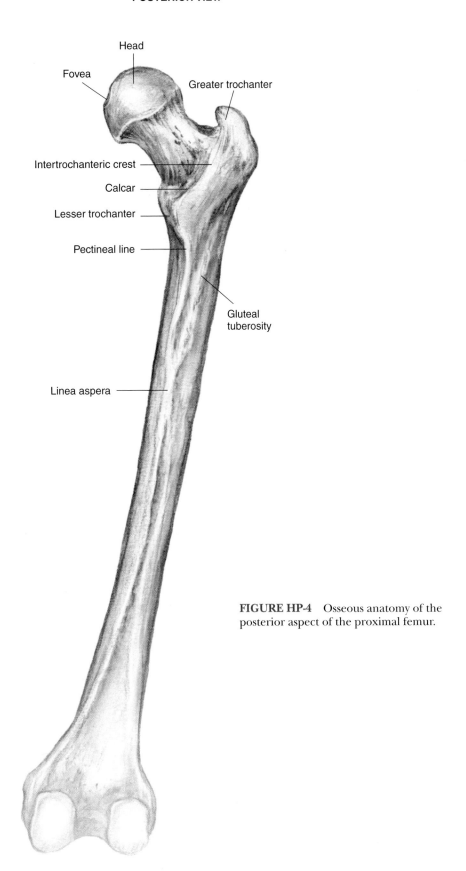

Head

Fovea

Greater trochanter

Intertrochanteric crest

Calcar

Lesser trochanter

Pectineal line

Gluteal tuberosity

Linea aspera

FIGURE HP-4   Osseous anatomy of the posterior aspect of the proximal femur.

Arthrology

- Hip joint (Figures HP-5, HP-6, and HP-7)
  - Ball and socket with only sliding—no translation
  - Static restraints
    - Ligaments
      - Hip stabilizing ligaments
        - Iliofemoral
        - Iliopectineal
        - Pubofemoral
        - Ischiofemoral
    - Labrum
    - Articular congruity
  - Dynamic restraints
    - Gluteus medius and minimus
    - Iliopsoas
    - External rotators
    - Iliotibial band

- Sacroiliac joint
  - Small translations of the joint
  - Largely stabilized by ligaments
    - Pelvis and sacroiliac ligament joint stabilizers
      - Sacrotuberous ligament (connects posterior inferior iliac spine and lateral aspect of sacrum to coccyx and ischial tuberosity)
      - Sacrospinous (connects the lateral part of the sacrum and the coccyx to the spine of the ischium)
      - Anterior sacral ligaments
      - Posterior sacral ligaments
      - Iliolumbar ligaments (transverse process of lower lumbar vertebrae to the ilium)

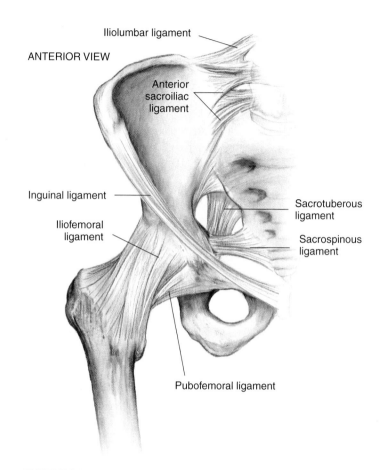

FIGURE HP-5   Anterior aspect of the hip capsule showing the iliofemoral and pubofemoral ligaments.

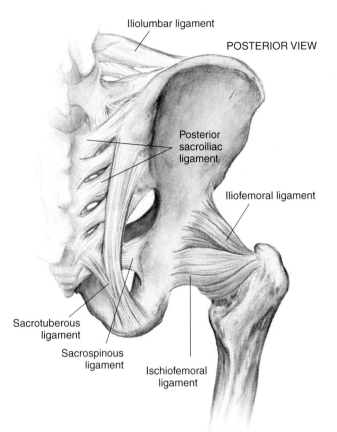

Iliolumbar ligament

POSTERIOR VIEW

Posterior sacroiliac ligament

Iliofemoral ligament

Sacrotuberous ligament

Sacrospinous ligament

Ischiofemoral ligament

FIGURE HP-6 Posterior aspect of the hip capsule showing the iliofemoral and ischiofemoral ligaments.

LATERAL VIEW

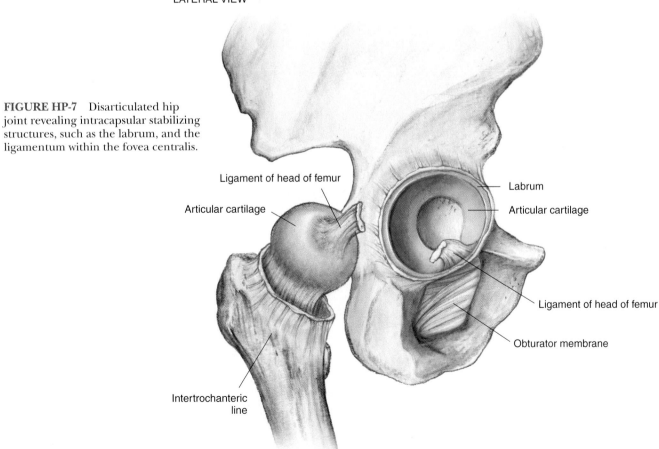

FIGURE HP-7 Disarticulated hip joint revealing intracapsular stabilizing structures, such as the labrum, and the ligamentum within the fovea centralis.

Ligament of head of femur

Articular cartilage

Labrum

Articular cartilage

Ligament of head of femur

Obturator membrane

Intertrochanteric line

Muscles

- **Pelvic origins
  (Figures HP-8 and HP-9)**

  ▪ Iliacus (intrapelvic)
  ▪ Sartorius (ASIS)
  ▪ Rectus femoris (anterior
    inferior iliac spine,
    anterior and lateral
    rim of acetabulum)
  ▪ Gluteus maximus
  ▪ Gluteus medius
  ▪ Gluteus minimus
  ▪ Tensor fascia lata
  ▪ Sartorius
  ▪ Superior gemellus
  ▪ Inferior gemellus
  ▪ Quadratus femoris
  ▪ Obturator internus
  ▪ Adductor magnus
  ▪ Long head of
    biceps femoris
  ▪ Semitendinosus
  ▪ Semimembranosus

- **Pelvis insertions**

  ▪ Rectus abdominis
  ▪ External oblique
  ▪ Internal oblique
  ▪ Transversalis

- **Proximal femur origins**

  ▪ Vastus lateralis
  ▪ Vastus medialis
  ▪ Vastus intermedius

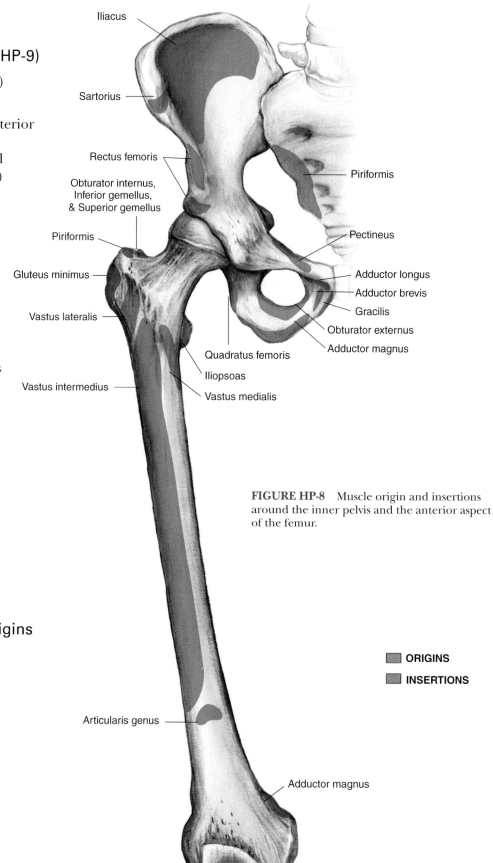

FIGURE HP-8 Muscle origin and insertions around the inner pelvis and the anterior aspect of the femur.

■ ORIGINS
■ INSERTIONS

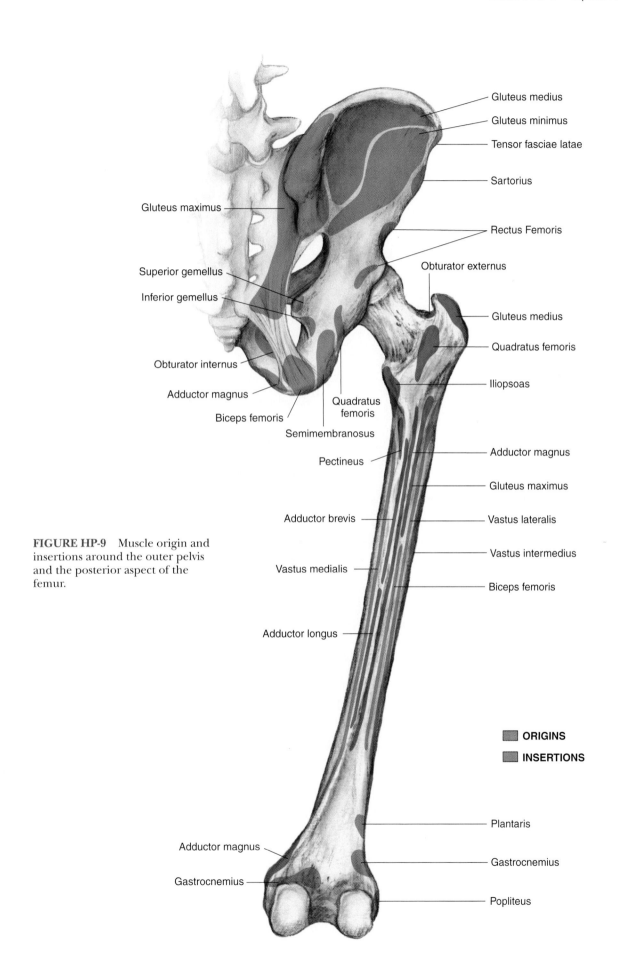

FIGURE HP-9 Muscle origin and insertions around the outer pelvis and the posterior aspect of the femur.

● Proximal femoral insertions (Figures HP-10 through HP-15)

- Piriformis
- Obturator internus
- Superior gemellus
- Inferior gemellus
- Gluteus medius
- Quadratus femoris
- Obturator externus
- Iliopsoas
- Gluteus maximus
- Pectineus

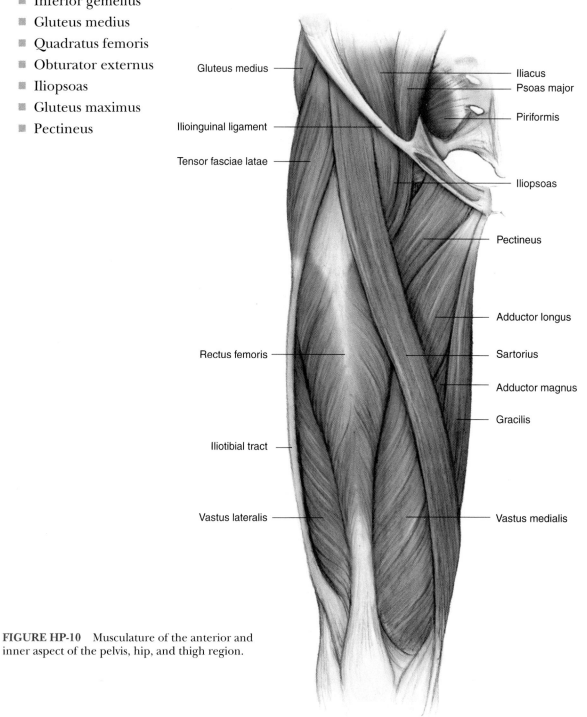

FIGURE HP-10 Musculature of the anterior and inner aspect of the pelvis, hip, and thigh region.

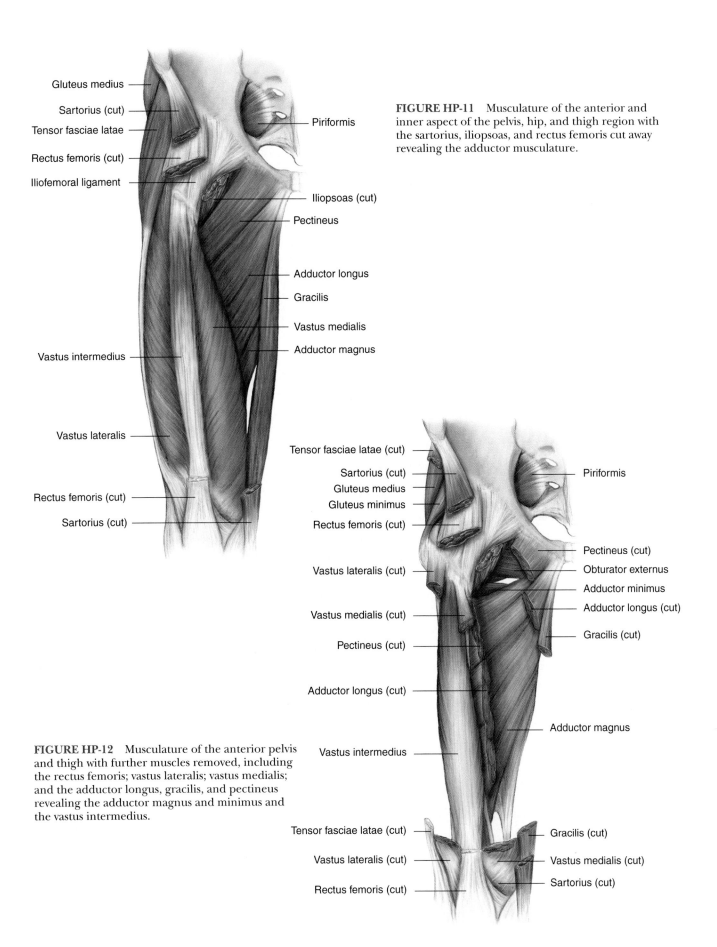

Gluteus medius

Sartorius (cut)

Tensor fasciae latae

Rectus femoris (cut)

Iliofemoral ligament

Piriformis

Iliopsoas (cut)

Pectineus

Adductor longus

Gracilis

Vastus medialis

Adductor magnus

Vastus intermedius

Vastus lateralis

Rectus femoris (cut)

Sartorius (cut)

FIGURE HP-11 Musculature of the anterior and inner aspect of the pelvis, hip, and thigh region with the sartorius, iliopsoas, and rectus femoris cut away revealing the adductor musculature.

Tensor fasciae latae (cut)

Sartorius (cut)

Gluteus medius

Gluteus minimus

Rectus femoris (cut)

Piriformis

Pectineus (cut)

Obturator externus

Adductor minimus

Adductor longus (cut)

Gracilis (cut)

Vastus lateralis (cut)

Vastus medialis (cut)

Pectineus (cut)

Adductor longus (cut)

Adductor magnus

Vastus intermedius

Tensor fasciae latae (cut)

Vastus lateralis (cut)

Rectus femoris (cut)

Gracilis (cut)

Vastus medialis (cut)

Sartorius (cut)

FIGURE HP-12 Musculature of the anterior pelvis and thigh with further muscles removed, including the rectus femoris; vastus lateralis; vastus medialis; and the adductor longus, gracilis, and pectineus revealing the adductor magnus and minimus and the vastus intermedius.

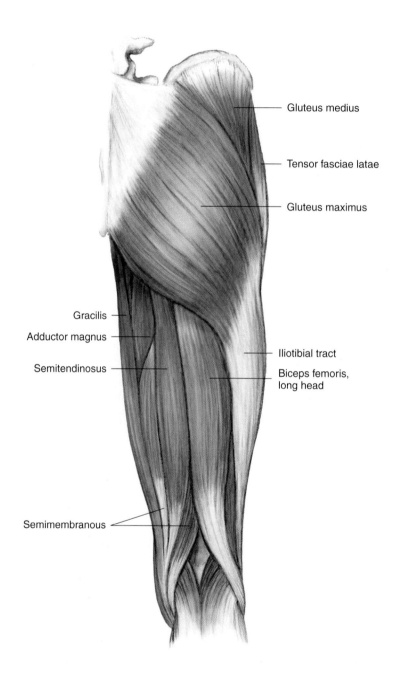

Gluteus medius

Tensor fasciae latae

Gluteus maximus

Gracilis

Adductor magnus

Semitendinosus

Iliotibial tract

Biceps femoris, long head

Semimembranous

FIGURE HP-13 Posterior musculature of the pelvis and thigh region.

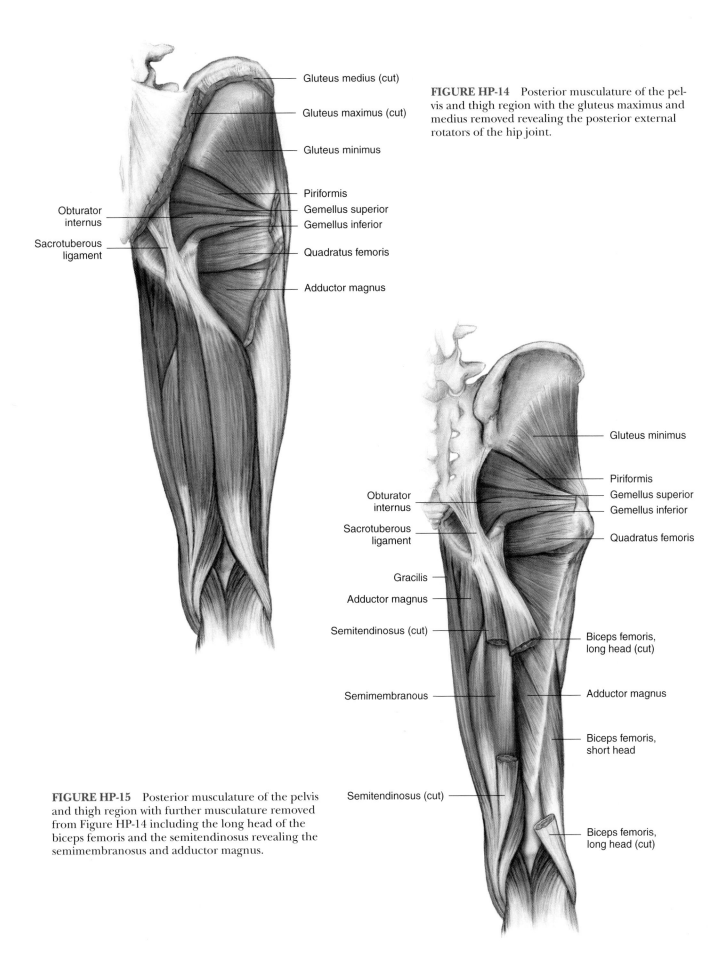

Gluteus medius (cut)

Gluteus maximus (cut)

Gluteus minimus

Piriformis
Gemellus superior
Gemellus inferior

Quadratus femoris

Adductor magnus

Obturator internus

Sacrotuberous ligament

FIGURE HP-14 Posterior musculature of the pelvis and thigh region with the gluteus maximus and medius removed revealing the posterior external rotators of the hip joint.

Gluteus minimus

Piriformis
Gemellus superior
Gemellus inferior

Quadratus femoris

Obturator internus

Sacrotuberous ligament

Gracilis

Adductor magnus

Semitendinosus (cut)

Biceps femoris, long head (cut)

Adductor magnus

Semimembranous

Biceps femoris, short head

Semitendinosus (cut)

Biceps femoris, long head (cut)

FIGURE HP-15 Posterior musculature of the pelvis and thigh region with further musculature removed from Figure HP-14 including the long head of the biceps femoris and the semitendinosus revealing the semimembranosus and adductor magnus.

Nerves

- **Extension of nerves from lumbosacral plexus (Figure HP-16)**
  - Branches of sacral plexus
    - Sciatic nerve (L4 and L5 and S1, S2, and S3)—greater sciatic notch
      - Tibial portion—long head of biceps femoris, semitendinosus, adductor magnus, gastrocnemius, soleus, plantaris, popliteus, tibialis posterior, flexor digitorum longus, flexor hallucis longus, sural nerve branches to the skin
      - Common peroneal portion—short head of biceps femoris, tibialis anterior, extensor hallucis longus, extensor digitorum brevis, peroneus tertius, extensor digitorum longus, peroneus brevis, peroneus longus
    - Superior gluteal (gluteus medius, gluteus minimus, and tensor fasciae latae muscles)
    - Inferior gluteal (gluteus maximus)
    - Nerve to quadratus femoris and inferior gemellus
    - Nerve to obturator internus and superior gemellus
    - Posterior femoral cutaneous (skin of buttock and posterior aspect of the thigh)
    - Nerve to piriformis
    - Pudendal nerve (S2, S3, and S4)—exits via greater sciatic foramen and enters via lesser sciatic foramen
    - Dorsal nerve of penis or clitoris
    - Perineal and posterior (labral or scrotal) nerves
  - Branches of the lumbar plexus
    - Lumbosacral trunk—involves contributions from L4 and L5
    - Lateral femoral cutaneous
    - Obturator nerve
    - Femoral nerve (largest branch L2, L3, and L4)
      - Anterior division—medial and intermediate cutaneous nerves of the thigh
      - Posterior division—saphenous nerve, branch to rectus femoris, and quadriceps
    - Accessory obturator

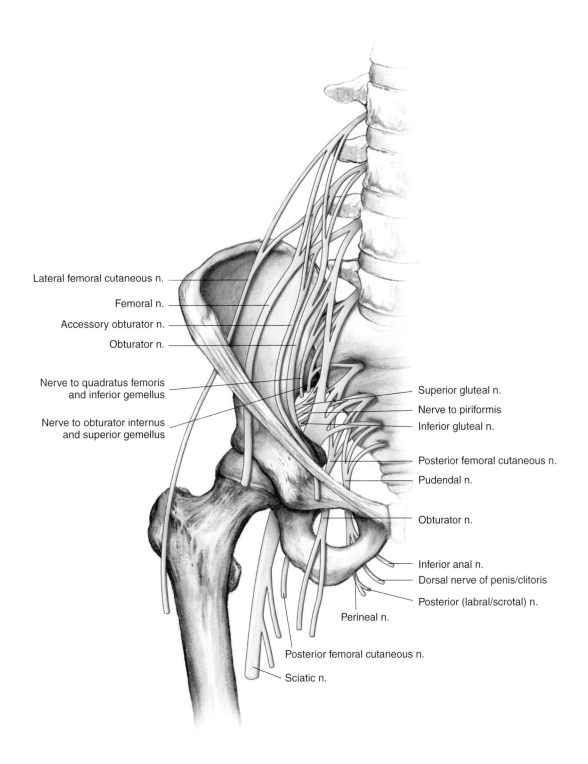

Lateral femoral cutaneous n.

Femoral n.

Accessory obturator n.

Obturator n.

Nerve to quadratus femoris
and inferior gemellus

Nerve to obturator internus
and superior gemellus

Superior gluteal n.

Nerve to piriformis

Inferior gluteal n.

Posterior femoral cutaneous n.

Pudendal n.

Obturator n.

Inferior anal n.

Dorsal nerve of penis/clitoris

Posterior (labral/scrotal) n.

Perineal n.

Posterior femoral cutaneous n.

Sciatic n.

FIGURE HP-16   Divisions of the lumbosacral plexus.

Vascularity (Figure HP-17)

- Internal iliac
  - Superior gluteal
  - Inferior gluteal
  - Internal pudendal
  - Middle rectal
  - Uterine
  - Obturator

- External iliac artery and vein
  - Deep circumflex iliac artery

- Femoral artery
  - Deep femoral
    - Lateral femoral circumflex
      - Ascending
      - Descending
      - Transverse
    - Medial femoral circumflex
      - Lateral ascending branch-femoral branch
    - Perforating branches
  - Superficial femoral

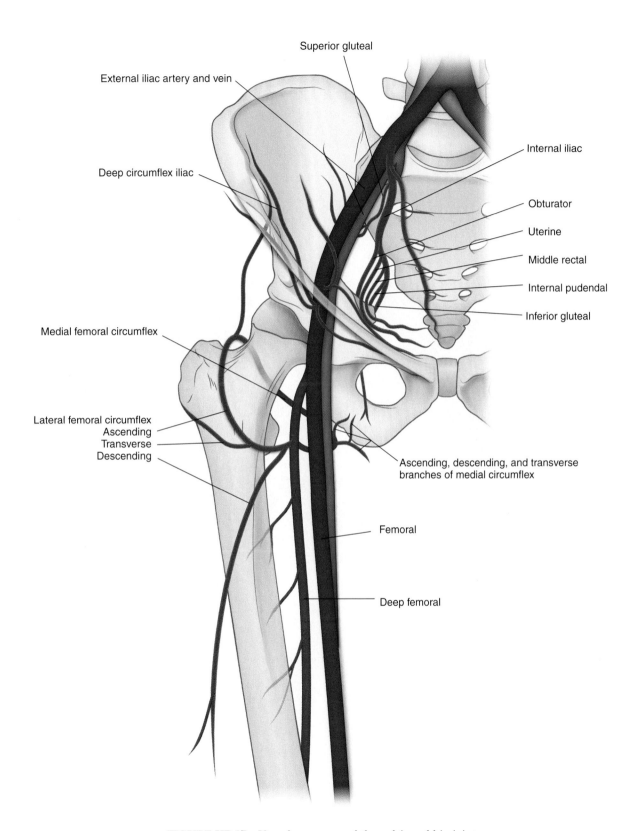

FIGURE HP-17   Vasculature around the pelvis and hip joint.

CROSS-SECTIONAL ANATOMY (Figures HP-18 through HP-23)

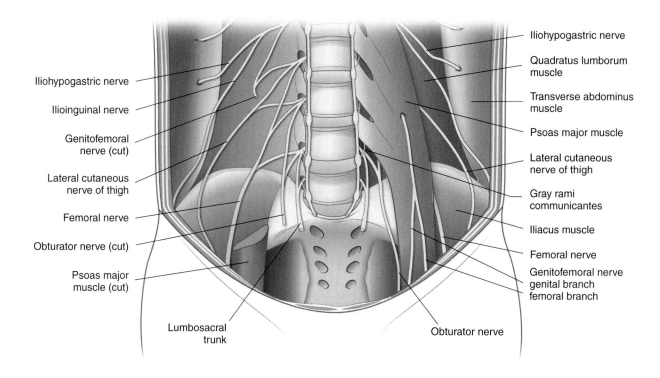

Iliohypogastric nerve

Ilioinguinal nerve

Genitofemoral nerve (cut)

Lateral cutaneous nerve of thigh

Femoral nerve

Obturator nerve (cut)

Psoas major muscle (cut)

Lumbosacral trunk

Iliohypogastric nerve

Quadratus lumborum muscle

Transverse abdominus muscle

Psoas major muscle

Lateral cutaneous nerve of thigh

Gray rami communicantes

Iliacus muscle

Femoral nerve

Genitofemoral nerve genital branch femoral branch

Obturator nerve

FIGURE HP-18 Cross-sectional coronal anatomy of the pelvis and lumbar sacral region.

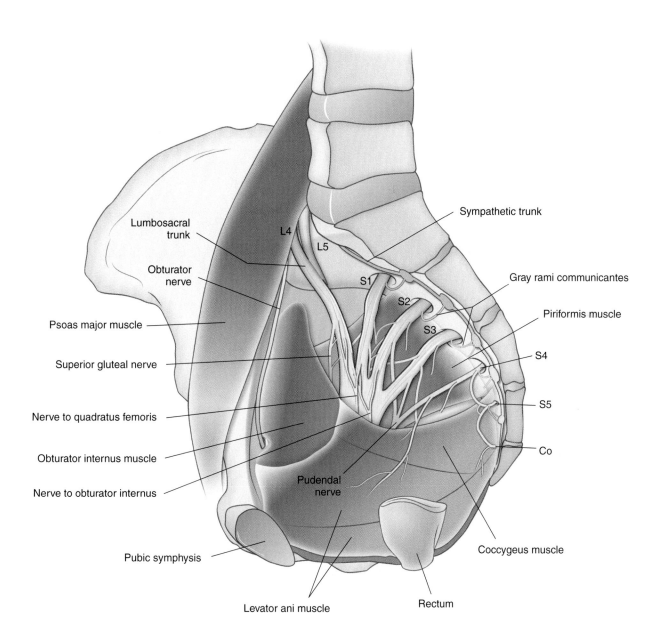

FIGURE HP-19   Cross-sectional sagittal anatomy of the pelvis and lumbar sacral region.

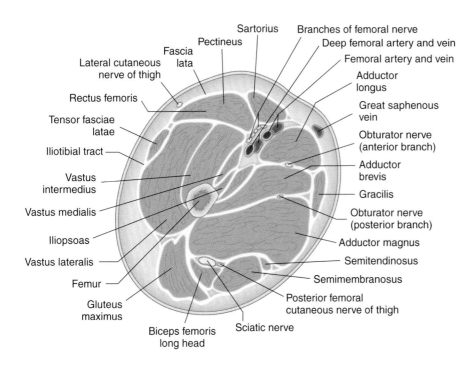

FIGURE HP-20   Cross-sectional transverse anatomy of the thigh region.

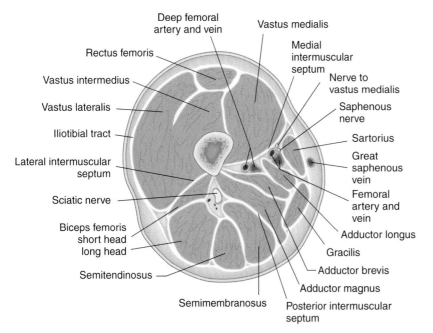

FIGURE HP-21   Cross-sectional transverse anatomy of the thigh region.

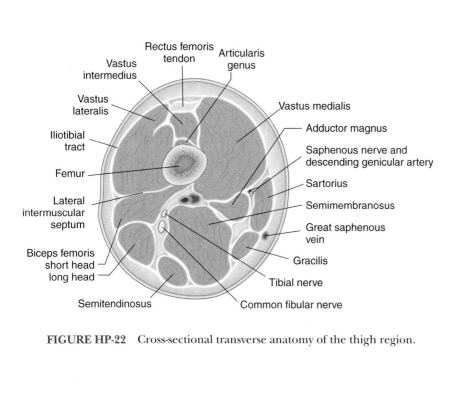

FIGURE HP-22   Cross-sectional transverse anatomy of the thigh region.

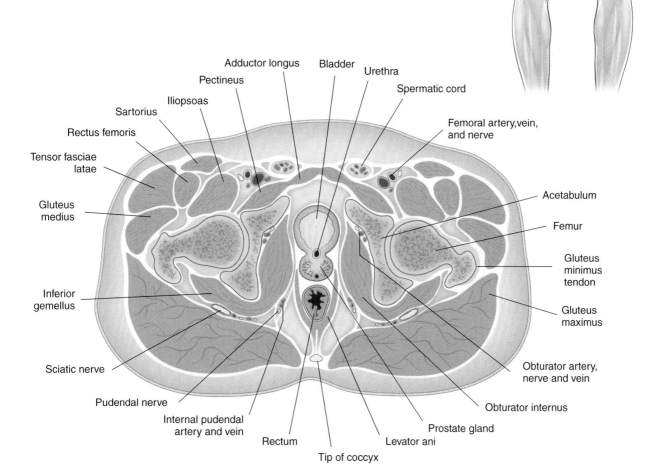

FIGURE HP-23   Cross-sectional transverse anatomy of the proximal femur and pelvis at the level of the hip joint.

HAZARDS (Figures HP-24 and HP-25)

- **Femoral triangle**
  - Bordered by the inguinal ligament, sartorius and the adductor longus, the structures from lateral to medial consist of the femoral nerve, artery, vein, and lymphatics, (see Figure HP-24)

Nerves

- Sciatic nerve: Exits from the greater sciatic notch and from the inferior surface of the piriformis and over the external rotators of the hip. Variations of its course around the piriformis exist

- Femoral nerve: At risk from direct injury in an anterior approach to the hip or ilioinguinal approach. Indirect injury from retractor placement can occur

- Obturator nerve: Direct or indirect injury may occur along the inferior aspect of the acetabulum

- Superior gluteal nerve: Located between the gluteus minimus and medius 3 to 5 cm superior to the tip of the greater trochanter

- Inferior gluteal nerve: Exits the greater sciatic notch inferior to the sciatic nerve and enters the gluteus maximus

- Lateral femoral cutaneous nerve: Arises from the fascia just medial to the anterior superior iliac spine. Variations exist where the nerve may arise out of the fascia over, under or through the sartorius muscle

- Posterior femoral cutaneous nerve: This nerve travels with the posterior aspect of the sciatic nerve until it travels superficial to this nerve at the biceps femoris

Vascular

- Femoral artery: Direct injury during an ilioinguinal approach or indirect injury from retractor placement during hip approaches

- Superior gluteal artery: Exits the superior border of the piriformis and enters the gluteus medius. If damaged may retract necessitating an intrapelvic approach for hemostasis

- Inferior gluteal artery: Exits the pelvis underneath the piriformis and supplies the deep aspects of the gluteus maximus. If the muscle is split too superiorly it may damage the main trunk

- Ascending branch of the lateral femoral circumflex: Lies within the intermuscular septum of the sartorius and tensor fascia

Bladder

- Injury may occur indirectly through bone during hip approaches or directly during pelvic approaches

ANTERIOR VIEW

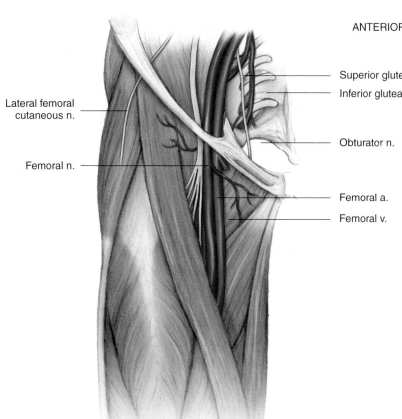

Lateral femoral cutaneous n.

Femoral n.

Superior gluteal a.

Inferior gluteal a.

Obturator n.

Femoral a.

Femoral v.

FIGURE HP-24   Hazards around the hip and pelvis including neurovasculature and hollow structures. Anteriorly, the neurovascular bundle from lateral to medial contains structures that form the mnemonic "NAVEL" (femoral *N*erve over the psoas, femoral *A*rtery, femoral *V*ein, *E*mpty space, and *L*ymphatics). The bladder lies directly behind the superior pubic rami behind the potential space of Retzius (see Figure HP-35).

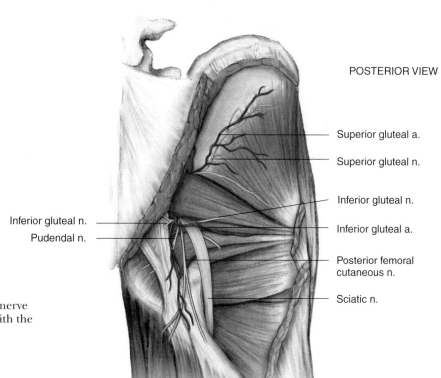

POSTERIOR VIEW

Superior gluteal a.

Superior gluteal n.

Inferior gluteal n.

Inferior gluteal a.

Posterior femoral cutaneous n.

Sciatic n.

Inferior gluteal n.

Pudendal n.

FIGURE HP-25   Posteriorly, the sciatic nerve exits through the greater sciatic notch with the superior gluteal artery.

LANDMARKS (Figures HP-26 and HP-27)

ASIS

PSIS

Iliac Crest

Pubic Symphysis

Pubic Tubercle

Ischial Tuberosity

Greater Trochanter

Surgical Approaches to the Pelvis

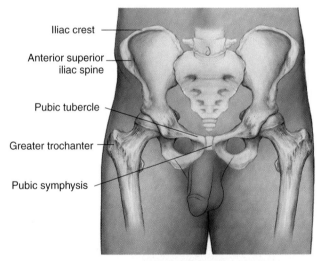

Iliac crest

Anterior superior
iliac spine

Pubic tubercle

Greater trochanter

Pubic symphysis

FIGURE HP-26 Bony landmarks around the pelvis and the hip joint. Anteriorly, these include the pubic symphysis, pubic tubercles, ASIS, and iliac crest.

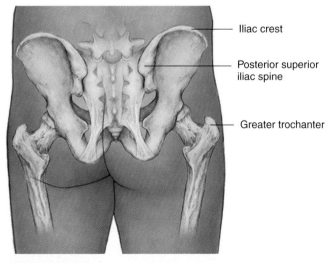

Iliac crest

Posterior superior
iliac spine

Greater trochanter

FIGURE HP-27 Posterior bony landmarks around the hip and pelvis. These include the PSIS, iliac crest, and greater trochanter.

POSTERIOR APPROACH TO THE SACROILIAC JOINT

Indications: Fixation of disruption to the sacroiliac joint, fractures of the ilium adjacent to the sacroiliac joint, irrigation and débridement of infection to the area

POSITIONING (FIGURE HP-28)

- Prone
- Bolsters and padding in place to allow expansion of the chest and abdomen without restriction
- Isolation of the anus from the field with an isolation type of drape
- Radiolucent table used for fluoroscopic assistance is advised

DANGERS

- Structures
  - Inferior gluteal nerve
  - Superior gluteal nerve
  - Sacral nerve roots (from screw fixation)
  - Superior cluneal nerves

- Vessels
  - Branches of the superior and inferior gluteal arteries are in danger and should be cauterized

LANDMARKS

- Posterior iliac crest and PSIS

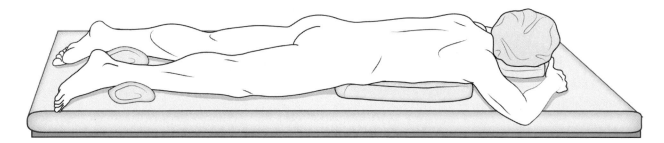

FIGURE HP-28   Prone illustration with bumps to pad all prominences. For the posterior approach to the sacroiliac joint, the bony prominences are well padded, and the chest and abdomen are free to expand by being suspended by longitudinal padding along the sides of the patient.

INCISION (FIGURE HP-29)

- 8-12 cm centered 2-3 cm above and lateral to the PSIS (Figure HP-30)

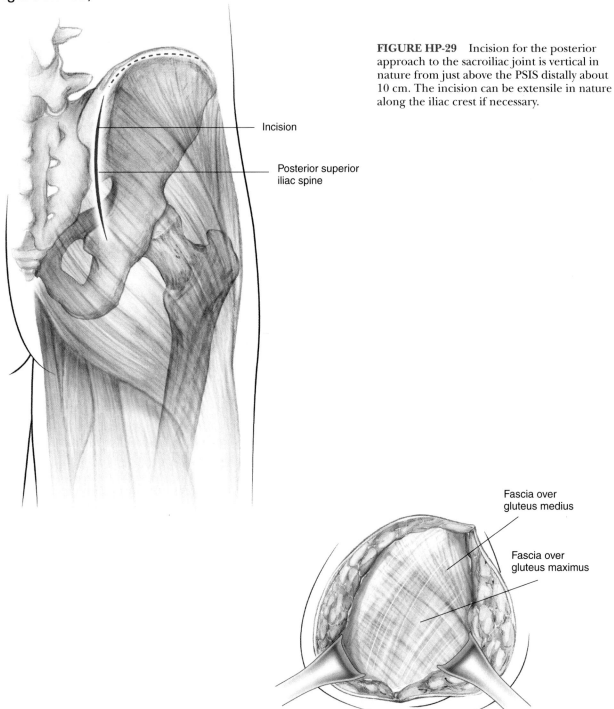

Incision

Posterior superior
iliac spine

FIGURE HP-29   Incision for the posterior approach to the sacroiliac joint is vertical in nature from just above the PSIS distally about 10 cm. The incision can be extensile in nature along the iliac crest if necessary.

Fascia over
gluteus medius

Fascia over
gluteus maximus

FIGURE HP-30   Superficial dissection is carried down the PSIS and the fascia of the gluteus maximus, and the fascia capsule over the sacroiliac joint is uncovered.

• Superficial dissection

- ▣ No true internervous plane
- ▣ Subcutaneous tissue is incised in line with the incision uncovering the fascia of the gluteus maximus and medius
- ▣ Incise the fascia of the maximus over the crest of the ilium
- ▣ Reflect the gluteus maximus subperiosteally downward and laterally (branches of the inferior gluteal artery may be present)
- ▣ This uncovers the gluteus medius and the piriformis emerging from the greater sciatic notch (superior gluteal nerve and artery emerging as well) (Figure HP-31)

• Deep dissection

- ▣ In trauma cases, the sacroiliac joint capsule may be disrupted and easily visualized; otherwise, it may need to be incised to visualize the reduction
- ▣ The gluteus medius cannot be elevated far anteriorly because the neurovascular bundle to the muscle is present (superior gluteal nerve and artery)

• Extensile measures

- ▣ The incision superiorly can be carried in a curving fashion along the crest of the ilium superiorly and anteriorly to uncover the wing of the ilium

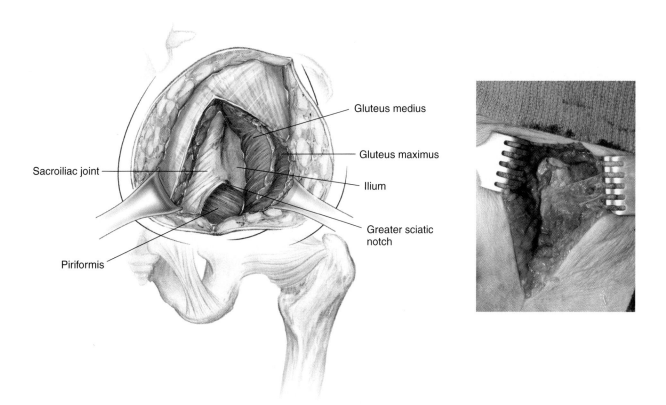

FIGURE HP-31 Deeper dissection involves incising the gluteus maximus fascia and subperiosteally elevating the maximus off of the ilium just lateral to the PSIS. The joint capsule of the sacroiliac joint, if not traumatically disrupted, may need to be incised for anatomical reduction of the joint surface.

ANTERIOR APPROACH TO THE PUBIC SYMPHYSIS

Indication: Plating of pubic symphysis diastasis

POSITIONING

- Supine (Figure HP-32)
- Foley catheter in place

DANGERS

- Structures
  - ▓ Bladder

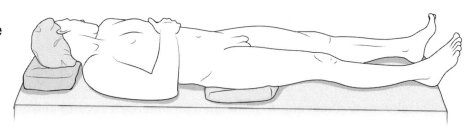

FIGURE HP-32   Supine positioning of the patient for approach to the pubic symphysis.

- Vessels
  - ▓ Superficial epigastric artery and vein

LANDMARKS

- Pubic symphysis and pubic tubercles

INCISION

- ▓ 8-16 cm centered at the pubic symphysis
- ▓ In line with skin crease and about 1 cm above the pubic symphysis and superior rami (Figure HP-33)

SUPERFICIAL DISSECTION

- ▓ No true internervous plane
- ▓ Subcutaneous tissue is incised in line with the incision uncovering the rectus sheath
- ▓ Ligation of the superficial epigastric artery and vein as they run across the field from inferior to superior may be necessary (Figure HP-34)

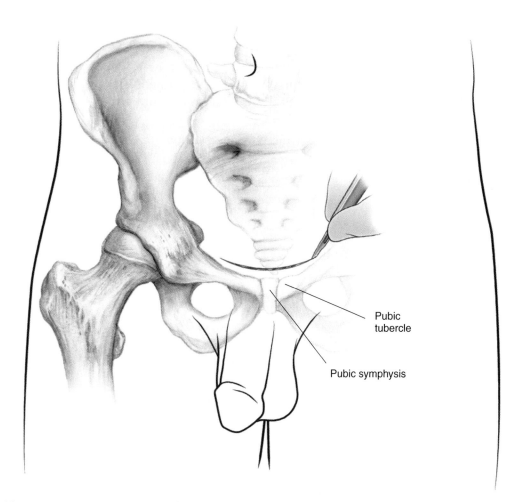

FIGURE HP-33 Incision for the approach to the pubic symphysis. The landmarks are the pubic tubercles, pubic symphysis, and superior rami. The incision is centered around the pubic symphysis just above the superior edge of the rami. The dissection is taken to the underlying fascia. Note the Foley catheter in place to decompress the bladder during the procedure.

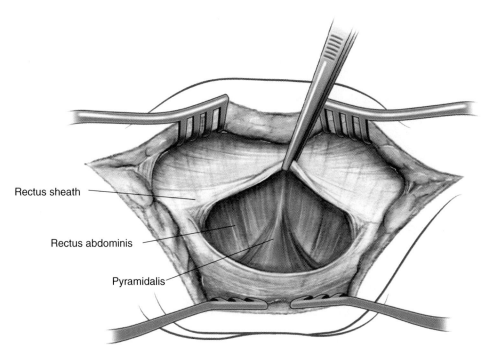

FIGURE HP-34 Ligation of the superficial epigastric artery and vein as they run across the field from inferior to superior may be necessary.

DEEP DISSECTION MIDLINE

- Care should be taken to maintain the rectus abdominis attachment if possible; this may mean you have to work under the rectus attachment to the ramus
- Often one side of the rectus insertion is avulsed in an anterior displaced pelvis disruption
- Retract the abdominis laterally and superiorly
- A layer of extraperitoneal fat may be present between the rectus abdominis and the bladder
- The posterior aspect of the superior rami and pubic symphysis can be accomplished digitally (preperitoneal space of Retzius) (Figures HP-35 and HP-36)

CLOSURE

- Repair of the rectus abdominis and its sheath should be done separately
- Subcutaneous and skin closure accomplished in the normal fashion

EXTENSILE MEASURES

- Can be used in conjunction with the ilioinguinal approach

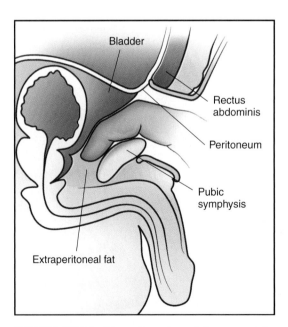

FIGURE HP-35 Blunt dissection of the potential space of Retzius should be performed to ensure the bladder is protected.

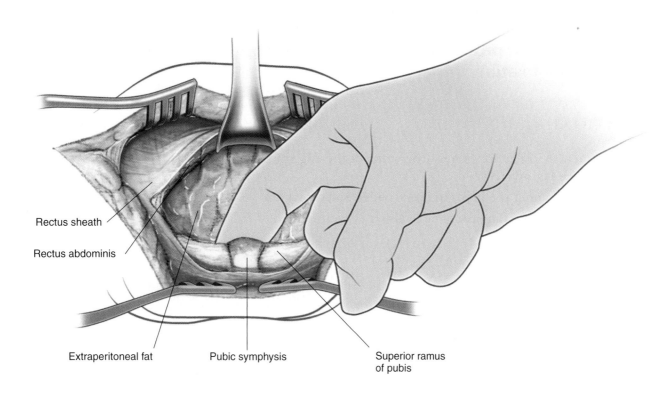

Rectus sheath

Rectus abdominis

Extraperitoneal fat

Pubic symphysis

Superior ramus
of pubis

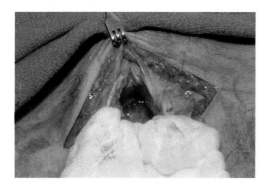
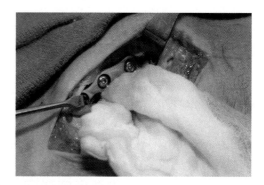

FIGURE HP-36 Deep dissection of the underlying fascia after ligation of the superior epigastric artery and vein. The rectus may be avulsed from one or both sides from the traumatic disruption, but otherwise splitting the muscle interval midline may be accomplished to expose the symphysis and the rami.

ILIOINGUINAL APPROACH TO THE PELVIS

Indications: Anterior column, some transverse and many both column fracture open reduction and internal fixation of the acetabulum, protrusio acetabuli fracture open reduction and internal fixation

POSITIONING

- Supine with ipsilateral greater trochanter at the edge of the operative table (see Figure HP-32)
- Soft bump under the pelvis in obese patients may be helpful
- Radiolucent operating room table also may be useful

DANGERS

- Structures
  - Bladder
  - Spermatic cord
  - Round ligament

- Nerves
  - Femoral nerve
  - Lateral femoral cutaneous nerve usually 1-3 cm medial to the ASIS

- Vessels
  - Femoral artery and vein
  - Inferior epigastric artery and vein
  - Damage to neurovascular sheath with hematoma formation if not properly handled
  - Lymphatics with possible postoperative lymphedema

LANDMARKS

- Pubic tubercle, ASIS, iliac crest

INCISION

- Medial 1 cm above the pubic tubercle curving to a lateral landmark
  4-5 cm from the ASIS 1 cm above the iliac crest (Figure HP-37)

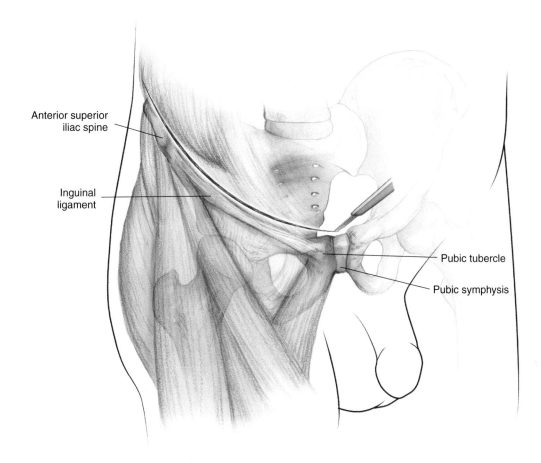

FIGURE HP-37   Incision for ilioinguinal approach. The incision is based 1 cm medial to the pubic tubercle curving to a lateral landmark 4-5 cm from the ASIS and 1 cm above the iliac crest.

SUPERFICIAL DISSECTION

▪ Subcutaneous tissue dissected in line with the incision exposing external oblique fascia

▪ Avoid the lateral femoral cutaneous nerve along the lateral aspect of the incision, which is usually 1-2 cm medial to ASIS (Figure HP-38)

▪ Divide the external oblique fascia in line with its fibers from the inguinal ring to the ASIS (Figure HP-39)

▪ Identify the round ligament (women) or the spermatic cord (men) medially; isolate and protect these structures

DEEP SURGICAL DISSECTION

▪ Incise the rectus sheath medially 1 cm above the pubic tubercle

▪ Laterally subperiosteally strip the iliacus off the iliac wing

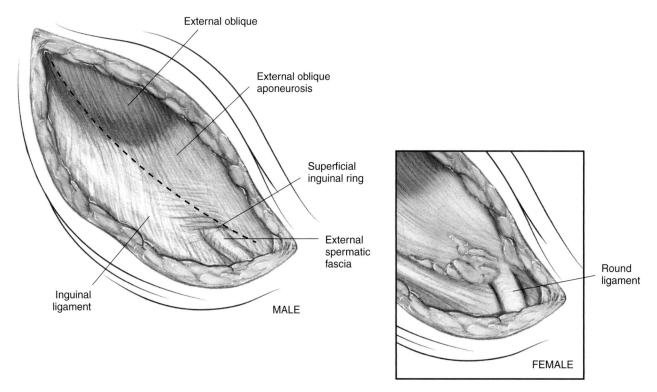

FIGURE HP-38   A and **B,** The superficial dissection of the ilioinguinal approach down to underlying external oblique fascia. Take care not to injure the lateral femoral cutaneous nerve usually 1 cm medial to the ASIS arising from the fascia distal to this point.

■ Medially incise the rectus abdominis muscle 1 cm above the pubic symphysis, and develop the space of Retzius with digital blunt dissection (Figure HP-40)

■ Incise the internal oblique and transversus abdominis because they form the posterior aspect of the inguinal canal

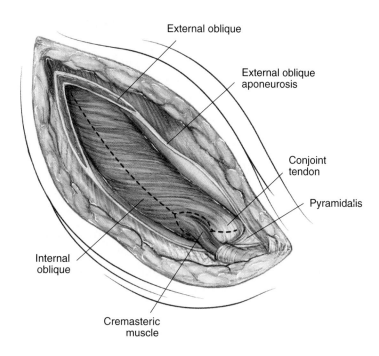

FIGURE HP-39   Further dissection through the external oblique fascia and around the inguinal ring.

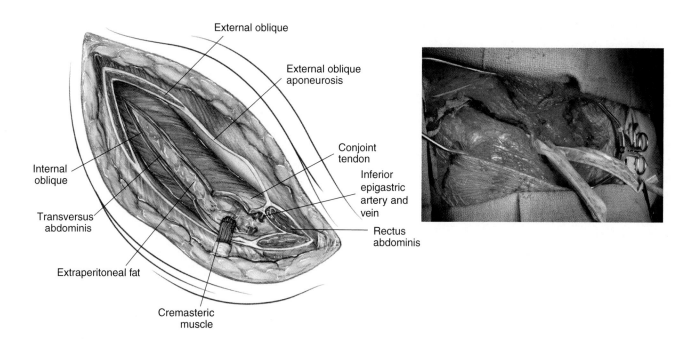

FIGURE HP-40   Deeper dissection includes the transverse abdominis muscle in line with the superficial dissection around the spermatic cord (males) or round ligament (females). Medially, the rectus abdominis fascia is incised as in the approach to the pubic symphysis if medial dissection is necessary.

- Ligate the inferior epigastric artery and vein as they cross the field at the medial edge of the inguinal ring
- Incise the transversalis muscle and fascia in line with the lateral aspect of the dissection
- Push the peritoneal fat upward with a lap pad, and expose the femoral nerve and vessels and tendon of the iliopsoas
- Isolate these structures within the femoral sheath (care should be taken not to create bleeding within the sheath), and protect with a Penrose drain
- Avoid excessive dissection of the vessels so as not to damage their sheath or the lymphatic structures, which can cause postoperative lymphedema
- The psoas and femoral nerve are isolated together and protected in a Penrose drain as well

- **This leaves 3 windows to work between (Figure HP-41)**
  - A lateral window from the psoas and femoral nerve to the lateral aspect of the incision through which the iliac wing and sacroiliac joint is exposed
  - A middle window between the psoas and the femoral vessels for the anterior column and medial wall of acetabulum and iliopubic eminence
  - A medial window between the femoral vessels and medial aspect of the incision to the pubic symphysis exposing the superior rami; care should be taken to retract and protect the bladder in this window

CLOSURE

- Meticulous care must be taken to repair the transversalis and external oblique muscle and fascia and the inguinal ring to prevent herniation
- Rectus abdominis and fascia also should be repaired accordingly

EXTENSILE MEASURES

- The medial aspect can be extended to the approach to the pubic symphysis when indicated
- Posteriorly, can be extended to expose the anterior aspect of the sacroiliac joint

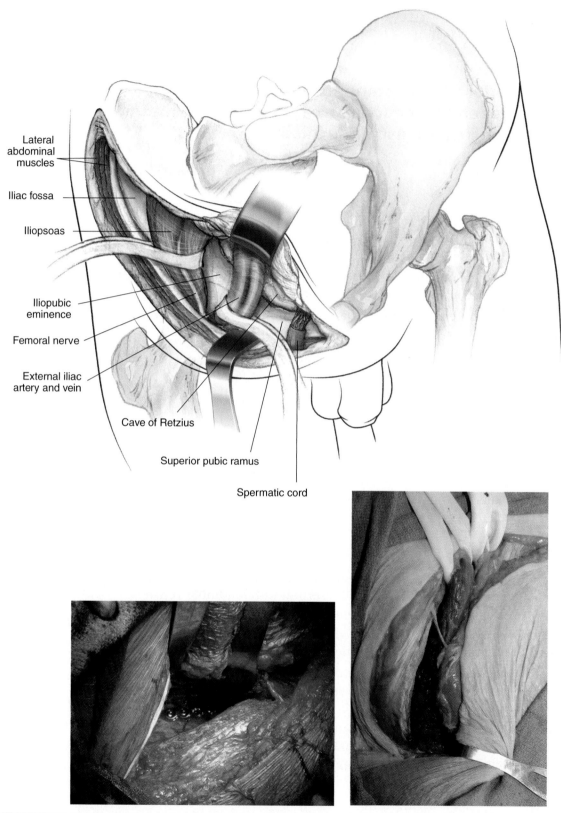

Lateral
abdominal
muscles

Iliac fossa

Iliopsoas

Iliopubic
eminence

Femoral nerve

External iliac
artery and vein

Cave of Retzius

Superior pubic ramus

Spermatic cord

FIGURE HP-41   Three windows are developed by placing Penrose drains or vessel loops around the femoral nerve and iliopsoas and the femoral artery, vein, and lymphatics. This creates a lateral window, which exposes the inner aspect of the ilium and can expose the anterior aspect of the sacroiliac joint and the inner aspect of the anterior column. The middle window lies between the iliopsoas and the vascular bundle exposing the iliopubic eminence. The medial window exposes the superior rami to the pubic symphysis.

POSTERIOR APPROACH TO THE ACETABULUM (KOCHER-LANGENBACH)

Indications: Posterior wall, posterior column, and some tranverse column acetabular fracture treatment; the approach differs slightly from arthroplasty indications

POSITIONING

- Lateral positioning is often used for simple posterior wall fractures; however, prone positioning may be used on a radiolucent table to allow treatment of transverse and combined component fractures by posterior approach

- Prone position allows oblique fluoroscopic views to be obtained to assist indirect anterior column reduction and anterior column screw fixation

- The disadvantage of prone positioning is that there may be difficulty dislocating the hip, unless a specialized pelvis traction table is available (Judet-Tasserit, Matta type, or equivalent) (Figure HP-42)

DANGERS

- Sciatic nerve

  - This is generally directly exposed and protected in most fractures with posterior column displacement. In the prone position, the hip is extended, and care is taken to maintain knee flexion to take tension off of the nerve

- Blood supply to the femoral head (lateral ascending branch of the medial femoral circumflex)

  - This is generally preserved by dividing the piriformis, obturator tendons, and external rotators 1-2 cm posterior to femoral insertion with tendinous repair instead of off the bone as in arthroplasty approaches

  - Superior gluteal artery and nerve enter the gluteus medius from the undersurface of the muscle, and retraction can damage these structures

  - Inferior gluteal artery may be damaged from the traumatic injury if being performed for a fracture, but the vessel leaves the pelvis and travels along the undersurface of the piriformis

    - If the artery is damaged during the surgical approach, it may retract into the pelvis necessitating rolling the patient over and control of the bleeding performed through a retroperitoneal approach and tying off of the external iliac artery

LANDMARKS

● Greater trochanter, iliac crest, posterior and anterior iliac
spine

INCISION

■ Incision extends from just below the posterior third of the iliac crest longitudinally
over the center of the greater trochanter extending 8-10 cm past this landmark
(Figure HP-43A)

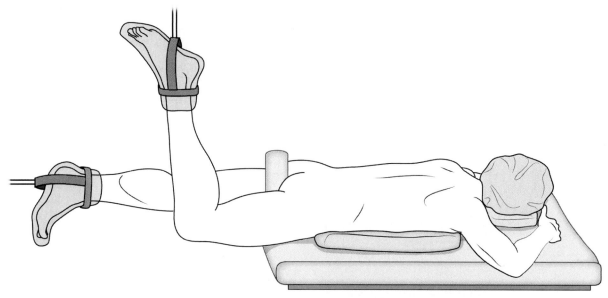

FIGURE HP-42   Prone position for the posterior approach to the acetabulum can be done without traction (see Figure HP-28) or with use of a traction table such a Judet-Tasserit or Matta type of table. All prominences are padded, and the abdomen and chest are left free to expand with longitudinal bumps along the lateral aspect of the torso.

SUPERFICIAL DISSECTION

■ Carry the incision through subcutaneous tissue down to the fascia of the gluteus
maximus on its anterior border and to the fascia lata distally (Figure HP-43B)

■ Incise the fascia in a line along the anterior border of the gluteus maximus and
fascia lata

■ Retract these incised fascial edges to expose the abductors and external rotators
(Figure HP-44A)

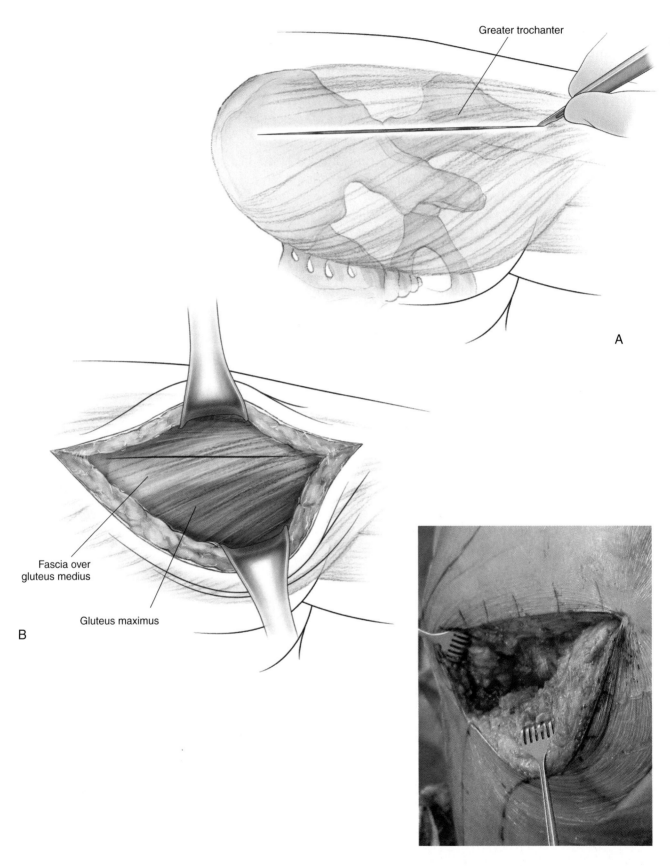

FIGURE HP-43 **A,** Incision extends from just below the posterior third of the iliac crest longitudinally over the center of the greater trochanter extending 8-10 cm past this landmark. **B,** Superficial dissection is carried down to the gluteus maximus and iliotibial band.

DEEP DISSECTION

- Make sure that tension is off of the sciatic nerve by extending the hip and flexing the ipsilateral knee
- Place tension on the external rotators by internally rotating the hip
- External rotators (piriformis, gemellus, obturator internus) are detached 1 cm off of the bone in their tendinous portions (protecting the capsular and femoral head blood supply) (Figure HP-44B)
- The sciatic nerve is located and may be protected by placing a vessel loop around it
- Posterior capsular attachments may be traumatically disrupted, but if needed the traumatic arthrotomy may be extended for visualization and anatomical reduction of the fracture

EXTENSILE MEASURES

- Distally, the incision may be extended to a lateral approach to the femur

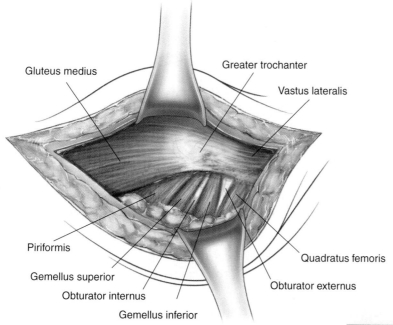

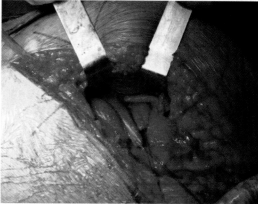

FIGURE HP-44   A, The maximus and iliotibial band are retracted to expose the external rotators.

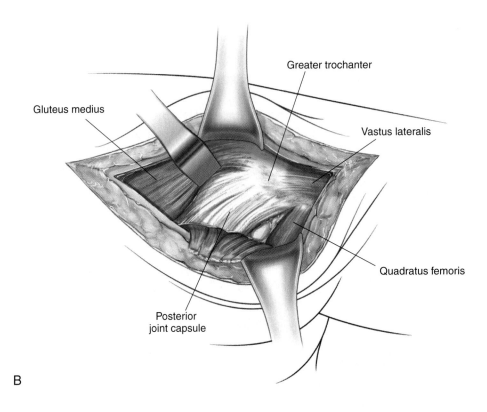

Greater trochanter

Gluteus medius

Vastus lateralis

Quadratus femoris

Posterior
joint capsule

B

FIGURE HP-44 (cont'd) **B,** The external rotators (piriformis, gemellae, obturator internus) are detached 1 cm off of the bone in their tendinous portions to protect the capsule and blood supply to the femoral head. These may be tagged with sutures to aid in retraction and protection of the sciatic nerve and for repair at the end of the case.

- Proximal dissection needs to make sure the superior gluteal nerve and artery are protected leaving the greater sciatic notch and the sciatic nerve

- For added exposure proximally, a greater trochanteric osteotomy may be performed to retract the abductors for better exposure

CLOSURE

- External rotators are repaired through tendon-to-tendon repair making sure no sutures are tenting the sciatic nerve

SURGICAL APPROACHES TO THE HIP

Overview of the Four Basic Approaches to the Hip (Figures HP-45 and HP-46)

- Anterior approach

  - Sartorius (femoral nerve) and tensor fasciae latae (superior gluteal nerve) interval

  - This approach has gained popularity for use in minimally invasive total hip replacement surgery

  - It also provides excellent exposure to the hip joint for fractures of the femoral head (Pipken type)

- Lateral approach (no true internervous plane)

  - This approach takes advantage of lifting the anterior structures of the hip off of the proximal femur to gain access into the hip joint

  - It has been used for total hip replacement and modified for a minimally invasive surgery (MIS) approach

- Posterior approach (no true internervous plane)

  - This approach takes advantage of accessing the hip by taking down the short external rotators to gain access to the hip joint

  - It is a popular approach for total joint replacement and can be modified for MIS approach

- Medial approach (no true internervous plane)

  - Adductor interval has obturator innervation as compartment, but proximal innervation allows the interval to be used

  - It is mainly used for approaches to gain access to the medial proximal femur and in pediatric cases for open reduction of congenital dislocation of the hip

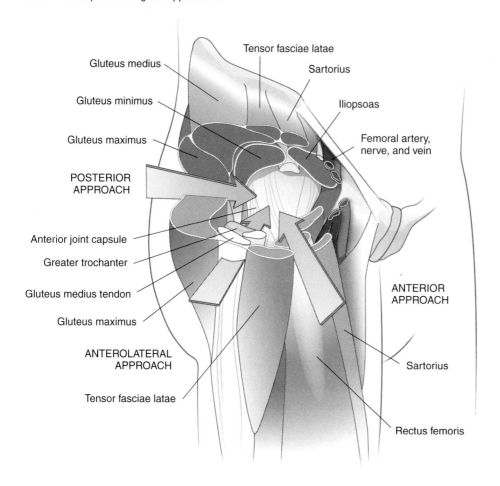

Gluteus medius

Gluteus minimus

Gluteus maximus

POSTERIOR APPROACH

Anterior joint capsule

Greater trochanter

Gluteus medius tendon

Gluteus maximus

ANTEROLATERAL APPROACH

Tensor fasciae latae

Tensor fasciae latae

Sartorius

Iliopsoas

Femoral artery, nerve, and vein

ANTERIOR APPROACH

Sartorius

Rectus femoris

FIGURE HP-45 Synopsis of the anterior, lateral, and posterior approaches to the hip joint and the anatomical planes that are exploited for each approach as depicted by the blue arrows.

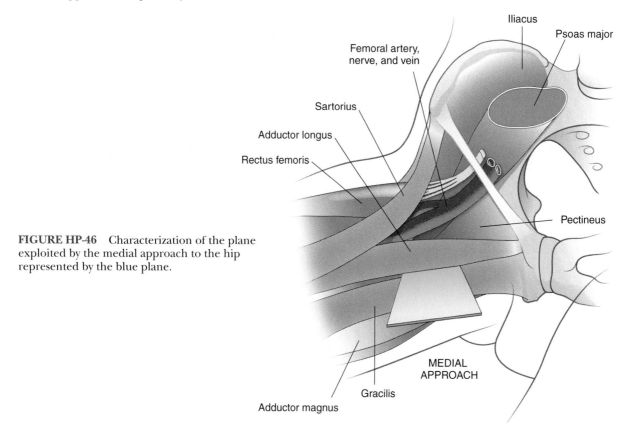

Iliacus

Psoas major

Femoral artery, nerve, and vein

Sartorius

Adductor longus

Rectus femoris

Pectineus

MEDIAL APPROACH

Gracilis

Adductor magnus

FIGURE HP-46 Characterization of the plane exploited by the medial approach to the hip represented by the blue plane.

ANTERIOR APPROACH TO THE HIP (SMITH-PETERSEN)

Indications: Pelvic osteotomies, hip fusion, open reduction of hip dislocation, femoral head fracture open reduction, total hip replacement, hemiarthroplasty of the hip, tumor biopsy and excision

POSITIONING

- Supine (see Figure HP-32)

DANGERS

- Nerves
  - Lateral femoral cutaneous, usually located 1-3 cm medial to the ASIS; patients should be warned of the possibility of damage to this structure
  - Femoral nerve—from retraction or direct injury
- Vessels
  - Ascending branch of the lateral femoral circumflex artery, which is ligated during the procedure
  - Femoral artery and vein from overzealous retraction during the procedure

LANDMARKS

- ASIS, iliac crest

INCISION

- Inferior aspect of iliac crest just below the ASIS
- From the ASIS landmark the incision is taken distally about 10 cm (Figure HP-47)

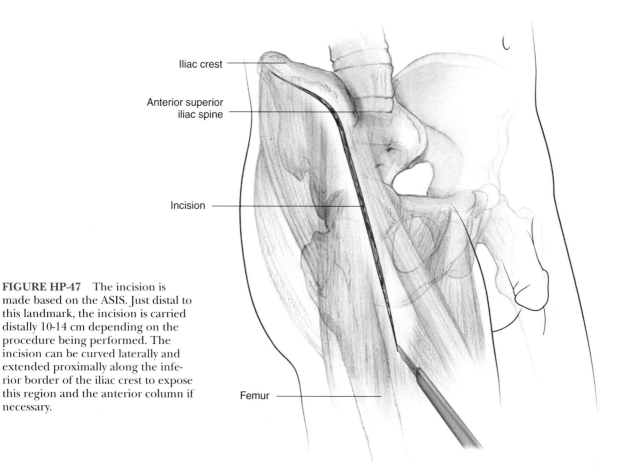

Iliac crest

Anterior superior
iliac spine

Incision

Femur

FIGURE HP-47   The incision is made based on the ASIS. Just distal to this landmark, the incision is carried distally 10-14 cm depending on the procedure being performed. The incision can be curved laterally and extended proximally along the inferior border of the iliac crest to expose this region and the anterior column if necessary.

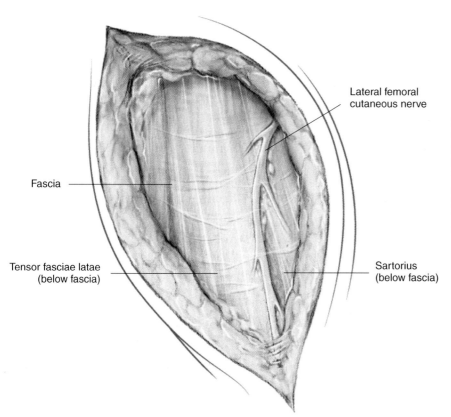

Lateral femoral
cutaneous nerve

Fascia

Tensor fasciae latae
(below fascia)

Sartorius
(below fascia)

FIGURE HP-48   The lateral femoral cutaneous nerve is found in the superficial dissection as it emerges from the superficial fascia just medial and distal to the ASIS. The interval between the sartorius and the tensor fasciae latae is identified and incised retracting the tensor laterally and the sartorius medially.

SUPERFICIAL DISSECTION

▤ Subcutaneous dissection is taken in line with the incision to underlying fascia of tensor and sartorius muscles

▤ The lateral femoral cutaneous nerve emerges from the fascia just distal and medial to the ASIS over the sartorius fascia

▤ Externally rotate the lower extremity to place the sartorius under a passive stretch to aid in dissection at this interval

▤ Identify the interval between the sartorius (femoral nerve) and the tensor fasciae latae (superior gluteal nerve) because this is the internervous plane (Figure HP-48)

DEEP DISSECTION

▤ Incise the fascia in this intermuscular plane between the sartorius and the tensor fasciae latae.

▤ Retract the sartorius medial and upward while the tensor is retracted laterally

▤ Tensor can be detached from the iliac crest if necessary

▤ The ascending branch of the lateral femoral circumflex lies in this interval and should be ligated in a controlled fashion (Figure HP-49)

▤ Rectus femoris and gluteus medius muscles are now exposed in the field

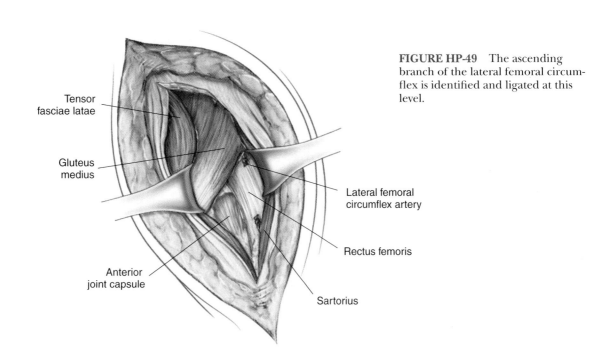

FIGURE HP-49   The ascending branch of the lateral femoral circumflex is identified and ligated at this level.

Tensor fasciae latae

Gluteus medius

Anterior joint capsule

Lateral femoral circumflex artery

Rectus femoris

Sartorius

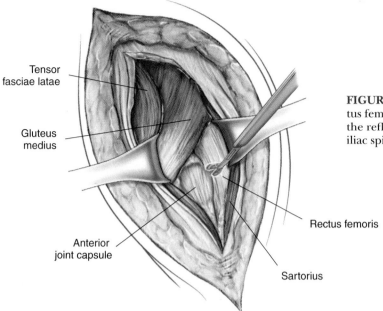

FIGURE HP-50   The anterior joint capsule and the rectus femoris are identified, and the rectus attachment from the reflected head is released from the anterior inferior iliac spine and the anterior lip of the acetabulum.

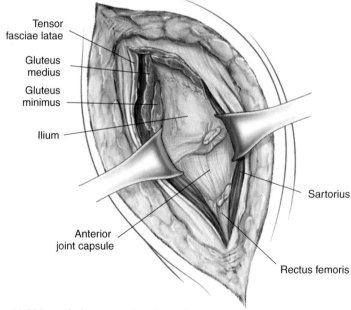

FIGURE HP-51   The hip capsule is cleared off with an elevator and properly identified by internally and externally rotating the hip joint.

- Detach the rectus femoris from its origin (ASIS and the anterior lip of the acetabulum and capsule) (Figures HP-50 and HP-51)
- The hip capsule is now exposed and can be tensed by externally rotating and extending the hip
- The capsule can be incised according to the necessity of the procedure being performed (Figure HP-52)

CLOSURE

- Capsule is repaired according to the procedure being performed

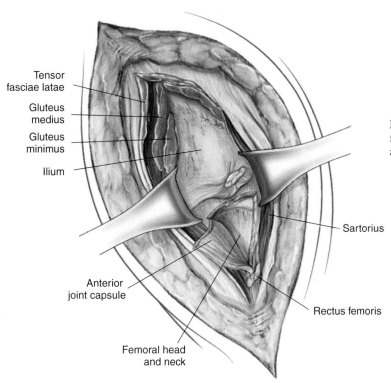

Tensor
fasciae latae

Gluteus
medius

Gluteus
minimus

Ilium

Sartorius

Anterior
joint capsule

Rectus femoris

Femoral head
and neck

FIGURE HP-52   The hip capsule is fully exposed at this juncture, and an arthrotomy is performed.

■ Superficial fascial interval is repaired
■ Subcutaneous tissue and skin are closed accordingly

EXTENSILE MEASURES

■ Distally, the interval between the rectus femoris and the vastus lateralis can be used to expose the shaft of the femur

■ Proximally, the iliac crest can be exposed for bone graft as necessary

■ The anterior column of the acetabulum and the ilium can be exposed in a subperiosteal manner by extending the proximal incision along the iliac crest (Figure HP-53)

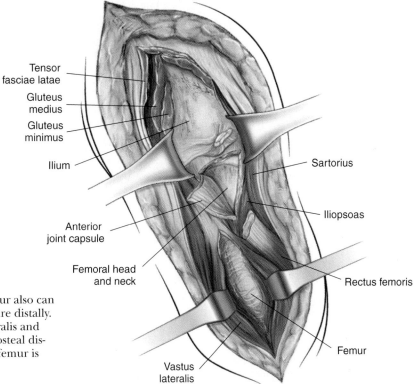

Tensor
fasciae latae

Gluteus
medius

Gluteus
minimus

Ilium

Sartorius

Iliopsoas

Anterior
joint capsule

Femoral head
and neck

Rectus femoris

Femur

Vastus
lateralis

FIGURE HP-53   The proximal femur also can be exposed with an extensile exposure distally. This is done through the vastus lateralis and rectus femoris interval, and subperiosteal dissection of the proximal shaft of the femur is performed.

MIS TOTAL HIP REPLACEMENT CONSIDERATIONS (HOZAK) (FIGURE HP-54)

■ This approach has been used for the MIS approach for total hip replacement, but the authors caution that expertise should be obtained before its use

■ The approach is useful for reaming of the acetabulum and is used as the acetabular approach for the 2-incision MIS approach for total hip replacement

■ The femoral preparation can be done by using a fracture table with the ipsilateral lower extremity in the extended and externally rotated position

■ Using a femoral neck elevator or bone hook to visualize the femur better allows preparation for the femoral component

■ Lateral capsule must be released to ensure that the femur can be delivered out of the incision for exposure to prepare the femur during total hip arthroplasty, especially if a fracture table is not used

■ The superficial dissection can be taken down to the sartorius tensor fascia interval (see Figure HP-54)

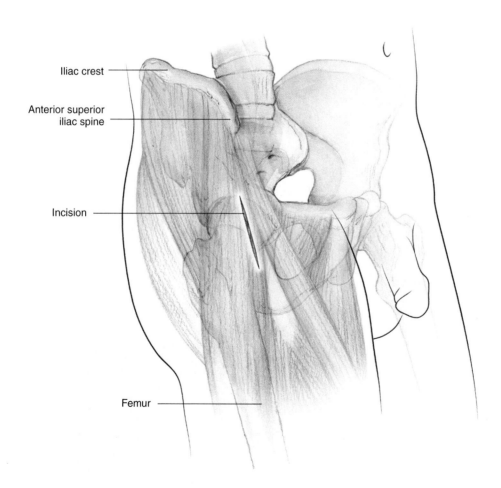

Iliac crest

Anterior superior iliac spine

Incision

Femur

FIGURE HP-54 The anterior MIS approach uses an 8-10 cm incision centered over the anterior portion of the hip joint in line with the ASIS; 4-6 cm distally from this point is used as the proximal extent of the incision.

- The tensor fascia can be incised, and blunt dissection along the interval of the sartorius medially can be performed

- Ligation of the ascending branch of the lateral femoral circumflex should be carried out

- Release of the rectus femoris off of the capsule is done, and the capsule is cleared off with an elevator

- This exposes the joint capsule, which can be incised for exposure of the joint

- The approach should include adequate exposure for visualization of all pertinent anatomical structures to prepare the femur and the acetabulum adequately for implant stability

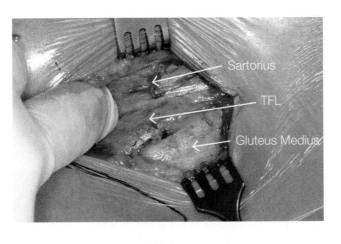

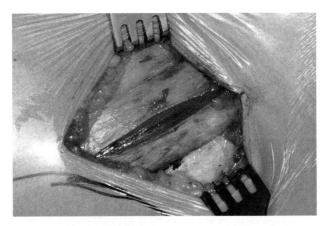

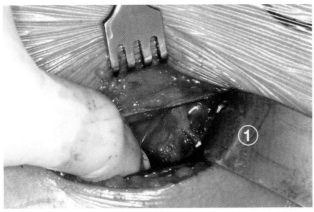

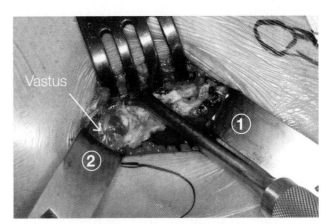

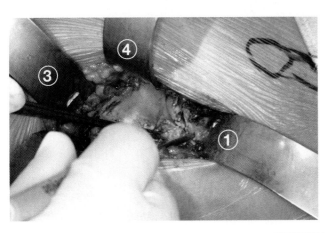

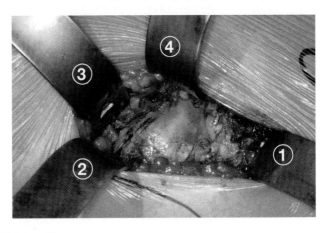

FIGURE HP-54, cont'd

Posterior Approach to the Hip

Indications: Total hip arthroplasty, hemiarthroplasty of the hip, posterior wall and column acetabular fracture open reduction and internal fixation, open reduction of posterior hip dislocations, hip arthrotomy

POSITIONING

- Lateral decubitus with an axillary roll (Figure HP-55)
- Kidney rests are used, and all bony prominences are padded

DANGERS

- Nerves

    - Sciatic nerve from direct injury or retraction or during repair of external rotators and capsule when closing
    - Femoral nerve from retraction and displacement of the proximal femur during reaming of the acetabulum or retractor placement
    - Obturator nerve from retraction or retractor placement

- Vessels

    - Inferior gluteal artery from direct injury or retraction
    - Medial femoral circumflex during the takedown of external rotators from the bone of the posterior proximal femur
    - Obturator artery (retractor in inferior aspect of the acetabulum)

LANDMARKS

- Greater trochanter, shaft of the proximal femur

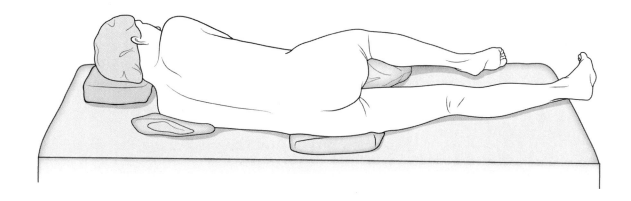

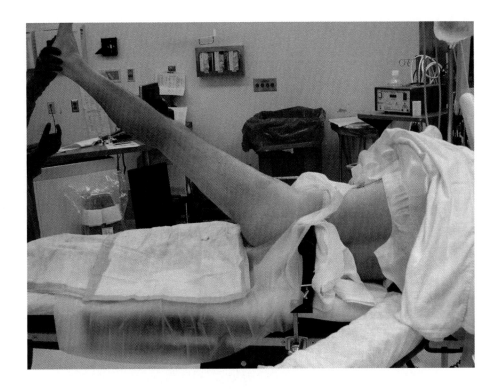

FIGURE HP-55   Lateral positioning of the patient with padding of bony prominences and an axillary roll in place.

INCISION

- ▨ Use the greater trochanter and femoral shaft as landmarks (Figure HP-56)
- ▨ Curved incision 12-16 cm in length with the apex centered at the posterior aspect of the trochanter starting on the lateral aspect of the proximal femur

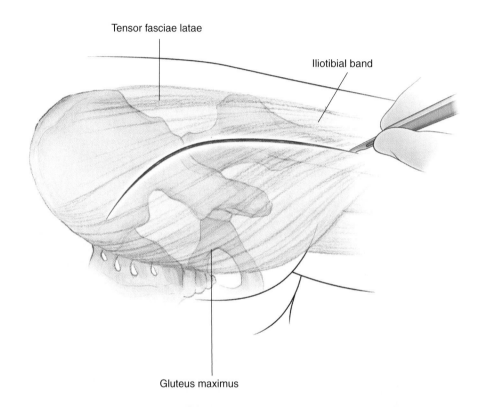

Tensor fasciae latae

Iliotibial band

Gluteus maximus

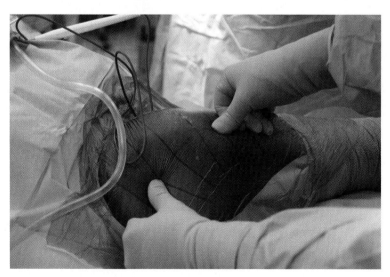

FIGURE HP-56   The incision is placed in the posterior third of the greater trochanteric prominence in a curvilinear fashion along the posterior aspect of the femoral shaft distally and curved in line with the gluteus maximus muscle fibers proximally. Alternatively, the hip can be flexed to 90 degrees, and a straight line along the posterior third of the posterior trochanteric prominence can be drawn. The incision is curved appropriately when the hip is extended into neutral position.

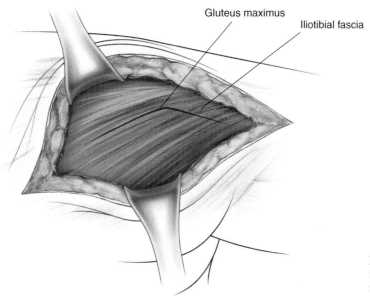

Gluteus maximus

Iliotibial fascia

FIGURE HP-57   Superficial dissection is carried down to the underlying gluteus maximus and iliotibial band fascia.

SUPERFICIAL DISSECTION

- Subcutaneous tissue is dissected in line with the incision
- Palpate as you go through subcutaneous layers, especially in obese patients, to make sure you do not slide posteriorly
- Uncover the tensor fascia and the gluteus maximus fascia around and posterior to the greater trochanter (Figure HP-57)

DEEP DISSECTION

- Incise the fascia lata laterally, and extend into the gluteus maximus fascia in line with the muscle fibers
- Bluntly dissect the gluteus maximus muscle fibers watching for intramuscular small vessels, and coagulate them along the way
- With a lap pad, bluntly sweep any underlying fat from the posterior aspect of the hip posteriorly (Figures HP-58 and HP-59)
- Identify the piriformis tendon insertion into the piriformis fossa
- Internally rotate the lower extremity at the hip to aid in exposure of the external rotator tendons

FIGURE HP-58 The iliotibial band is incised along with the gluteus maximus fascia, and the muscle fibers are bluntly dissected or dissected with controlled hemostasis to coagulate intramuscular bleeders as they appear.

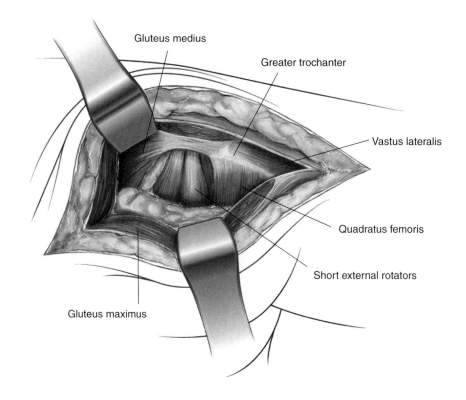

FIGURE HP-59 The external rotators are exposed along the posterior border of the proximal femur at this juncture.

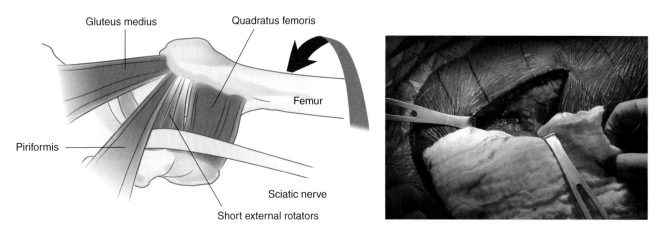

- Dissect the piriformis tendon from the fossa and the obturator externus and inferior and superior gemellae tendons (tag these with sutures for closure repair)

- The quadratus femoris is taken down leaving a cuff of tissue on the femur for repair

- Care should be taken to identify by site or palpation the position of the sciatic nerve as it exits beneath the piriformis muscle because its placement can vary, and it should be protected during the procedure

- The joint capsule is exposed, and the arthrotomy is done according to the procedure being performed (Figure HP-60)

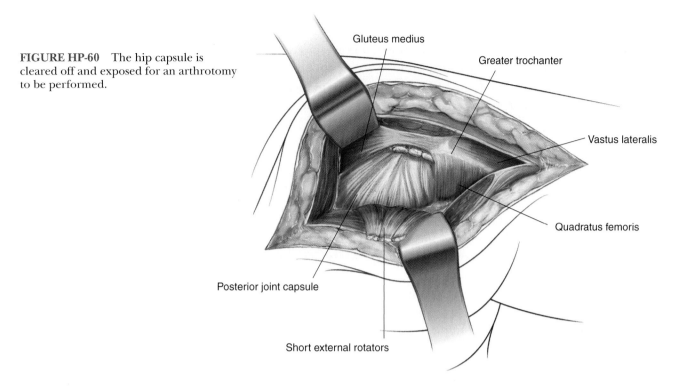

FIGURE HP-60 The hip capsule is cleared off and exposed for an arthrotomy to be performed.

Gluteus medius

Greater trochanter

Vastus lateralis

Quadratus femoris

Posterior joint capsule

Short external rotators

CLOSURE

- External rotator and capsule should be repaired through drill holes in the posterior aspect of the greater trochanter
- Sciatic nerve position should be confirmed so that no repair sutures are piercing or tenting the sciatic nerve
- The quadratus femoris is repaired back to its cuff of tissue on the femur, making sure that sutures are not deep and compromising the sciatic nerve as well

EXTENSILE MEASURES

- Posterior wall and column fractures
- Revision total hip arthroplasty with acetabular cage replacement
- Trochanteric osteotomy
  - Femoral component revision in total hip replacement
  - Acetabular exposure revision in total hip replacement
- Distal to expose femur as a lateral approach

MIS TOTAL HIP REPLACEMENT CONSIDERATIONS

- This approach can be amenable to a minimal incision technique, but the incision should be large enough to allow proper visualization of all anatomical structures involved in the applicable surgical procedure

- A smaller incision can be used with subcutaneous flap development, which allows for a mobile surgical window to be obtained

- The quadratus can be left attached, but care should be taken to ensure this is not under excessive force, which may avulse the muscle from its origin

- The use of lighted retractors allows for better visualization

- Anterior capsular release for adequate retraction of the femoral neck for acetabular reaming and the use of an offset reamer can aid in this step

- The approach should include the detachment of the piriformis tendon from the fossa on the femur because of its anatomical relationship and possible increased force on the sciatic nerve as the leg is manipulated for the procedure

- The approach should include adequate exposure for visualization of all pertinent anatomical structures to prepare the femur and the acetabulum adequately for implants (Figure HP-61)

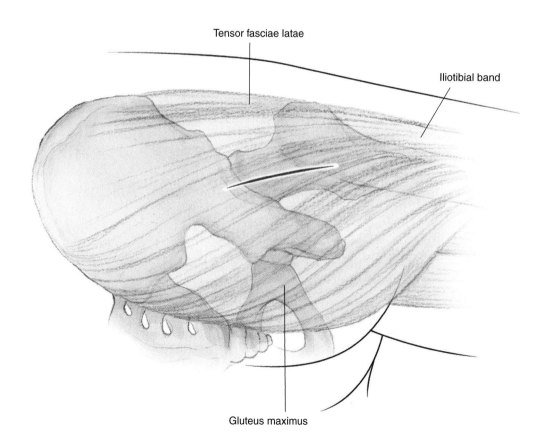

Tensor fasciae latae

Iliotibial band

Gluteus maximus

FIGURE HP-61 Posterior MIS approach incision is 10-12 cm and uses the upper limb of the curvilinear standard incision.

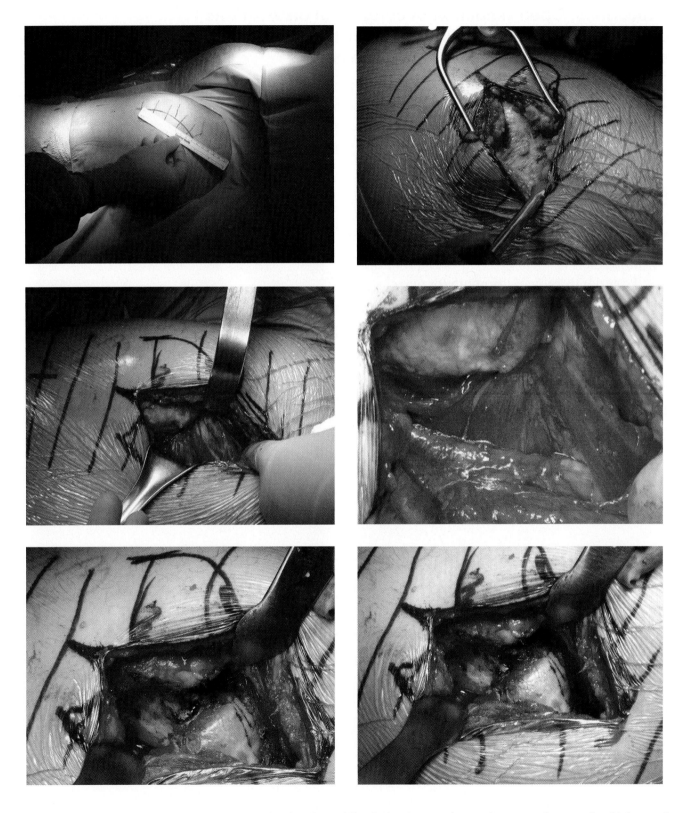

FIGURE HP-61, cont'd   A 12 cm incision is utilized and a mobile window is created to perform an arthrotomy in which a total hip procedure can be performed with excellent visualization.

MEDIAL APPROACH TO THE HIP

Indications: Open reduction of congenital dislocations of the hip, psoas release, inferior neck biopsy, obturator neurectomy and decompression

POSITIONING

- Supine (Figure HP-62)

DANGERS

- Nerves

  - Anterior division of the obturator nerve
  - Posterior division of the obturator nerve
  - No internervous plane is exploited by the approach, but the above-listed nerves supply muscles proximal to the dissection

- Vessels

  - Medial femoral circumflex artery

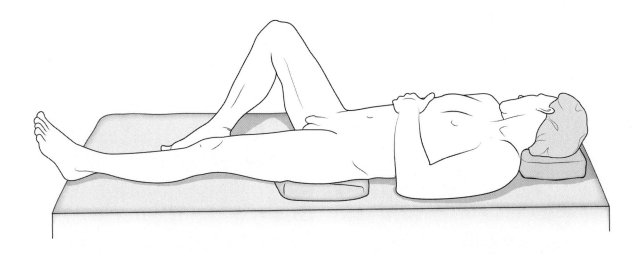

FIGURE HP-62   Positioning the patient for the medial approach to the hip. The patient is supine, and the hip is isolated to be able to flex, adduct, and rotate the hip if necessary during the procedure. Care should be taken to isolate the groin and perineum because this approach places the surgical field close to this area of contamination.

LANDMARKS

- Pubic tubercle, adductor tendons

INCISION (FIGURE HP-63)

- Palpate the tendon of the adductor longus, and mark its location
- Mark the pubic tubercle

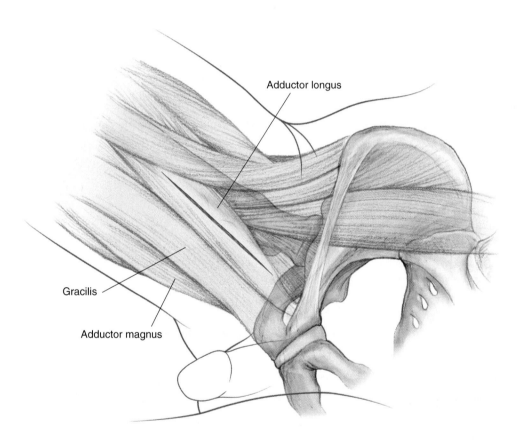

FIGURE HP-63   The landmarks for the medial approach incision are the pubic tubercle and the adductor longus (anterior) and the gracilis (posterior) attachments to the pubis. The incision is started 2-3 cm from the pubic tubercle and extends along the adductor tendon and muscles distally. The amount of the distal exposure and the length of the incision depends on the procedure being performed.

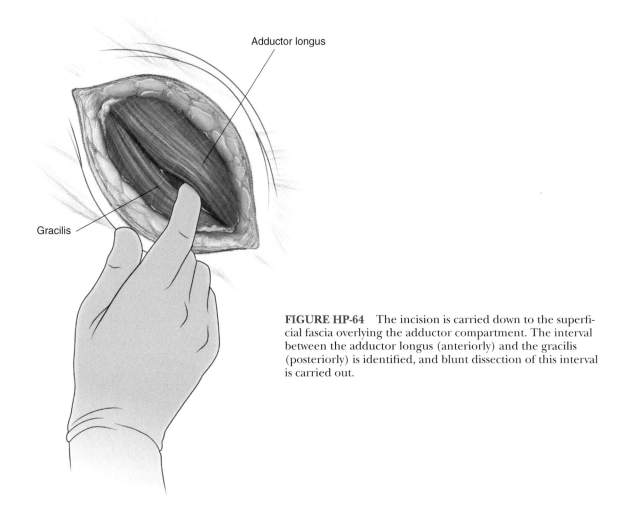

FIGURE HP-64 The incision is carried down to the superficial fascia overlying the adductor compartment. The interval between the adductor longus (anteriorly) and the gracilis (posteriorly) is identified, and blunt dissection of this interval is carried out.

- Medial incision based 2-3 cm from the pubic tubercle over the tendon of the adductor longus (Figure HP-64)

SUPERFICIAL DISSECTION

- Incise the skin and subcutaneous tissue to the underlying fascia of the adductor longus and gracilis muscles
- The superficial dissection can be developed by blunt dissection using the fascial plane between the adductor longus and the gracilis muscle

DEEP DISSECTION (FIGURE HP-65)

- Deeper in this plane, the dissection is continued between the adductor magnus posteriorly and the adductor brevis anteriorly

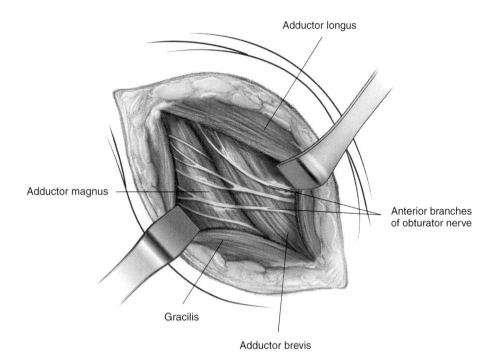

FIGURE HP-65 Retract the adductor longus anteriorly and the gracilis posteriorly to reveal the adductor magnus (posteriorly) and the adductor brevis (anteriorly). The anterior branch of the obturator nerve is present over the adductor brevis.

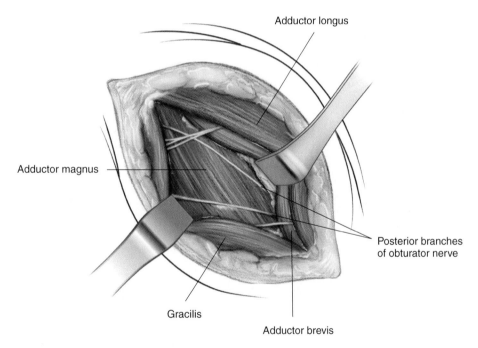

FIGURE HP-66 The adductor brevis is retracted anteriorly revealing the posterior branches of the obturator nerve over the adductor magnus. The lesser trochanter is revealed in the superior aspect of the surgical field.

■ The anterior branch of the obturator nerve has segmental branches that innervate the adductor magnus muscle at this level, and care should be taken not to have excessive retraction at this level

■ Lesser trochanter is now visible with the psoas tendon (Figure HP-66)

■ The medial aspect of the hip capsule can now be bluntly cleared off and prepared for an arthrotomy depending on the procedure being performed (Figures HP-67, HP-68, and HP-69)

■ The proximal 5 cm of the subtrochanteric aspect of the femoral shaft also can be exposed at this level

CLOSURE

■ Because intermuscular planes are used deeply, only the superficial fascia and subcutaneous tissues need to be repaired, aside from any procedure-specific capsular closure if violated

EXTENSILE MEASURES

■ Usually not extensile in nature

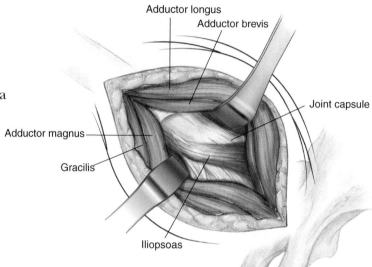

FIGURE HP-67   The lesser trochanter with its attachments of the iliacus and the iliopsoas tendons is isolated, and these tendons can be retracted off of the joint capsule posteriorly.

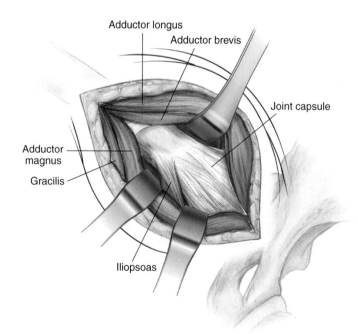

FIGURE HP-68   The joint capsule along the medial aspect of the femoral neck and calcar region can be bluntly cleared off and exposed.

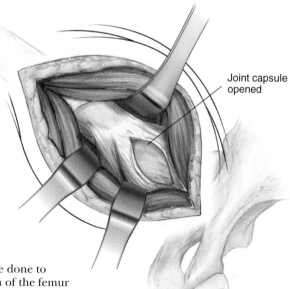

FIGURE HP-69   If necessary for the procedure, an arthrotomy can be done to expose the hip joint. The proximal 5 cm of the subtrochanteric region of the femur also can be exposed and may necessitate the release of the iliacus and the iliopsoas through this approach, but extensile exposure is impossible past these measures.

LATERAL APPROACH TO THE HIP

Indications: Total hip arthroplasty, hemiarthroplasty of the hip, open reduction and internal fixation of femoral neck fractures, open reduction and internal fixation of femoral head fractures, hip arthrotomy, intracapsular biopsy

POSITIONING (FIGURE HP-70; SEE ALSO FIGURE HP-55)

- The patient can be placed either supine on the operative table with the operative side buttocks just over the edge (see Figure HP-70) or in the lateral decubitus position (see Figure HP-55) with the operative side up
- In the supine position, a bump also may be used under the operative side in the buttocks region

DANGERS

- Nerves
  - Superior gluteal nerve if the dissection is carried too far proximally; the nerve lies between the gluteus medius and gluteus minimus and is located 3-5 cm above the tip of the greater trochanter
  - Femoral nerve (from inappropriately placed retractors anteriorly)

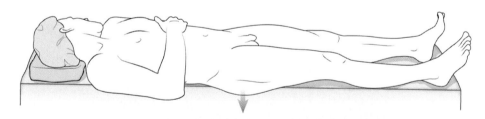

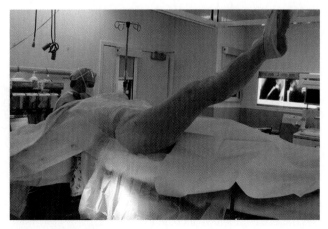

FIGURE HP-70   Supine positioning of the patient with the foot in a stirrup so that the extremity can be prepared. Alternately, the patient may be placed in the lateral position or a slightly rotated position with a bump or bean bag on the operative side under the buttocks region.

- Vessels

  - Femoral artery and vein (from inappropriately placed retractors anteriorly)
  - Lateral femoral circumflex artery transverse branch must be ligated during the approach when the vastus lateralis is mobilized off of the femur

LANDMARKS

- Greater trochanter, femoral shaft

INCISION (FIGURE HP-71)

- Direct lateral incision 12-20 cm made 5 cm from the proximal tip of the greater trochanter along the lateral aspect of the femoral shaft

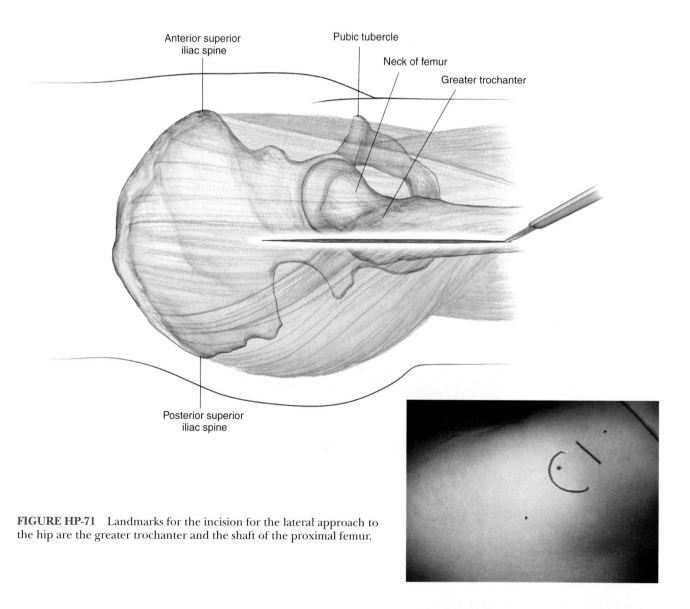

FIGURE HP-71 Landmarks for the incision for the lateral approach to the hip are the greater trochanter and the shaft of the proximal femur.

SUPERFICIAL DISSECTION

- Sharply dissect the subcutaneous tissue down to the fascia of the iliotibial band, the tensor fasciae latae superiorly and anteriorly, and the gluteus maximus superiorly and posteriorly

DEEP DISSECTION

- Incise the fascia over the tensor and the gluteus maximus to retract the tensor fascia anteriorly and the gluteus maximus muscle posteriorly
- Gluteus medius and vastus lateralis are exposed
- A self-retaining retraction system can be used after the superficial dissection is completed (Figure HP-72)
- Split the medius no more than 3 cm above the tip of the greater trochanter and carry this 2-3 cm into the vastus lateralis muscle

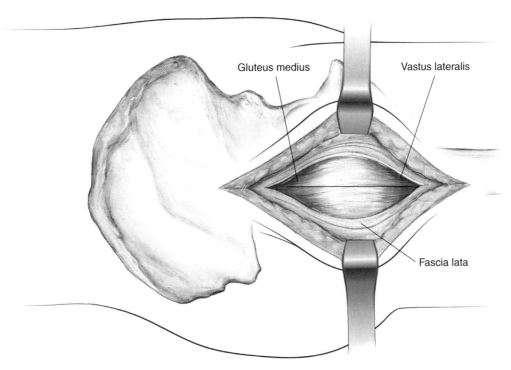

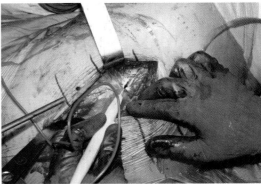

FIGURE HP-72   The superficial dissection is carried down the underlying gluteus maximus and iliotibial band fascia.

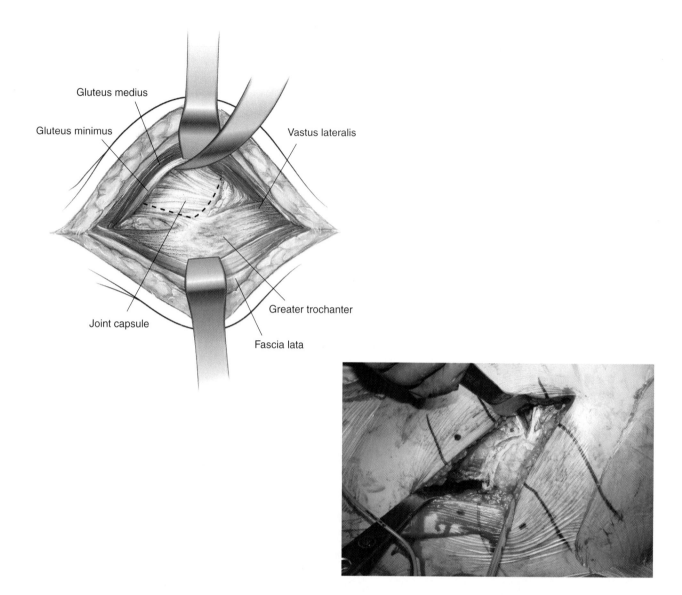

FIGURE HP-73 The gluteus medius and vastus lateralis sling of tissue is exposed. The incision is carried 3 cm from the tip of the trochanter and distally into the muscle 2-3 cm past its proximal origin; this sleeve is kept as a sling of tissue. This sling includes the gluteus minimus insertion taken off of the insertion on the anterior aspect of the proximal femur and exposes the joint capsule. Alternatively, the insertion of the minimus can be taken with an osteotome and a sliver of bone to enhance healing at the time of closure.

- This deep dissection creates an anterior flap consisting of the gluteus medius, the gluteus minimus tendon, and the vastus lateralis; alternatively, this can be taken with a broad osteotome to take a flake of bone off with the attachment of the minimus, vastus, and medius (Figure HP-73)

- Place a blunt retractor to dissect this flap from the anterior capsule to expose it

- The capsulotomy can be performed with release from the femoral attachment and a "T" into the acetabular rim. Blunt retractors can be placed around the neck of the femur to expose the joint better (Figures HP-74 and HP-75)

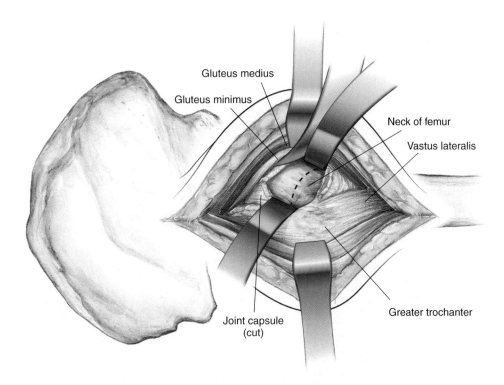

Gluteus medius

Gluteus minimus

Neck of femur

Vastus lateralis

Joint capsule
(cut)

Greater trochanter

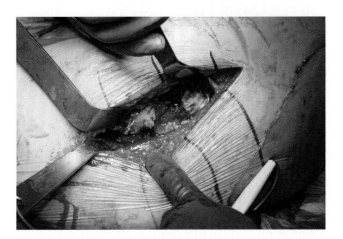

FIGURE HP-74   The joint capsule is exposed, and an arthrotomy can be performed depending on the surgical procedure at hand. An in situ osteotomy of the femoral neck also can be performed, and the femoral head can be removed with the aid of a corkscrew.

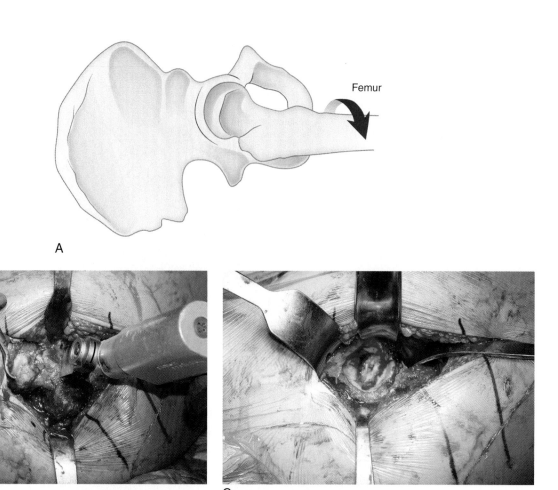

FIGURE HP-75 If the hip is to be dislocated, this can be facilitated by externally rotating and adducting the hip (**A**). A bone hook also can be used to aid in dislocation (**B**). If the acetabulum is exposed, the femur is retracted posteriorly with a retractor placed in the posterior inferior aspect of the lip of the acetabulum (**C**).

CLOSURE

- Capsular closure can be accomplished with large absorbable or nonabsorbable suture according to preference
- The anterior flap, including the medius, minimus, and vastus, is reattached to the trochanter with or without the flake of bone by drill holes and large absorbable or nonabsorbable suture to reattach this layer of tendinous structures anatomically to the trochanter
- Iliotibial band and gluteus maximus fascia lata interval are closed, and the subcutaneous tissue and skin are closed in the normal fashion

EXTENSILE MEASURES

- ▨ Distally to expose shaft of femur (lateral approach to femur)
- ▨ Not extended proximally

MIS TOTAL HIP REPLACEMENT CONSIDERATIONS (FIGURE HP-76)

- ▨ This approach can be amenable to a minimal incision technique, but the incision should be large enough to allow proper visualization of all anatomical structures involved in the applicable surgical procedure
- ▨ A smaller incision can be used (≤12 cm) with subcutaneous flap development, which allows for a mobile surgical window to be obtained
- ▨ The use of lighted retractors allows for better visualization
- ▨ Capsular release anterior and inferior for adequate retraction of the femoral neck can aid in this step of the procedure
- ▨ The approach should include adequate exposure for visualization of all pertinent anatomical structures to prepare the femur and the acetabulum adequately for implants

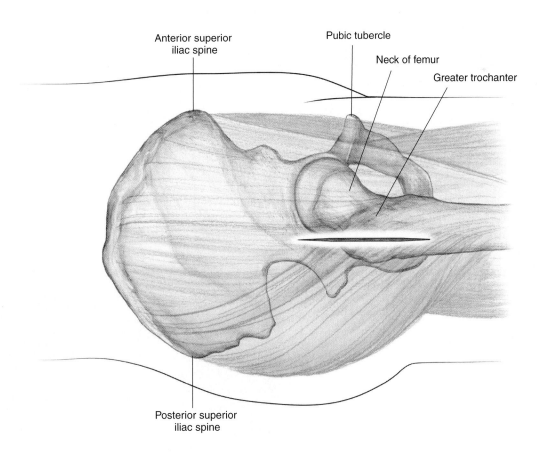

FIGURE HP-76   MIS approach simply shortens the incision from 4-5 cm above the tip of the trochanter to 7-8 cm distal to this landmark.

ANTEROLATERAL APPROACH TO THE HIP

Indications: Total hip arthroplasty, hemiarthroplasty of the hip, open reduction and internal fixation of femoral neck fractures, open reduction and internal fixation of femoral head fractures, hip arthrotomy, intracapsular biopsy

POSITIONING (FIGURE HP-77; SEE FIGURE HP-32)

- Operative side to the edge of the table
- Bump under the operative side buttocks region

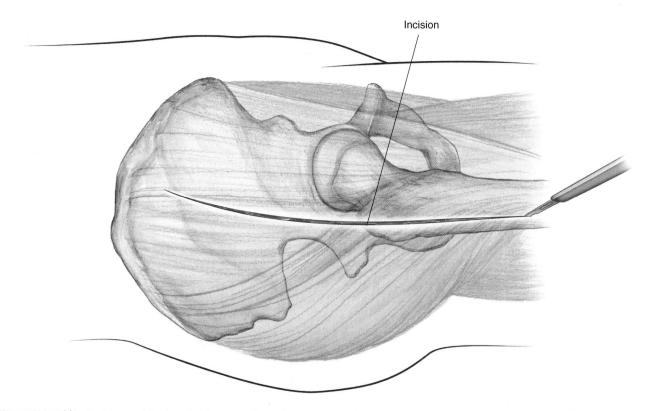

Incision

FIGURE HP-77 Patient positioning for the anterolateral approach can vary according to the surgeon's preference. Variations including the supine position, the supine position and bumped with a bean bag on the operative side, and the lateral position (depicted in photo) can be used.

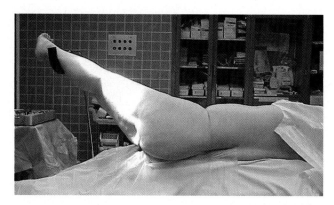

DANGERS

- Neurovascular structures enter the thigh anteriorly beneath the inguinal ligament. From lateral to medial, the femoral nerve lies over the iliopsoas, the artery is medial to the nerve and the vein, and lymphatics are even more medial; the mnemonic "NAVEL" aids in remembering the location of these structures from lateral to medial

● Nerves

- Femoral nerve (anterior retraction or inappropriately placed retractors)

● Vessels

- Profunda femoris artery
- Femoral artery and vein (anterior retraction or inappropriately placed retractors)

LANDMARKS

- Proximal shaft of the femur, greater trochanter, ASIS

INCISION

- Mark anterior and posterior aspects of the greater trochanter and the proximal femoral shaft
- Palpate and mark the ASIS
- The incision is marked from the mid aspect of the femoral shaft to the posterior aspect of the femur and 8-10 cm in the direction of the ASIS (Figures HP-77 and HP-78)

SUPERFICIAL DISSECTION

- Sharp dissection carried down to the superficial fascia of the tensor fasciae latae and iliotibial band
- Iliotibial band is incised in the posterior aspect of the incision to the posterior aspect of the greater trochanter (Figure HP-79)
- This exposes the medius and the vastus lateralis

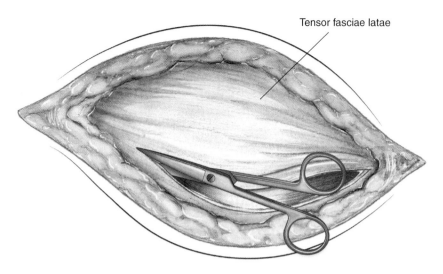

Tensor fasciae latae

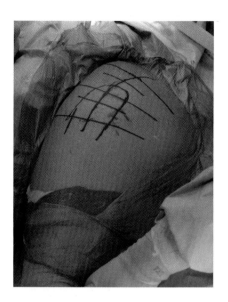

FIGURE HP-78 To mark the incision in the classic manner, the anterior and posterior aspects of the greater trochanter and the proximal femoral shaft are located along with the ASIS. The incision is marked from mid aspect of the femoral shaft to the posterior aspect of the femur and 8-10 cm in the direction of the ASIS.

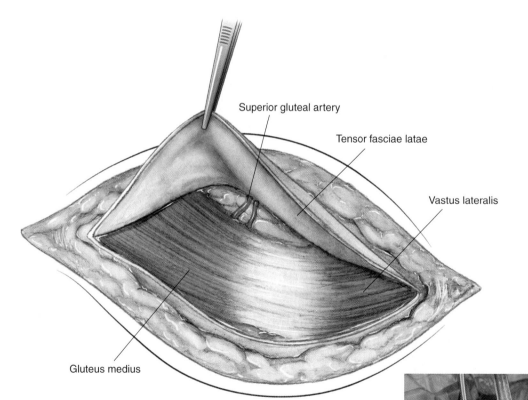

Superior gluteal artery

Tensor fasciae latae

Vastus lateralis

Gluteus medius

FIGURE HP-79 Superficial dissection involves carrying the incision down to the underlying tensor fasciae latae. The tensor fasciae latae is incised along the posterior aspect of the fascia lata in the surgical field and carried anteriorly at the tip of the trochanter.

DEEP DISSECTION

■ Anterior third of the medius is isolated to split the fibers
(Figure HP-80)

■ The medius and minimus can be taken together or layer by layer

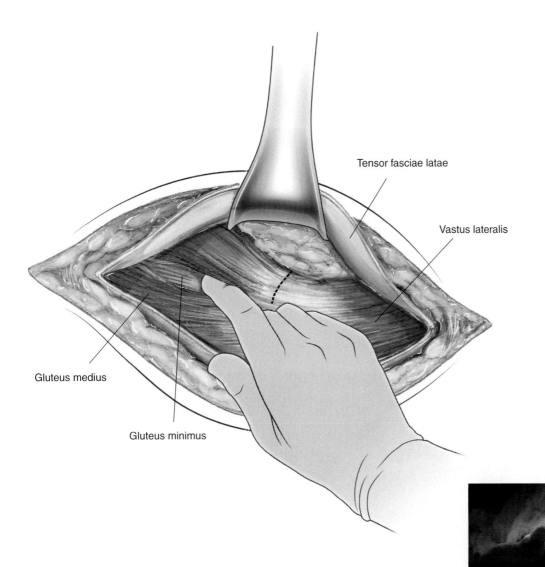

Tensor fasciae latae

Vastus lateralis

Gluteus medius

Gluteus minimus

FIGURE HP-80   The anterior third of the gluteus medius is isolated and taken off with a cuff of tissue left for repair.

◾ If the anterior flap is taken together, the capsule can be left and uncovered by blunt dissection (Figure HP-81)

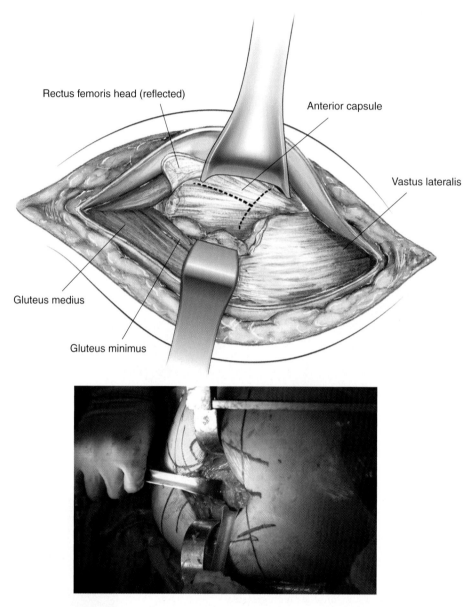

FIGURE HP-81 After release of the gluteus medius, this uncovers the gluteus minimus and underlying joint capsule. The gluteus minimus can be released off of its insertion on the proximal femur, and blunt dissection can be used to uncover the joint capsule and the reflected head of the rectus femoris anteriorly.

- The capsule is incised for a capsulotomy at the base of the neck of the femur and "T" made to the acetabular rim
- With external rotation, adduction maneuver, and aid of a bone hook, the femoral head can be dislocated (Figure HP-82)
- Anterior, posterior, and superior retractors are placed to expose the acetabulum (Figure HP-83)

CLOSURE

- Capsule is closed with large absorbable or nonabsorbable sutures by preference
- Minimus and medius are repaired anatomically by a running locking large absorbable suture through 2 drill holes in the femur
- Iliotibial band and tensor and gluteus interval are repaired
- Subcutaneous tissue and skin are closed in normal fashion

EXTENSILE MEASURES

- Distally to expose shaft of femur (lateral approach to femur)
- Not extended proximally

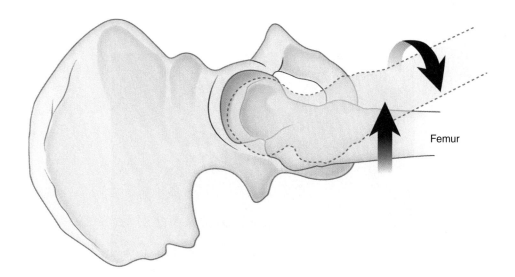

Femur

FIGURE HP-82   Arthrotomy of the hip joint can be performed exposing the joint with retractors placed around the femoral neck. The hip joint can be dislocated by external rotation and adduction of the hip and can be aided by a bone hook.

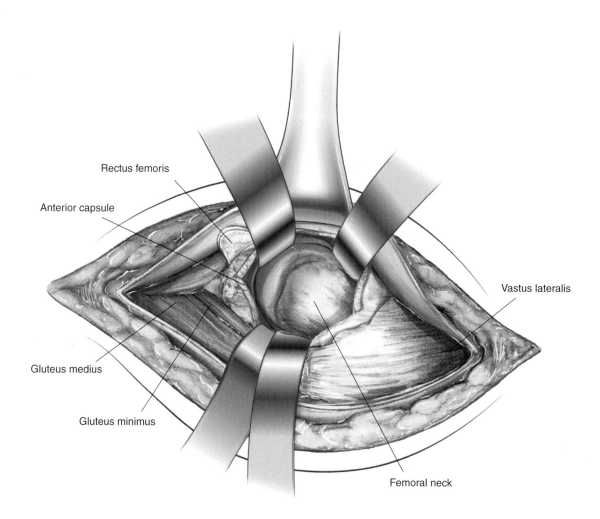

Rectus femoris

Anterior capsule

Vastus lateralis

Gluteus medius

Gluteus minimus

Femoral neck

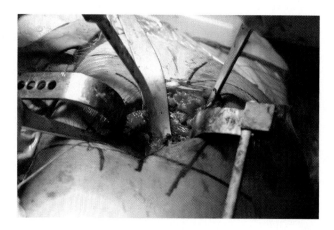

FIGURE HP-83 Retractor placement can be key for exposure and can include a Taylor type of retractor superiorly into the bone of the anterior lip of the acetabulum; a medial retractor around the anterior wall of the acetabulum, with similar retractor placement around the posterior wall of the acetabulum, can be helpful. In the clinical photo the femoral neck is fractured and the Mueller is lifting it as a femoral neck elevator.

MIS TOTAL HIP REPLACEMENT CONSIDERATIONS (FIGURE HP-84)

- Adequate exposure is always the goal for any approach, and it should not be compromised simply for length of incision
- Using the anterolateral approach with a smaller incision can present a problem with adequate exposure for the femoral preparation
- Curving the upper limb of the incision posteriorly can aid in the access to the femoral shaft for broaching
- Care should be taken to ensure that all skin edges are properly protected and not violated during the procedure, which may increase the chance for any vascular devitalization of the soft tissue edges of the incision

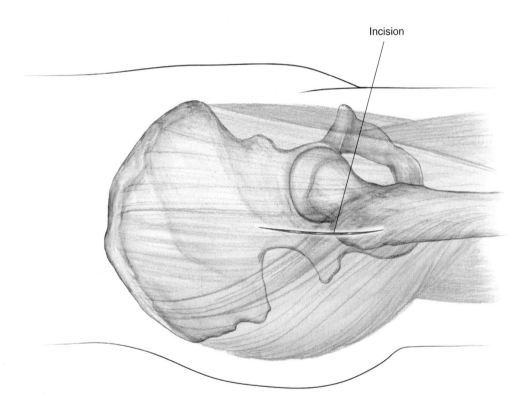

Incision

FIGURE HP-84 MIS anterolateral approach considerations. The incision can be curved slightly posterior along the superior limb to aid in broaching of the femur. This can help during the procedure because exposure of the acetabulum is not an issue using the lower half of the incision during the surgical approach.

Two-Incision Hip MIS Approach*

Indications: Total hip replacement

POSITIONING (SEE FIGURE HP-32)

- Supine with a bolster under the ipsilateral buttocks

DANGERS

- Nerves
  - Lateral femoral cutaneous
  - Femoral nerve—from retraction

- Vessels
  - Ascending branch of the lateral femoral circumflex

- Bone
  - Iatrogenic femur fracture
  - Component malposition

LANDMARKS

- Fluoroscopic assistance of identified landmarks may be useful to place incisions as described subsequently

FIGURE HP-85 The incision for the anterior approach to the acetabulum is similar to the direct anterior MIS approach and is 4-5 cm in length centered over the hip joint in the interval between the tensor fasciae latae and sartorius. The posterior incision is 4-5 cm in length in a longitudinal fashion and can be marked with the leg adducted in a line about 4 cm above the piriformis fossa and proximal posterior shaft of the femur.

INCISION (FIGURE HP-85)

- Using a metal marker and fluoroscopic imaging, a line is marked along the femoral neck axis from the head and neck junction to the base (about 4 cm)
- With the leg adducted, a line is marked (about 4 cm) in the lateral buttock region in line with the piriformis fossa and proximal posterior shaft of the femur

---

*The authors do not recommend use of this approach without proper experience and training before using the approach in the operating room.

SUPERFICIAL AND DEEP DISSECTION

● Acetabular incision

▨ Make the skin incision, and sharply dissect down to superficial fascia over the sartorius and tensor fasciae latae

▨ The sartorius is visualized in the superior medial aspect of the exposure and the tensor fasciae latae on the lateral aspect

▨ This interval is dissected retracting the tensor laterally and the sartorius medially (Figure HP-86)

▨ The rectus femoris is visualized, and the lateral edge is dissected and retracted medially with a blunt retractor, which exposes the capsule and the lateral circumflex vessels, which can be coagulated with electric cautery (Figure HP-87)

▨ The capsule can be incised or excised to preference, but stay sutures should be placed in the medial and lateral capsular tissue for retraction and aid at closure; this exposes the femoral neck and neck head junction (Figure HP-88)

▨ The femoral neck cut is performed in situ, and the femoral head is removed from the acetabulum allowing exposure for the acetabular preparation

▨ Lighted retractors and use of fluoroscopy are used for preparation of the acetabulum and femur

▨ Homan-type retractors are placed around the acetabulum with one superiorly, a second anteroinferior just in front of the transverse ligament, and a third over the posterior wall

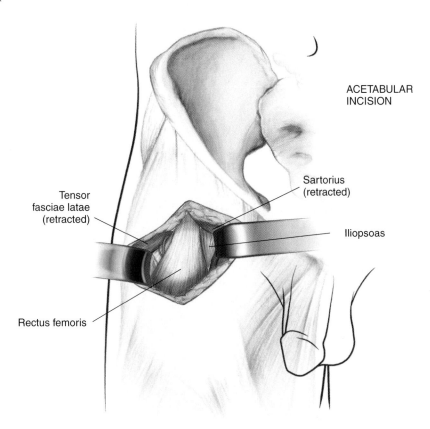

FIGURE HP-86   For the anterior incision, the interval between the sartorius and the tensor fasciae latae is developed. The rectus femoris is released, and the joint capsule is uncovered. The use of the lighted retractors can be helpful.

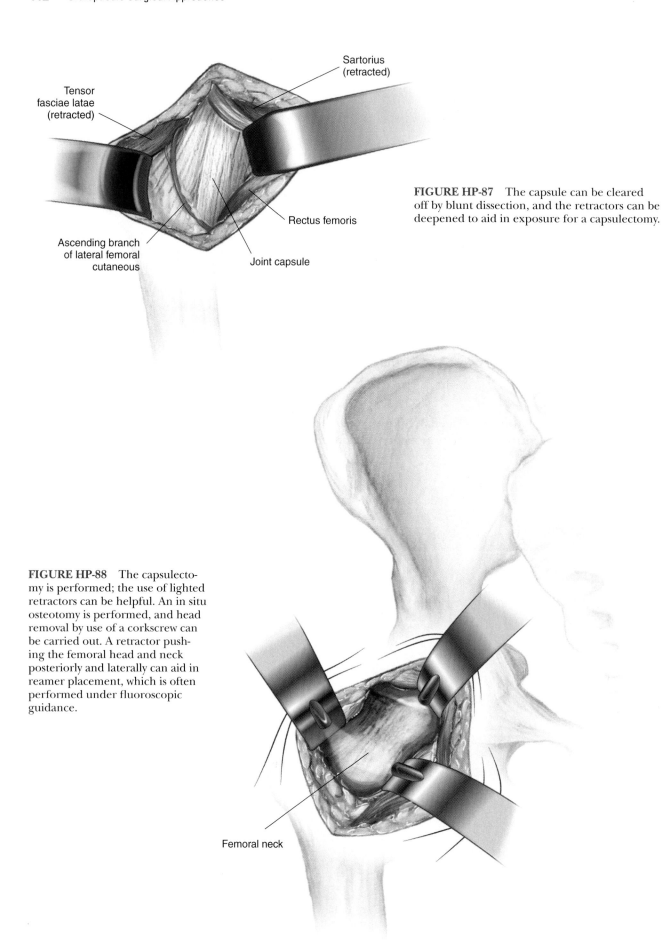

Tensor
fasciae latae
(retracted)

Sartorius
(retracted)

Ascending branch
of lateral femoral
cutaneous

Rectus femoris

Joint capsule

FIGURE HP-87 The capsule can be cleared off by blunt dissection, and the retractors can be deepened to aid in exposure for a capsulectomy.

FIGURE HP-88 The capsulectomy is performed; the use of lighted retractors can be helpful. An in situ osteotomy is performed, and head removal by use of a corkscrew can be carried out. A retractor pushing the femoral head and neck posteriorly and laterally can aid in reamer placement, which is often performed under fluoroscopic guidance.

Femoral neck

- Femoral preparation incision (Figure HP-89)

  - The skin incision is made, and blunt digital dissection is made to the proximal tip of the greater trochanter with feel of the piriformis insertion in the fossa
  - The preparation guide for the femur should be placed posterior to the abductors and anterior to the piriformis fossa and tendon
  - Specialized femoral preparation instruments and fluoroscopy are necessary to carry out the femoral preparation

CLOSURE

  - For the anterior incision, the limbs of the capsule can be closed by tying the stay sutures
  - The fascia is closed between the sartorius and the tensor fasciae latae
  - The posterior closure consists only of fascial closure of the gluteus maximus
  - Subcutaneous tissue and skin are closed in the normal fashion

EXTENSILE MEASURES

  - Anterior incision can be used for anterior approach to the hip
  - Lateral incision is not extensile

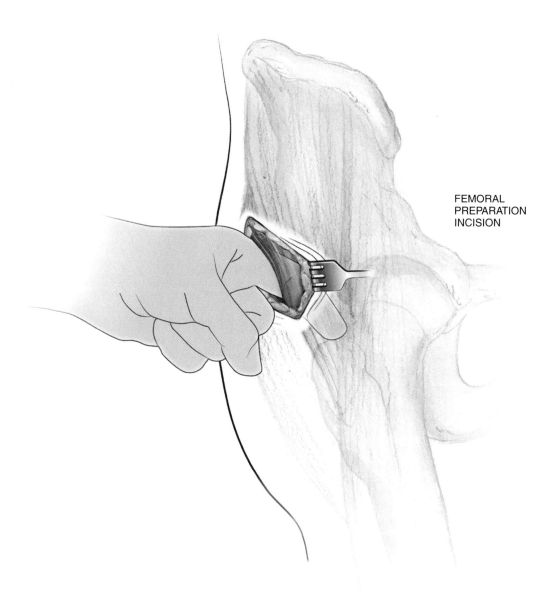

FEMORAL
PREPARATION
INCISION

FIGURE HP-89 The approach to the femur uses blunt dissection through the posterior incision. The broaching of the femur should be performed keeping the abductors anterior to the broach and the piriformis posterior to it during the procedure.

Hip Arthroscopy

Indications: Undiagnosed hip pain failing conservative management, labral tears, ligamentum teres injury, loose bodies, synovial disease, chondral injury or osteonecrosis, joint sepsis, instability, snapping hip syndrome, femoral acetabular impingement

POSITIONING (FIGURES HP-90 AND HP-91)

- Requires traction (usually with a fracture table) and fluoroscopy; 2 positioning options
  - Supine (illustrated in this section)
  - Lateral decubitus

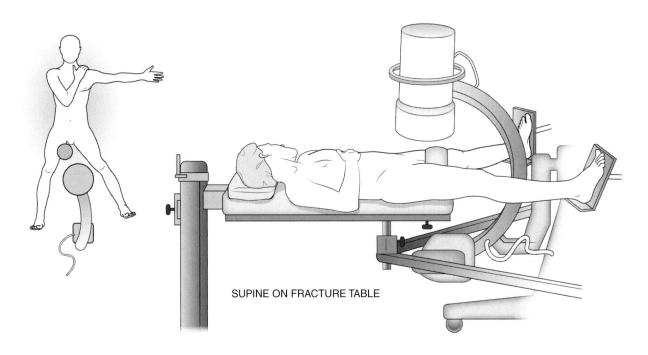

SUPINE ON FRACTURE TABLE

FIGURE HP-90 Hip arthroscopy patient positioning in a fracture table allowing for traction of the hip and better visualization of the hip joint. Supine positioning for hip arthroscopy on a fracture table using a padded perineal post with fluoroscopic assistance.

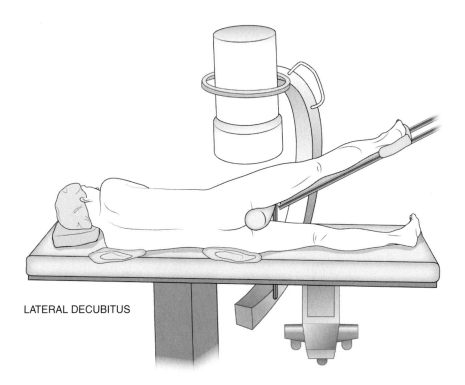

LATERAL DECUBITUS

FIGURE HP-91 Lateral position for a hip arthroscopy with the operative side in traction and a padded perineal post. Fluoroscopic assistance is used.

PORTALS (FIGURES HP-92 AND HP-93)

- **Anterolateral**
  - ▨ 1 cm superior and 1 cm anterior to the anterosuperior border of the greater trochanter
  - ▨ Usually established first with a cannulated needle; placement is confirmed fluoroscopically by injecting contrast medium into the joint

- **Posterolateral**
  - ▨ 1-2 cm posterior to posterosuperior border of the greater trochanter

- **Anterior**
  - ▨ Starting point is located at the intersection of a line extending from the greater trochanter anteriorly and a line extending distally from the ASIS
  - ▨ Placement is directed 45 degrees cephalad and 30 degrees medially into the joint

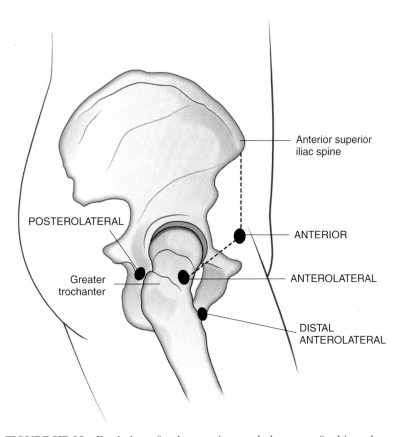

FIGURE HP-92   Depiction of arthroscopic portal placement for hip arthroscopy.

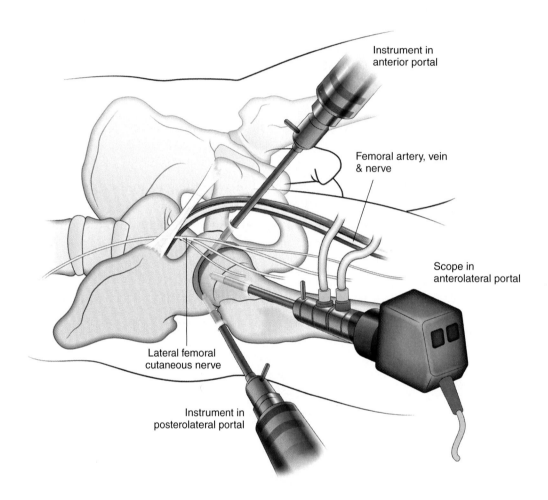

Instrument in
anterior portal

Femoral artery, vein
& nerve

Scope in
anterolateral portal

Lateral femoral
cutaneous nerve

Instrument in
posterolateral portal

FIGURE HP-93 Depiction of the femoral vessels and their relationship to the arthroscopic portals used. This relationship must be taken into consideration for safe placement of cannulas during the procedure.

VISUALIZATION (FIGURES HP-94 THROUGH HP-97)

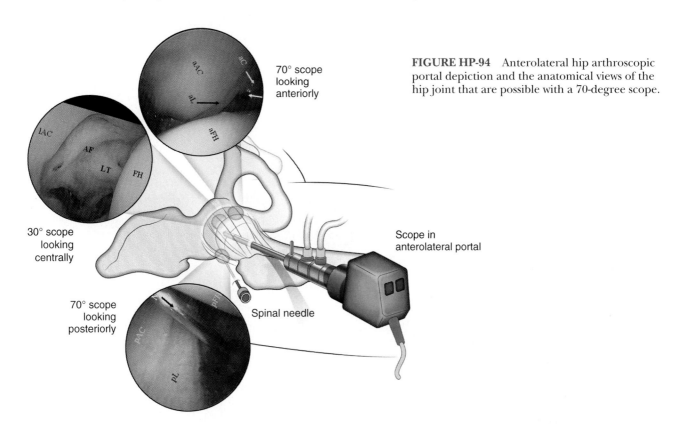

70° scope
looking
anteriorly

30° scope
looking
centrally

70° scope
looking
posteriorly

Spinal needle

Scope in
anterolateral portal

FIGURE HP-94 Anterolateral hip arthroscopic portal depiction and the anatomical views of the hip joint that are possible with a 70-degree scope.

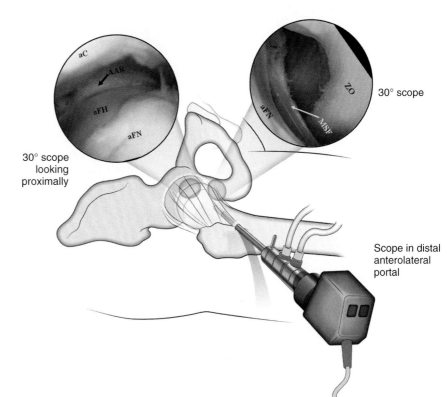

30° scope
looking
proximally

30° scope

FIGURE HP-95 Anterolateral hip arthroscopic portal depiction and the anatomical views of the hip joint that are possible with a 30 degree scope.

Scope in distal
anterolateral
portal

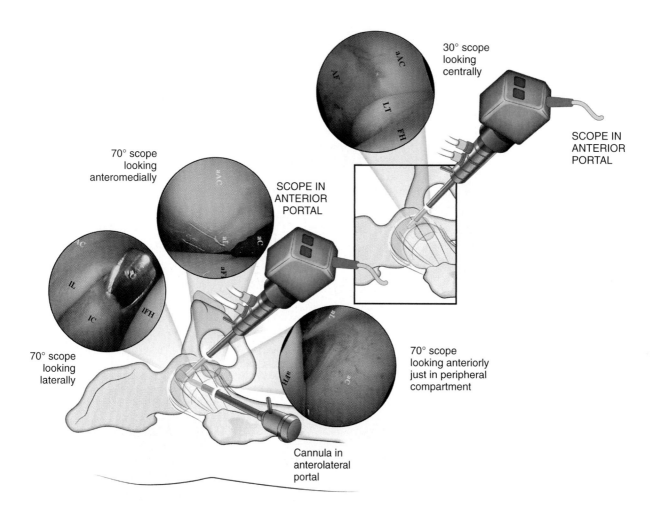

30° scope
looking
centrally

SCOPE IN
ANTERIOR
PORTAL

70° scope
looking
anteromedially

SCOPE IN
ANTERIOR
PORTAL

70° scope
looking
laterally

70° scope
looking anteriorly
just in peripheral
compartment

Cannula in
anterolateral
portal

FIGURE HP-96   Anterior hip arthroscopic portal depiction and the anatomical views of the hip joint that are possible with a 70 degree scope and a 30 degree scope.

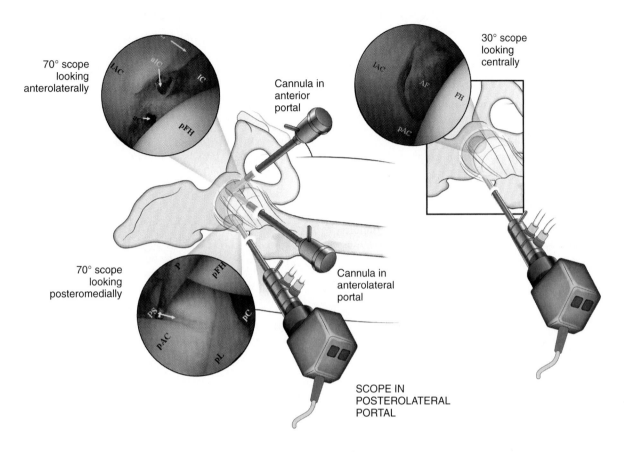

FIGURE HP-97   Posterior hip arthroscopic portal depiction and the anatomical views of the hip joint that are possible with a 70 degree scope and a 30 degree scope.

REFERENCES

Archibeck MJ, White RE Jr: Learning curve for the two-incision total hip replacement, Clin Orthop 429:232-238, 2004.

Berger RA: Total hip arthroplasty using the minimally invasive two-incision approach, Clin Orthop 417:232-241, 2003.

Berger RA: The technique of minimally invasive total hip arthroplasty using the two-incision approach, Instr Course Lect 53:149-155, 2004.

Byrd JW: Hip arthroscopy: The supine position, Clin Sports Med 20:703-731, 2001.

Byrd JW: Hip arthroscopy: The supine position, Instr Course Lect 52:721-730, 2003.

de Ridder VA, de Lange S, Popta JV: Anatomical variations of the lateral femoral cutaneous nerve and the consequences for surgery, J Orthop Trauma 13:207-211, 1999.

Glick JM: Hip arthroscopy: The lateral approach, Clin Sports Med 20:733-747, 2001.

Hospodar PP, Ashman ES, Traub JA: Anatomic study of the lateral femoral cutaneous nerve with respect to the ilioinguinal surgical dissection, J Orthop Trauma 13:17-19, 1999.

Juliano PJ, Bosse MJ, Edwards KJ: The superior gluteal artery in complex acetabular procedures: A cadaveric angiographic study, J Bone Joint Surg Am 76:244-248, 1994.

Karunakar MA, Le TT, Bosse MJ: The modified ilioinguinal approach, J Orthop Trauma 18:379-383, 2004.

Kloen P, Siebenrock KA, Ganz R: Modification of the ilioinguinal approach, J Orthop Trauma 16:586-593, 2002.

Matta JM: Operative treatment of acetabular fractures through the ilioinguinal approach: A 10-year perspective, J Orthop Trauma 20(1 Suppl):S20-S29, 2000.

Matta JM, Shahrdar C, Ferguson T: Single-incision anterior approach for total hip arthroplasty on an orthopaedic table, Clin Orthop 441:115-124, 2005.

O'Brien DA, Rorabeck CH: The mini-incision direct lateral approach in primary total hip arthroplasty, Clin Orthop 441:99-103, 2005.

Pagnano MW, Leone J, Lewallen DG, et al: Two-incision THA had modest outcomes and some substantial complications, Clin Orthop 441:86-90, 2005.

Pokorny D, Jahoda D, Veigl D: Topographic variations of the relationship of the sciatic nerve and the piriformis muscle and its relevance to palsy after total hip arthroplasty, Surg Radiol Anat 28:88-91, 2006.

Stiehl JB, Harlow M, Hackbarth D: Extensile triradiate approach for complex acetabular reconstruction in total hip arthroplasty, Clin Orthop 294:162-169, 1993.

Sweeney HJ: Arthroscopy of the hip: Anatomy and portals, Clin Sports Med 20:697-702, 2001.

Weber TG, Mast JW: The extended ilioinguinal approach for specific both column fractures, Clin Orthop 305:106-111, 1994.

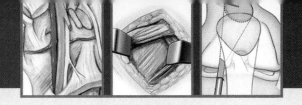

CHAPTER

7

KNEE AND LOWER LEG

—

MARK D. MILLER

REGIONAL ANATOMY

Osteology

- ● Distal femur (Figure KL-1)

  - ▪ The femur (largest bone in the body) flares distally and forms 2 condyles—a larger medial and a longer and more narrow lateral femoral condyle

  - ▪ The intercondylar area serves as the region for cruciate attachments—lateral, anterior cruciate ligament (ACL); medial, posterior cruciate ligament (PCL)

  - ▪ The medial epicondyle serves as an attachment for the medial collateral ligament (MCL). The medial patellofemoral ligament inserts on the medial epicondyle, and the adductor magnus tendon inserts on the adductor tubercle at the superior aspect of the medial epicondyle

  - ▪ The lateral condyle serves as an attachment for the lateral collateral ligament (LCL) at the lateral epicondyle, which is less prominent than the medial epicondyle. The popliteus tendon lies in a groove distal to the epicondyle

- ● Proximal tibia (Figure KL-2)

  - ▪ The tibia is the second longest bone in the body

  - ▪ The condylar areas match the corresponding femoral condyle

    - ● Medial tibial condyle is broad and concave

    - ● Lateral tibial condyle is smaller and convex

  - ▪ The tibial eminences (spines) define the borders of the cruciate ligament insertions

    - ● ACL lies between the eminences

    - ● PCL lies posterior to the eminences below the joint line. It originates in a sulcus that is bordered by 2 posterior tubercles (a larger medial tubercle and a smaller lateral tubercle)

  - ▪ The tubercles serve as attachments for tendons

    - ● Tibial tubercle (or tuberosity) serves as the patellar tendon attachment

    - ● Gerdy's tubercle serves as the iliotibial band attachment

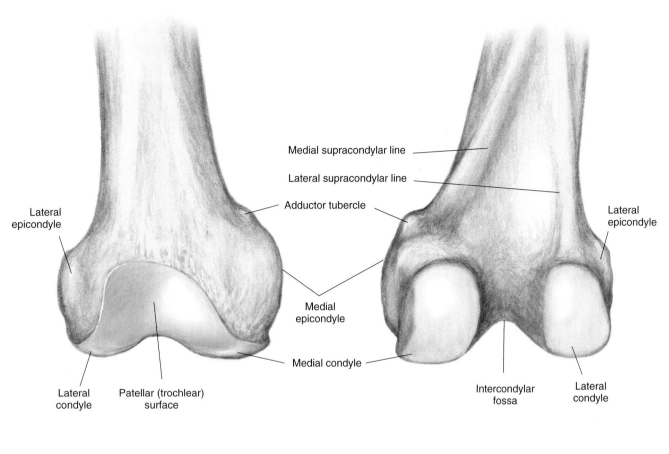

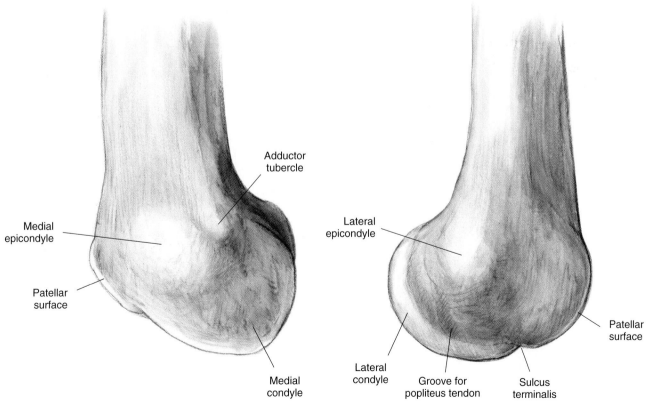

FIGURE KL-1   A-D, Bony architecture of the distal femur.

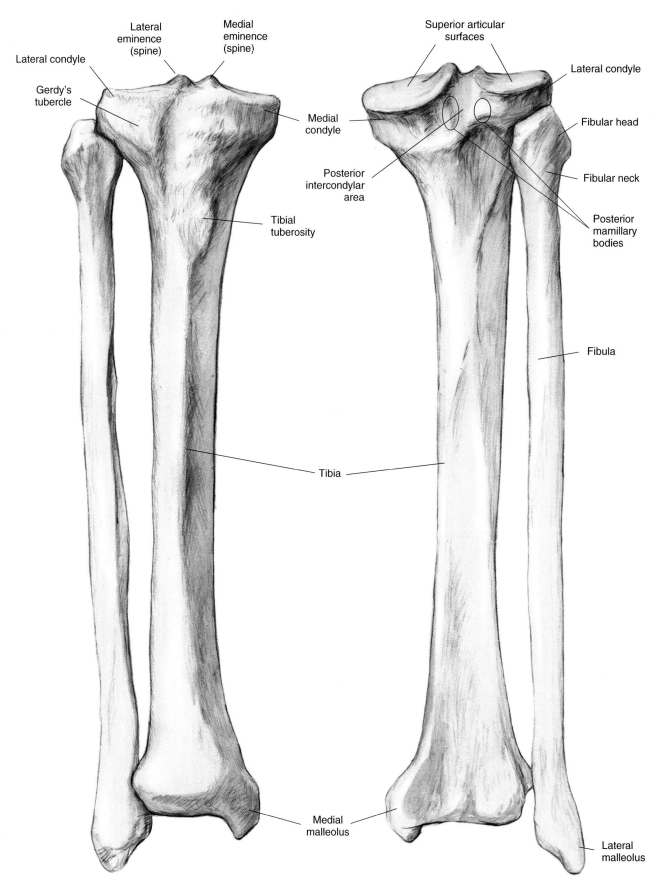

FIGURE KL-2 Bony architecture of the proximal tibia.

● Patella (Figure KL-3)

- ▪ Largest sesamoid bone in the body
- ▪ Thickest articular cartilage in the body
- ▪ Medial and lateral facets
  - ● Lateral facet is larger
  - ● Facets separated by a vertical ridge

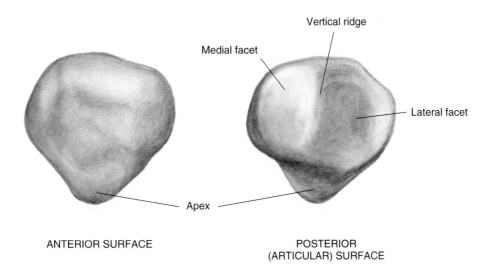

ANTERIOR SURFACE   POSTERIOR
                                   (ARTICULAR) SURFACE

FIGURE KL-3   Bony architecture of the patella.

Arthrology

- ● Knee joint (Figures KL-4 and KL-5)
  - ▨ Largest joint in the body
  - ▨ The knee joint is a ginglymus (hinge) joint that allows rolling and sliding
  - ▨ Static restraints
    - ● Ligaments
      - ○ ACL—resists anterior translation
      - ○ PCL—resists posterior translation
      - ○ MCL—resists valgus displacement
      - ○ LCL—resists varus displacement
      - ○ Posteromedial and posterolateral capsular structures—resist rotation
    - ● Menisci
      - ○ Medial—semicircular and broader posteriorly
      - ○ Lateral—more circular and covers a larger portion of the articular surface
    - ● Articular congruity
  - ▨ Dynamic restraints
    - ● Quadriceps muscles
    - ● Hamstring muscles

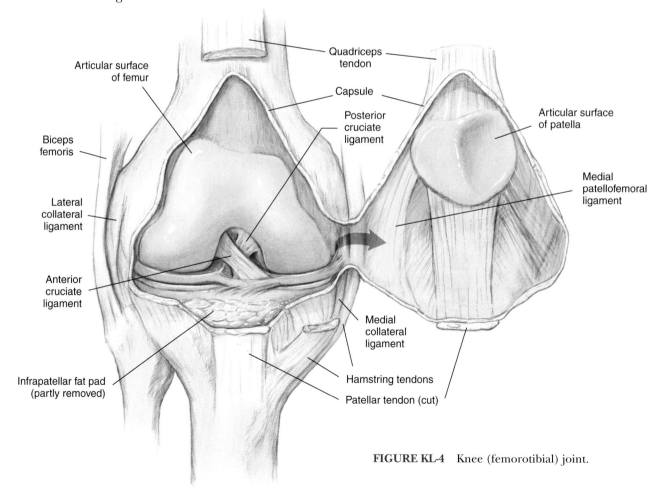

FIGURE KL-4   Knee (femorotibial) joint.

● Proximal tibiofibular joint

   ■ Plane gliding joint

   ■ Surrounded by thick capsule

   ■ Anterior and posterior ligaments of the head of the fibula stabilize the joint

● Patellofemoral joint

   ■ Plane (gliding) joint that stabilizes the patella in the trochlear groove of the femur and enhances the effect of the quadriceps muscles (fulcrum effect)

   ■ Medial patellofemoral ligament—primary restraint to lateral patellar displacement

   ■ Capsule/retinaculum

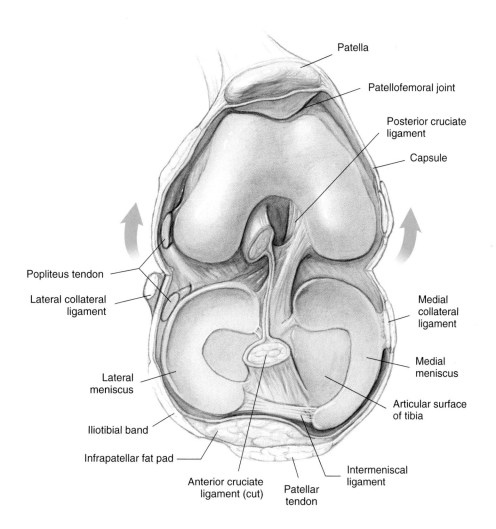

FIGURE KL-5 Knee joint (hinged open).

Muscles

- Knee and leg muscles are best considered in groups or compartments (Figures KL-6 and KL-7; Tables KL-1 and KL-2)
  - Anterior thigh
    - Quadriceps muscles
      - Vastus lateralis, intermedius, medialis, and rectus femoris
  - Posterior thigh
    - Hamstring muscles
      - Lateral—biceps femoris
      - Medial—semimembranosus, semitendinosus, sartorius, gracilis
    - Adductors—magnus, longus, brevis
  - Anterior leg
    - Tibialis anterior, extensor hallucis longus, extensor digitorum longus
  - Posterior leg
    - Gastrocnemius, soleus, plantaris, flexor hallucis longus, flexor digitorum longus, tibialis posterior (deep), popliteus
  - Lateral leg
    - Peroneus brevis, longus, and tertius (distally)

TABLE KL–1   Muscles of the Thigh

Muscle	Origin	Insertion	Innervation
Vastus lateralis	Iliotibial line/greater trochanter/lateral linea aspera	Lateral patella	Femoral
Vastus medialis	Iliotibial line/medial linea aspera/supracondylar line	Medial patella	Femoral
Vastus intermedius	Proximal anterior femoral shaft	Patella	Femoral
Biceps (long head)	Medial ischial tuberosity	Fibular head/lateral tibia	Tibial
Biceps (short head)	Lateral linea aspera/lateral intermuscular septum	Lateral tibial condyle	Peroneal
Semitendinosus	Distal medial ischial tuberosity	Anterior tibial crest	Tibial
Semimembranosus	Proximal lateral ischial tuberosity	Oblique popliteal ligament Posterior capsule Posterior/medial tibia Popliteus Medial meniscus	Tibial

TABLE KL–2   Muscles of the Leg

Muscle	Origin	Insertion	Action	Innervation
Anterior Compartment				
Tibialis anterior	Lateral tibia	Medial cuneiform, 1st metatarsal	Dorsiflex, invert foot	Deep peroneal (L4)
Extensor hallucis longus	Mid fibula	Great toe distal phalanx	Dorsiflex, extend toe	Deep peroneal (L5)
Extensor digitorum longus	Tibial condyle/fibula	Toe middle and distal phalanges	Dorsiflex, extend toes	Deep peroneal (L5)
Peroneus tertius	Fibula and extensor digitorum longus tendon	5th metatarsal	Evert, plantar flex, abduct foot	Deep peroneal (S1)
Lateral Compartment				
Peroneus longus	Proximal fibula	Medial cuneiform, 1st metatarsal	Evert, plantar flex, abduct foot	Superficial peroneal (S1)
Peroneus brevis	Distal fibula	Tuberosity of 5th metatarsal	Evert foot	Superficial peroneal (S1)
Superficial Posterior Compartment				
Gastrocnemius	Posterior, medial, and lateral femoral condyles	Calcaneus	Plantar flex foot	Tibial (S1)
Soleus	Fibula/tibia	Calcaneus	Plantar flex foot	Tibial (S1)
Plantaris	Lateral femoral condyle	Calcaneus	Plantar flex foot	Tibial (S1)
Deep Posterior Compartment				
Popliteus	Lateral femoral condyle, fibular head	Proximal tibia	Flex, IR knee	Tibial (L5, S1)
Flexor hallucis longus	Fibula	Great toe distal phalanx	Plantar flex great toe	Tibial (S1)
Flexor digitorum longus	Tibia	2nd-5th toe distal phalanges	Plantar flex toes, foot	Tibial (S1, S2)
Tibialis posterior	Tibia, fibula, interosseous membrane	Navicular, medial cuneiform	Invert/plantar flex foot	Tibial (L4, L5)

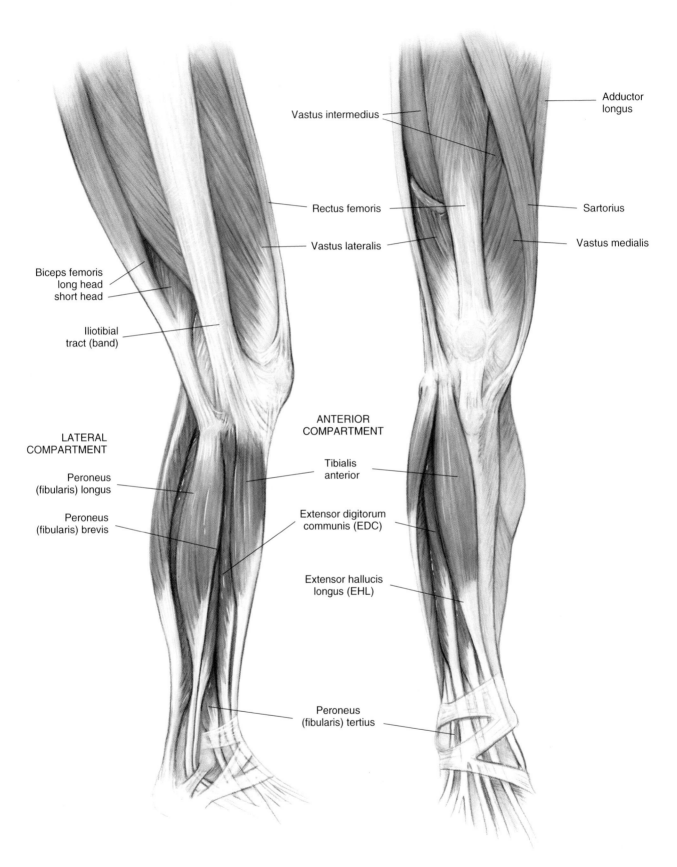

FIGURE KL-6 Muscles (anterior and lateral views).

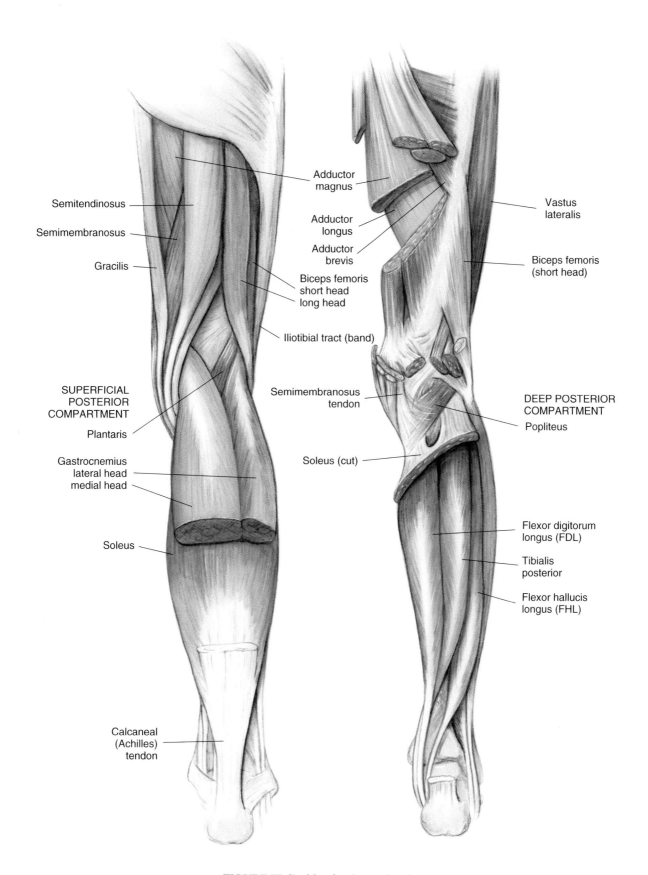

Semitendinosus

Semimembranosus

Gracilis

Adductor magnus

Adductor longus

Adductor brevis

Biceps femoris
short head
long head

Iliotibial tract (band)

Vastus lateralis

Biceps femoris (short head)

SUPERFICIAL POSTERIOR COMPARTMENT

Plantaris

Semimembranosus tendon

DEEP POSTERIOR COMPARTMENT

Popliteus

Gastrocnemius
lateral head
medial head

Soleus (cut)

Soleus

Flexor digitorum longus (FDL)

Tibialis posterior

Flexor hallucis longus (FHL)

Calcaneal (Achilles) tendon

FIGURE KL-7 Muscles (posterior view).

Nerves

- Extension of nerves from the lumbosacral plexus (Figure KL-8)

  - Sciatic nerve—divides in midthigh
    - Tibial division
    - Peroneal division
  - Femoral nerve
  - Obturator nerve

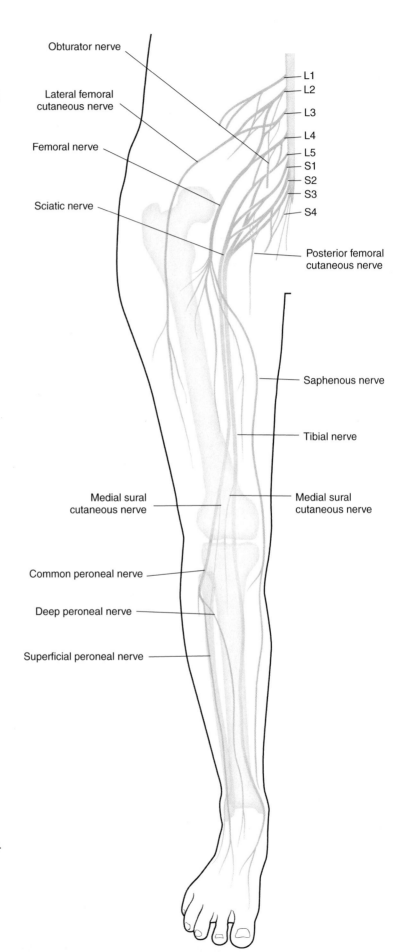

FIGURE KL-8 Major nerves of the thigh and leg.

Vascularity (Figure KL-9)

- **Femoral artery**
  - Thigh branches
  - Trifurcation
    - Anterior tibial artery
    - Posterior tibial artery
    - Peroneal artery (usually splits from posterior branch)

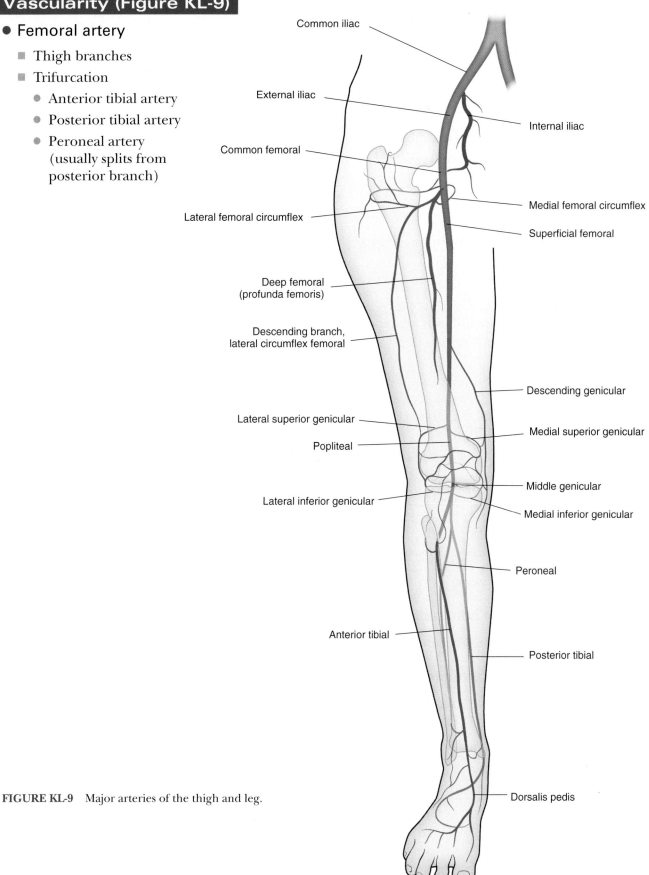

FIGURE KL-9 Major arteries of the thigh and leg.

CROSS-SECTIONAL ANATOMY (Figure KL-10)

Thigh

- **Anterior compartment**
  - Vastus medialis, vastus intermedius, vastus lateralis, rectus femoris, sartorius
  - Superficial femoral artery and vein
  - Saphenous nerve

- **Medial compartment**
  - Adductor longus, adductor brevis, adductor magnus, gracilis
  - Deep femoral artery and vein

- **Posterior compartment**
  - Biceps femoris, semitendinosus, semimembranosus
  - Sciatic nerve

Lower Leg

- **Anterior compartment**
  - Tibialis anterior, extensor hallucis longus, extensor digitorum longus
  - Deep peroneal nerve
  - Anterior tibial artery and vein

- **Lateral compartment**
  - Peroneus longus and brevis
  - Superficial peroneal nerve

- **Superficial posterior compartment**
  - Gastrocnemius, soleus, plantaris

- **Deep posterior compartment**
  - Flexor hallucis longus, flexor digitorum longus, tibialis posterior
  - Tibial nerve
  - Posterior tibial artery and vein

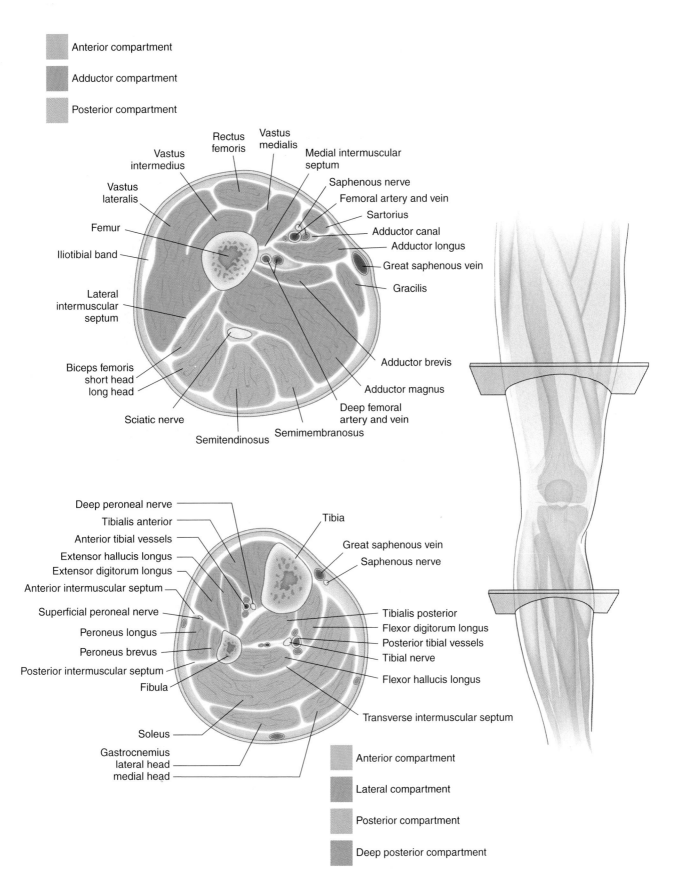

Anterior compartment

Adductor compartment

Posterior compartment

Rectus femoris
Vastus medialis
Vastus intermedius
Medial intermuscular septum
Vastus lateralis
Saphenous nerve
Femoral artery and vein
Femur
Sartorius
Iliotibial band
Adductor canal
Adductor longus
Lateral intermuscular septum
Great saphenous vein
Gracilis
Biceps femoris short head long head
Adductor brevis
Adductor magnus
Sciatic nerve
Deep femoral artery and vein
Semitendinosus
Semimembranosus

Deep peroneal nerve
Tibialis anterior
Tibia
Anterior tibial vessels
Great saphenous vein
Extensor hallucis longus
Saphenous nerve
Extensor digitorum longus
Anterior intermuscular septum
Superficial peroneal nerve
Peroneus longus
Tibialis posterior
Peroneus brevus
Flexor digitorum longus
Posterior tibial vessels
Posterior intermuscular septum
Tibial nerve
Fibula
Flexor hallucis longus
Soleus
Transverse intermuscular septum
Gastrocnemius lateral head medial head

Anterior compartment

Lateral compartment

Posterior compartment

Deep posterior compartment

FIGURE KL-10 Cross section of the thigh and lower leg.

SUPERFICIAL LANDMARKS (Figure KL-11)

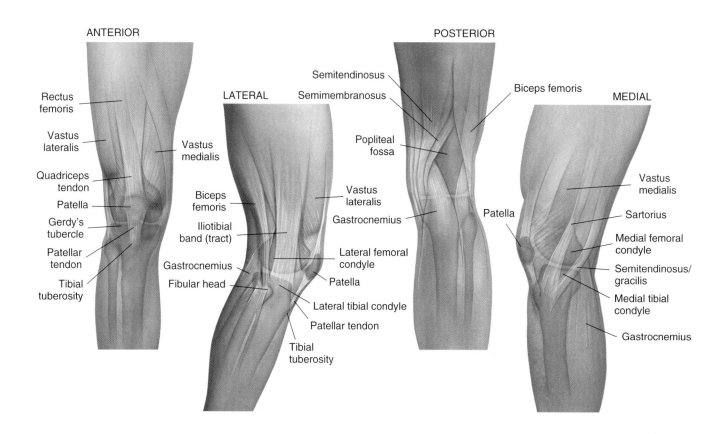

FIGURE KL-11   Superficial landmarks.

HAZARDS (Figure KL-12)

Sciatic Nerve

- Main nerve to lower extremity
- At risk
  - Dissection near ischium (proximal hamstring injuries)

Peroneal Nerve

- Branch of the sciatic nerve that crosses the fibula before dividing into superficial and deep branches
- At risk (peroneal nerve)
  - As it crosses the neck of the fibula
- At risk (superficial peroneal nerve)
  - During lower extremity compartment release approximately 12 cm proximal to the tip of the lateral malleolus

Tibial Nerve

- At risk
  - Popliteal dissection

Vascular

- Popliteal artery and vein
  - At risk
    - Popliteal dissection and PCL transtibial procedure
    - Knee arthroplasty especially in revision cases where bone loss extends posteriorly
- Geniculate arteries
  - At risk
    - Medial and lateral dissection

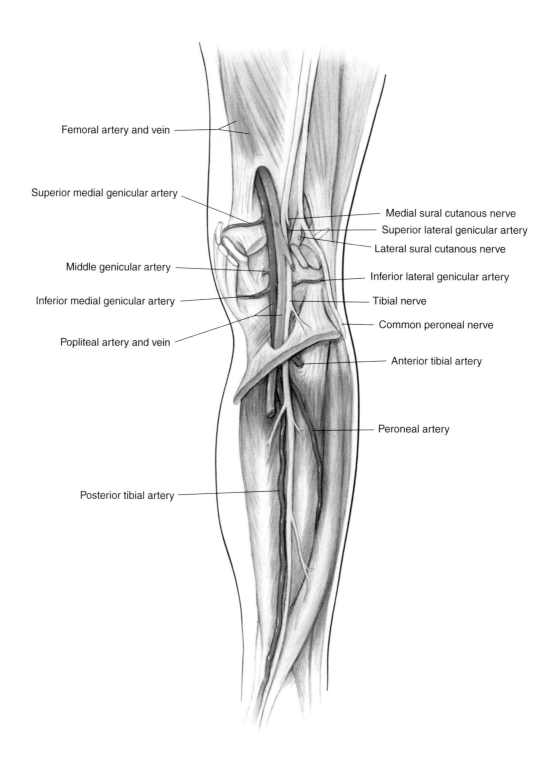

Femoral artery and vein

Superior medial genicular artery

Middle genicular artery

Inferior medial genicular artery

Popliteal artery and vein

Posterior tibial artery

Medial sural cutanous nerve

Superior lateral genicular artery

Lateral sural cutanous nerve

Inferior lateral genicular artery

Tibial nerve

Common peroneal nerve

Anterior tibial artery

Peroneal artery

FIGURE KL-12   Hazards in the thigh and leg.

ANTERIOR APPROACHES TO THE KNEE

Indications: Open ligament or cartilage procedures, knee arthroplasty

STANDARD APPROACH FOR TOTAL KNEE ARTHROPLASTY
(FIGURE KL-13)

- Positioning
  - Commercially available leg holders or positioners may be helpful
  - Supine

- Incision
  - Medial parapatellar incision (Figure KL-13A)
    - Traditional incision for knee arthroplasty
    - A 10-15 cm incision is made just medial to midline beginning several centimeters superior to the patella and extending to the tibial tubercle

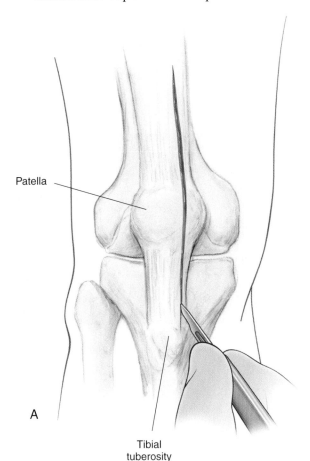

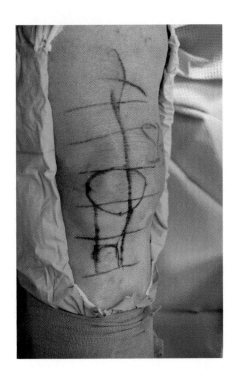

FIGURE KL-13   Standard anterior approach to the knee. **A,** Incision.

● Superficial and deep dissection (Figure KL-13B and C)

■ Subcutaneous tissue is dissected to expose the quadriceps tendon, patella, and patellar tendon

■ A vertical incision is made in the retinaculum leaving a 5 mm strip of tendon for later closure. The incision is curved around the patella and immediately adjacent to the patellar tendon

■ The patella can be everted, the knee flexed, and the joint exposed

■ Additional exposure of the proximal tibia can be accomplished by fat pad excision and subperiosteal dissection of the proximal medial tibia

■ Alternatives to the parapatellar incision include a midvastus or subvastus approach (Figure KL-13D)

● Closure

■ The extensor tendon and retinaculum are closed using heavy nonabsorbable suture

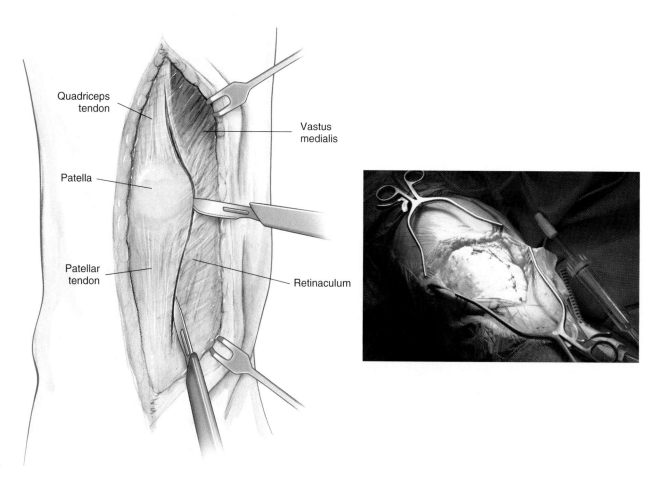

B

FIGURE KL-13, cont'd   B, Parapatellar dissection.

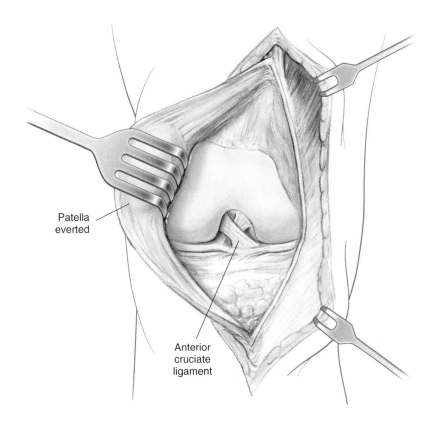

Patella
everted

Anterior
cruciate
ligament

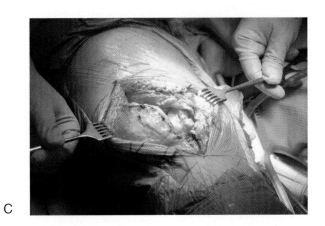

C

FIGURE KL-13, cont'd   C, Patella eversion.

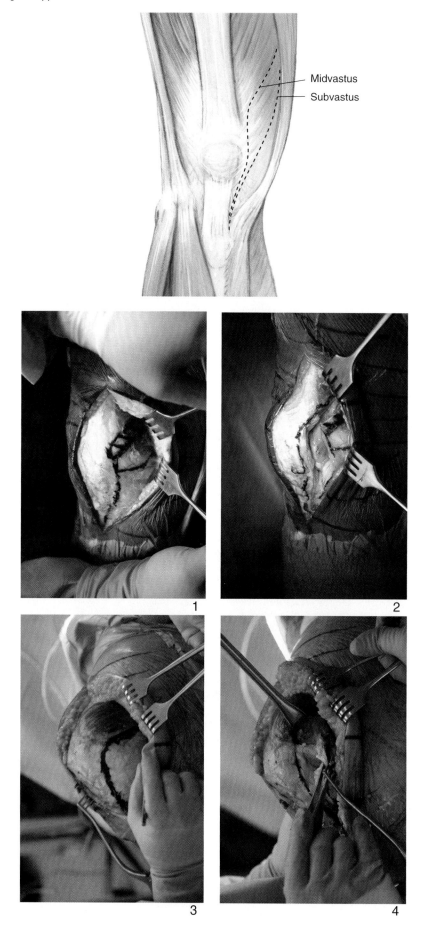

FIGURE KL-13, cont'd D, Midvastus (1 and 2) and subvastus (3 and 4) approaches.

LIMITED ANTERIOR INCISION (QUADRICEPS SPARING) (FIGURE KL-14A)

- Positioning
  - Commercially available leg holders or positioners may be helpful
  - Supine

- Incision
  - A 5 cm vertical incision is made starting distal to the quadriceps muscle

- Superficial and deep dissection (Figure KL-14B)
  - Subcutaneous tissue is dissected to expose the patella and patellar tendon
  - A vertical incision is made in the retinaculum leaving a 5 mm strip of tendon for later closure. The incision is curved around the patella and immediately adjacent to the patellar tendon
  - The dissection continues under the patella

- Closure
  - The extensor tendon and retinaculum are closed using heavy nonabsorbable suture

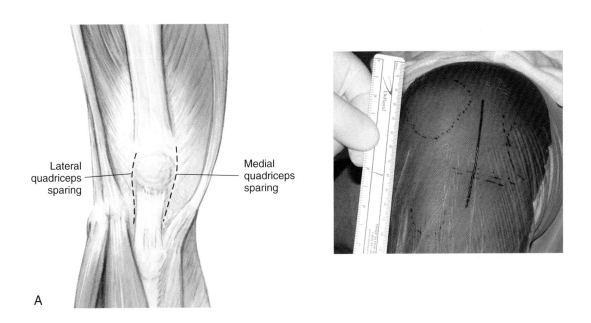

Lateral quadriceps sparing

Medial quadriceps sparing

A

FIGURE KL-14   Quadriceps sparing (limited) approach. **A,** Lateral and medial incision.

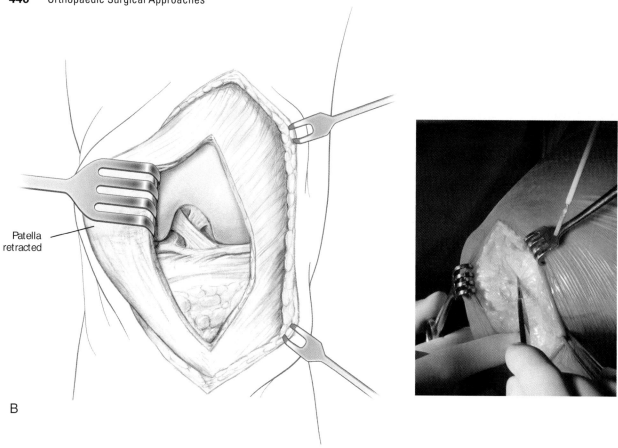

Patella
retracted

B

FIGURE KL-14, cont'd B, Patella retraction.

ANTERIOR APPROACH FOR PATELLA TENDON HARVEST

- **Positioning**

  - Commercially available leg holders or positioners may be helpful

  - End of the table is dropped to allow the knee to drop into flexion

- **Incision**

  - Only the inferior portion of the incision is made (from the midpatella to the tibial tuberosity)

- **Superficial and deep dissection (Figure KL-15)**

  - The paratenon is carefully dissected off the underlying tendon fibers

  - An appropriate graft is harvested with 25 mm of bone from the patella and the tibial tubercle

  - Bone graft is placed into the defect before closure

- **Closure**

  - Nonabsorbable suture is used to close the tissue over the patella and the patellar tendon paratenon, but not the tendon itself

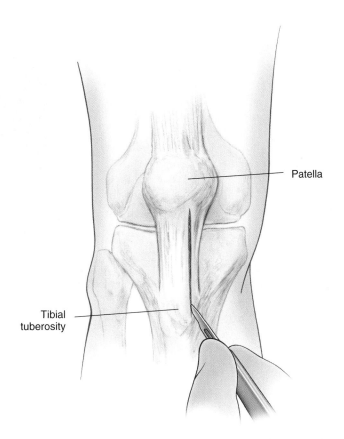

Patella

Tibial
tuberosity

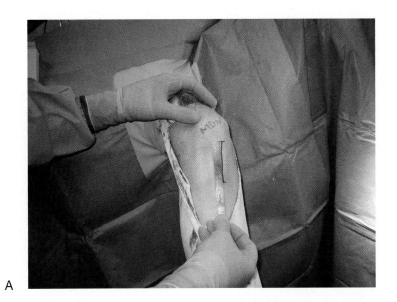

A

FIGURE KL-15   Patella tendon graft harvest. **A,** Skin incision.

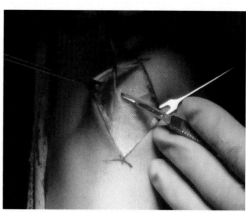

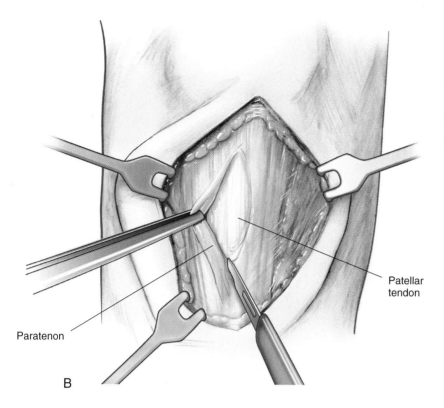

Patellar
tendon

Paratenon

B

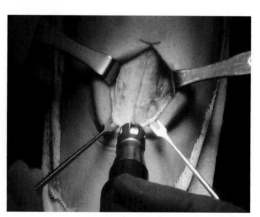

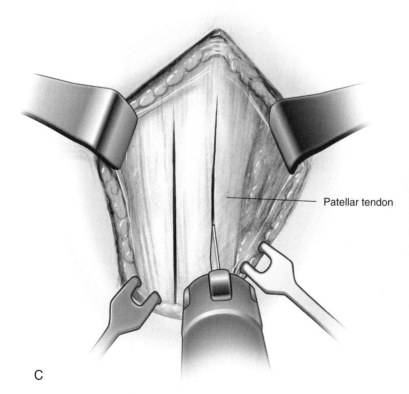

Patellar tendon

C

FIGURE KL-15, cont'd   **B,** Incision of paratenon to expose the patella tendon. **C,** Harvesting the middle third of the patella tendon.

INFEROMEDIAL APPROACH FOR HAMSTRING HARVEST

INCISION (FIGURE KL-16A)

- 3 cm vertical incision is centered 6 cm distal to the medial joint line adjacent to the tibial tubercle

SUPERFICIAL DISSECTION (FIGURE KL-16B)

- Skin and subcutaneous tissue dissected to expose the underlying sartorial fascia

DEEP DISSECTION (FIGURE KL-16C AND D)

- The sartorial fascia is carefully reflected off the underlying gracilis and semitendinosus tendons, which are then harvested
- Right-angle clamps are often helpful in identifying and dissecting these tendons
- Alternatively, the tendons can be harvested from the back side of the sartorial fascia by deep reflection
- Care should be taken to free up completely any attachments of the tendons (including major slips of the semitendinosus to the medial head of the gastrocnemius) before tendon harvesting

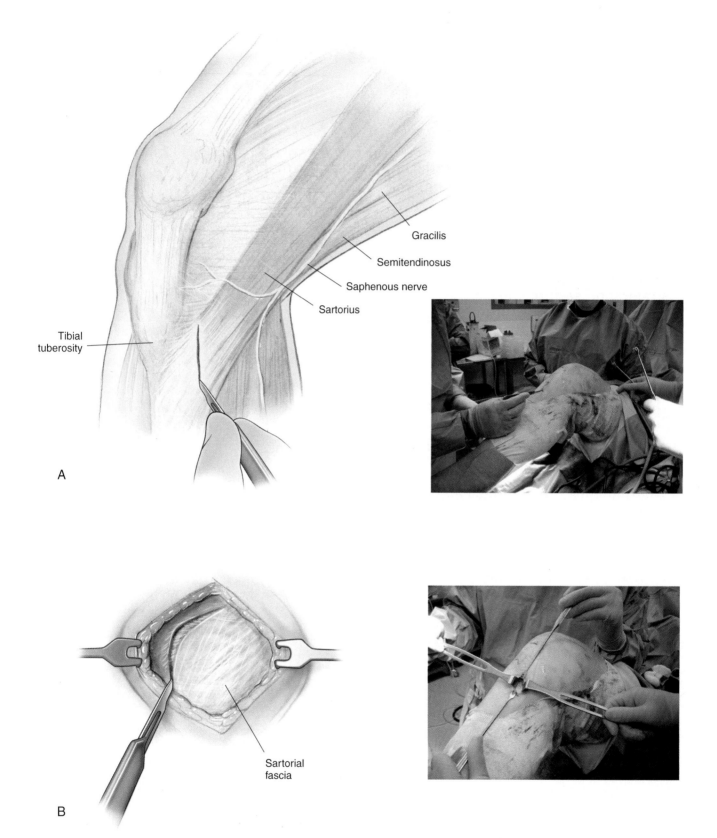

FIGURE KL-16   Inferomedial approach for hamstring harvest. **A,** Incision. **B,** Hockey-stick incision in the sartorial fascia.

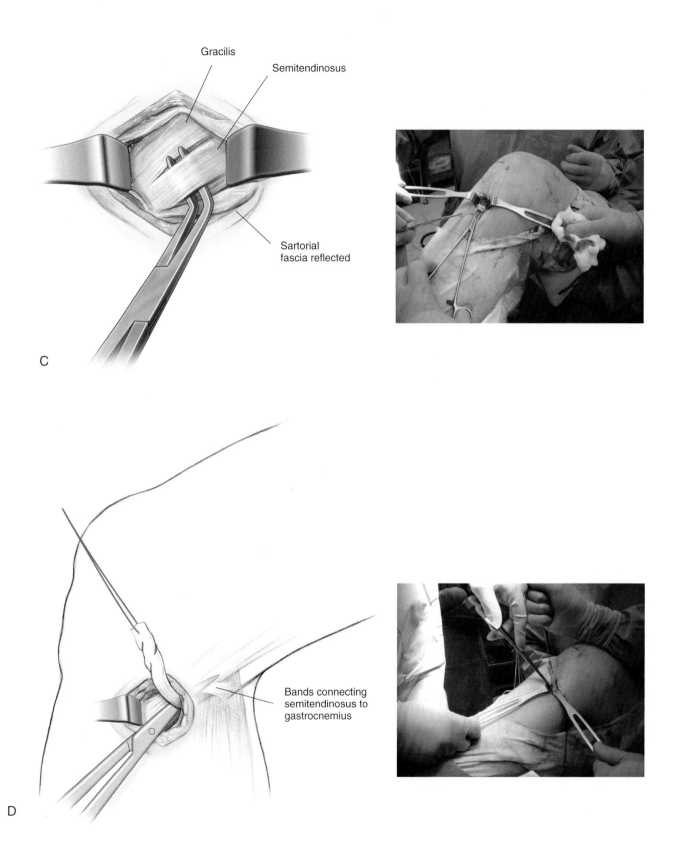

Gracilis

Semitendinosus

Sartorial
fascia reflected

C

Bands connecting
semitendinosus to
gastrocnemius

D

FIGURE KL-16, cont'd **C,** Right-angle clamp is used to grasp the tendon. **D,** Tendon is carefully freed of attachments.

MEDIAL APPROACH TO THE KNEE (Figure KL-17)

Indications: Medial collateral ligament repair or reconstruction, medial meniscal repair

POSITIONING

- ▧ Supine or knee holder
  - ● Can follow arthroscopy in this position

INCISION

- ● 8-10 cm vertical incision is centered on the posterior medial joint line
- ● Incision should be in the posterior half of the MCL

SUPERFICIAL DISSECTION

- ● Skin and subcutaneous tissues are dissected to expose the sartorial fascia
  - ▧ Identify and protect the saphenous and nerve branches
- ● Dissect the sartorial fascia, and make an incision along its fibers
  - ▧ Alternatively, the sartorial fascia can be reflected

DEEP DISSECTION

- ● Expose the MCL (the superficial fibers extend quite distal; the deep fibers are actually the thickened capsule in this area)
- ● A vertical incision can be made just posterior to the deep MCL to allow reefing of the posterior oblique ligament (capsular tissue that is posterior to the deep MCL)

CLOSURE

- ● Repair the sartorius using absorbable suture

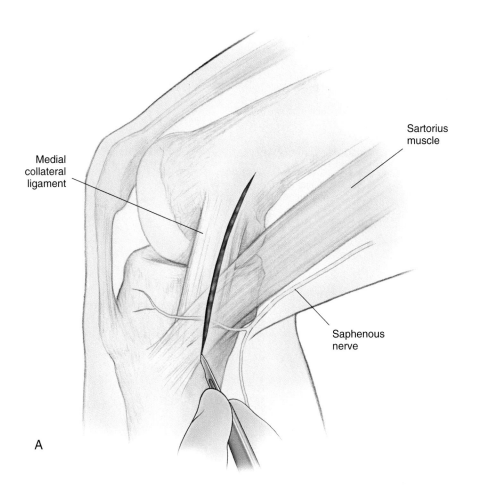

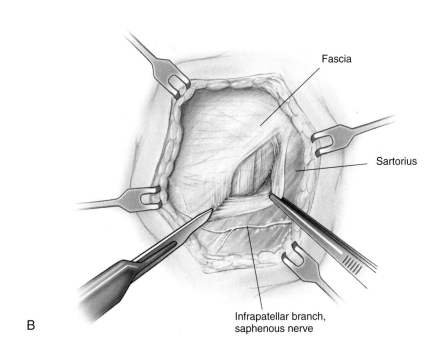

FIGURE KL-17   Medial approach to the knee. **A,** Incision. **B,** Superficial dissection.

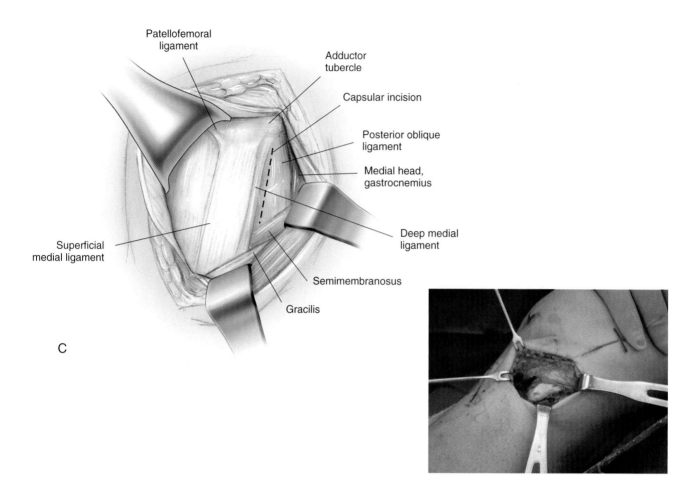

Patellofemoral ligament

Adductor tubercle

Capsular incision

Posterior oblique ligament

Medial head, gastrocnemius

Deep medial ligament

Superficial medial ligament

Semimembranosus

Gracilis

C

FIGURE KL-17, cont'd   C, Incision is made just posterior to the MCL.

MENISCAL REPAIR (FIGURE KL-18)

- For inside-out meniscal repair, a much smaller, 3 cm incision is made in the same area; most of the incision is below the joint line. The sartorial fascia is split or reflected, and the capsule is exposed. Posterior dissection, deep to the medial head of the gastrocnemius, is necessary for retractor placement

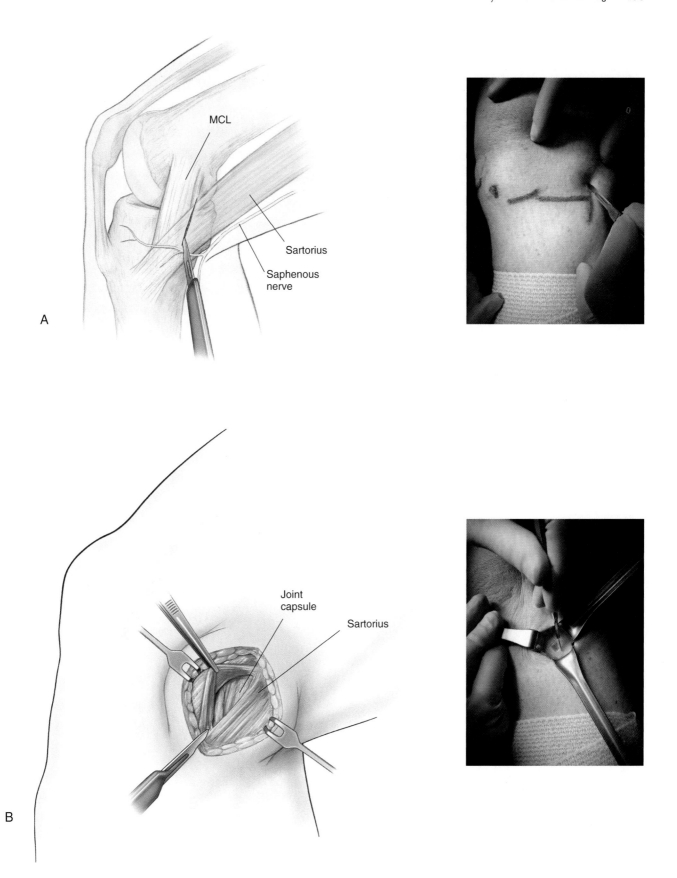

FIGURE KL-18   Medial meniscal repair. **A,** Incision. **B,** Sartorius is incised, and joint capsule is exposed.

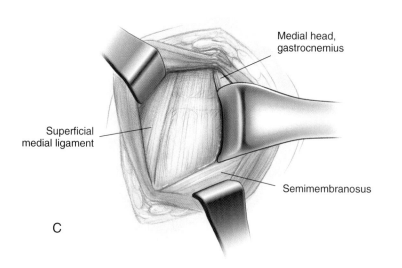

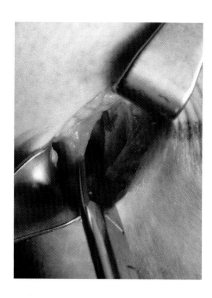

C

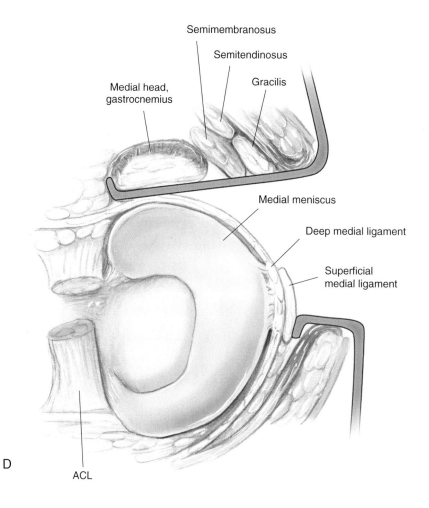

D

FIGURE KL-18, cont'd   **C,** Gastrocnemius is identified and retracted. **D,** Anatomy of the repair exposure.

LATERAL APPROACH TO THE KNEE (Figure KL-19)

Indications: Lateral or posterolateral repair or reconstruction, lateral meniscal repair

POSITIONING

- Supine or knee holder
  - Can follow arthroscopy in this position

INCISION

- 8-10 cm vertical incision is centered on the posterior lateral joint line
- Incision should be *behind the LCL* (palpable with the knee in the figure-4 position) and *anterior to the biceps tendon* (to protect the peroneal nerve)

SUPERFICIAL DISSECTION

- Skin and subcutaneous tissues are dissected to expose the iliotibial band and the biceps tendon

DEEP DISSECTION

- Identify and protect the peroneal nerve (just posterior to the biceps muscle); carefully dissect the nerve across the neck of the fibula
- Develop the interval between the iliotibial tract (posterior ⅓ of the iliotibial band) and the biceps (interval 1)
  - This allows identification of the LCL and popliteus tendon
- Develop the interval between the iliotibial band and tract (interval 2)
  - This allows identification of the lateral femoral epicondyle

CLOSURE

- Repair intervals 1 and 2 using absorbable suture

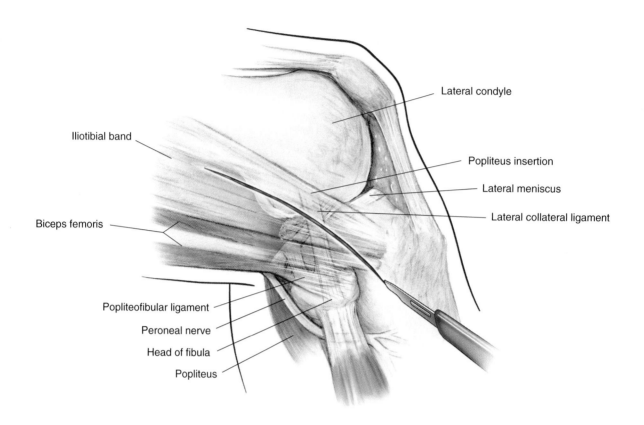

Lateral condyle

Iliotibial band

Popliteus insertion

Lateral meniscus

Lateral collateral ligament

Biceps femoris

Popliteofibular ligament

Peroneal nerve

Head of fibula

Popliteus

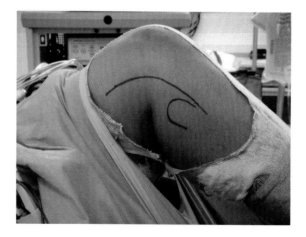

A

FIGURE KL-19 Lateral approach to the knee. **A,** Incision.

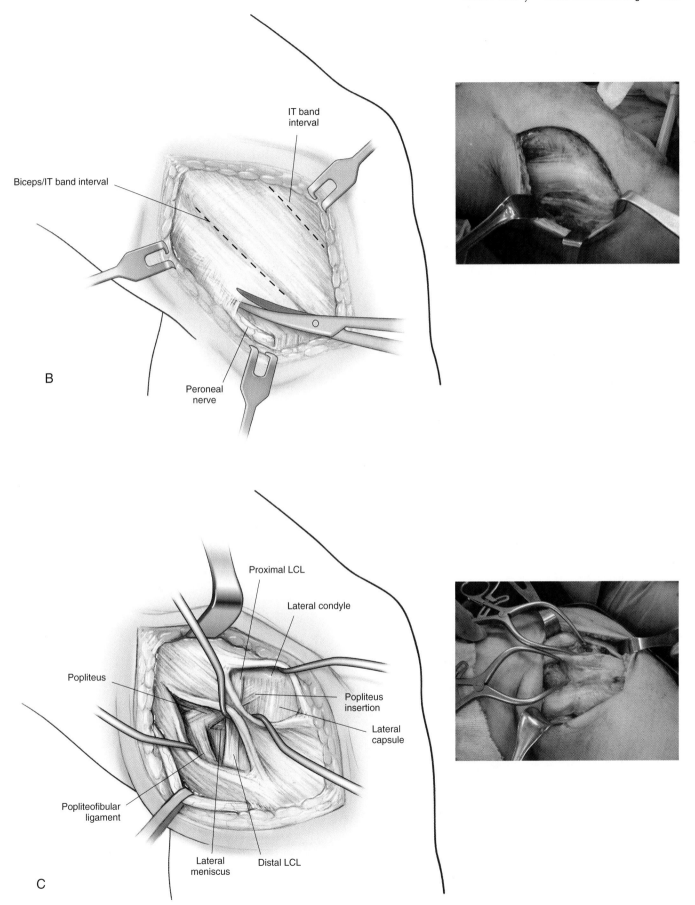

Biceps/IT band interval

IT band interval

Peroneal nerve

B

Proximal LCL

Lateral condyle

Popliteus

Popliteus insertion

Lateral capsule

Popliteofibular ligament

Lateral meniscus

Distal LCL

C

FIGURE KL-19, cont'd   B, Two intervals are identified. **C,** Deep dissection. IT, iliotibial.

MENISCAL REPAIR (FIGURE KL-20)

● For inside-out meniscal repair, a much smaller, 3 cm incision is made in the same area; most of the incision is below the joint line

● The biceps/iliotibibial band (interval 1) is developed, and the capsule is exposed. Posterior dissection, deep to the lateral head of the gastrocnemius, is necessary for retractor placement

● It is often necessary to dissect some fibers of the short head of the biceps femoris off the capsule

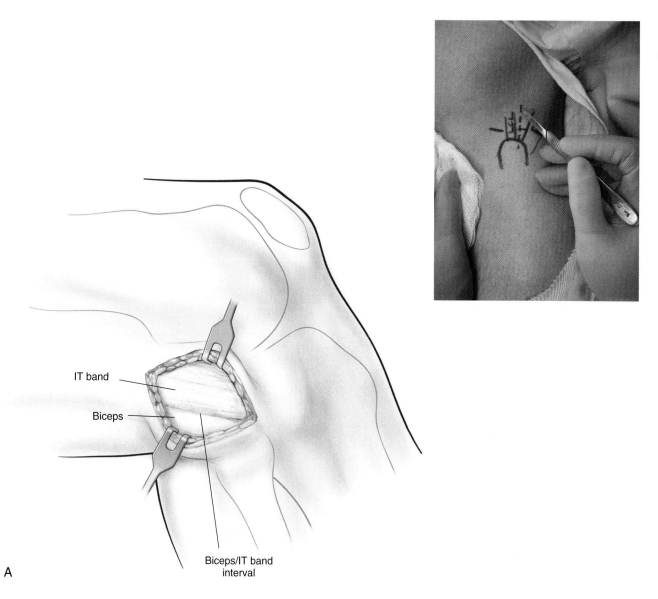

IT band

Biceps

Biceps/IT band interval

A

FIGURE KL-20   Lateral meniscal repair. **A,** Incision.

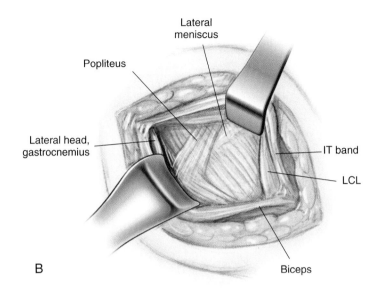

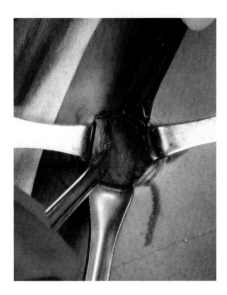

B, Interval between the biceps and iliotibial (IT) band is developed.

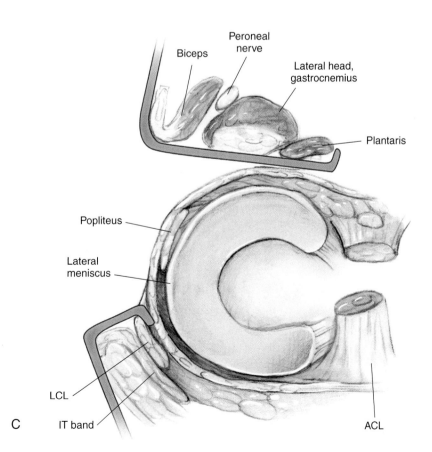

FIGURE KL-20, cont'd   B, Interval between the biceps and iliotibial (IT) band is developed. **C,** Anatomy of the repair.

POSTERIOR APPROACH TO THE KNEE (Figures KL-21 and KL-22)

Indications: PCL repair or reconstruction (tibial inlay technique)

POSITIONING

- Lateral decubitus or prone

INCISION

- Traditional approach
  - ▨ A long vertical S-shaped incision is made from proximal to distal, beginning laterally running obliquely across the popliteal fossa and then extending medially

- Inlay approach
  - ▨ 10 cm medial hockey-stick incision is made beginning in the popliteal crease horizontally and curving distally on the medial border of the calf

- Modified inlay approach
  - ▨ 6 cm horizontal incision is made in the popliteal crease

SUPERFICIAL DISSECTION

- Traditional approach
  - ▨ Subcutaneous tissues are dissected to expose the popliteal and gastrocnemius fascia
  - ▨ The small saphenous nerve and vein are identified distally and traced proximally

- Inlay approach
  - ▨ The gastrocnemius fascia is dissected in line with the incision
  - ▨ Interval between the medial head of the gastrocnemius is developed, and the gastrocnemius is mobilized laterally

- Modified inlay approach
  - ▨ The gastrocnemius fascia is incised horizontally and distally with subcutaneous retraction

DEEP DISSECTION

- Traditional approach

- **Inlay and modified inlay approach**
  - The medial head of the gastrocnemius is retracted laterally and held in place with ³⁄₃₂ Steinmann pins
  - The popliteal fascia and muscle belly are split exposing the back of the tibia
  - The 2 posterior eminences are palpated, and the PCL sulcus is identified and exposed

CLOSURE

- No deep closure is necessary
- It is often helpful to place a drain under the medial head of the gastrocnemius
- The skin and subcutaneous tissues are closed in the standard fashion

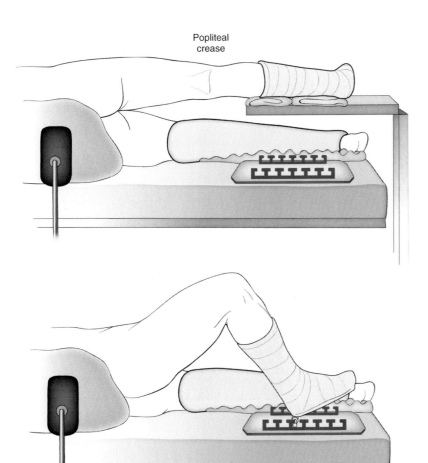

Popliteal crease

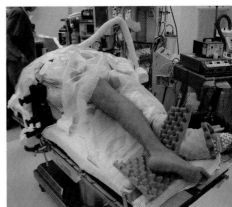

A

FIGURE KL-21   Posterior approach to the knee (modified inlay technique). **A,** Positioning.

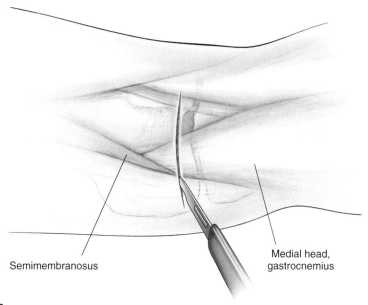

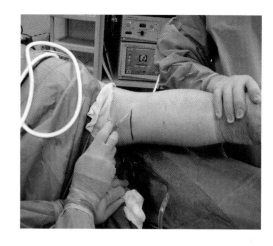

Semimembranosus

Medial head,
gastrocnemius

B

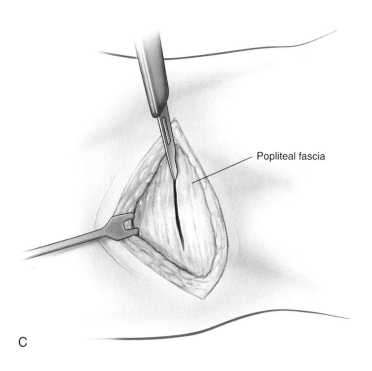

Popliteal fascia

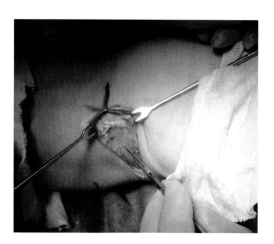

C

FIGURE KL-21, cont'd B, Incision. **C,** Popliteal fascia is excised.

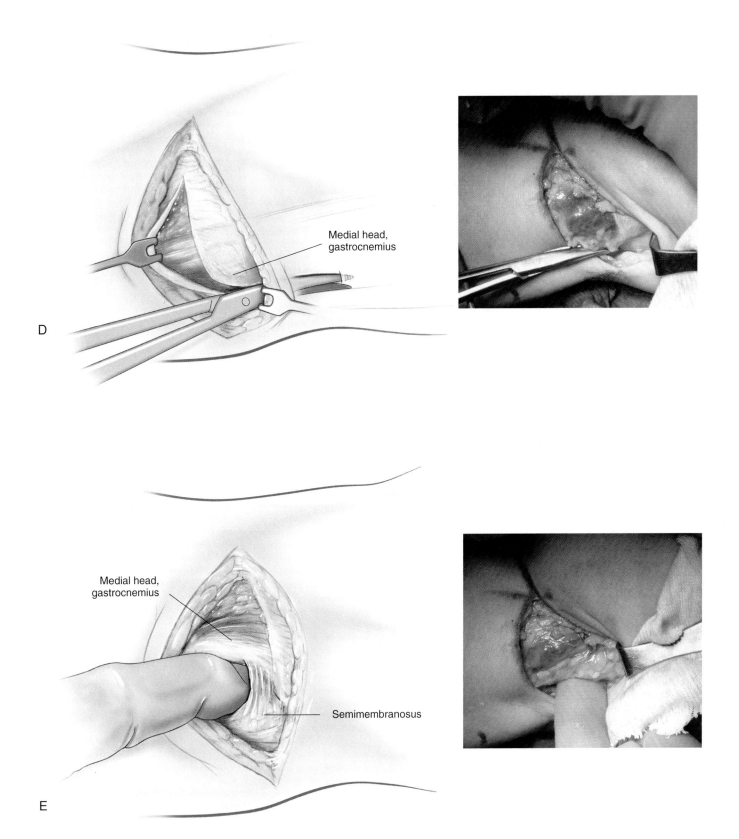

FIGURE KL-21, cont'd   D, Medial head of gastrocnemius exposed. **E,** Interval identified between the medial head of the gastrocnemius and the semimembranosus.

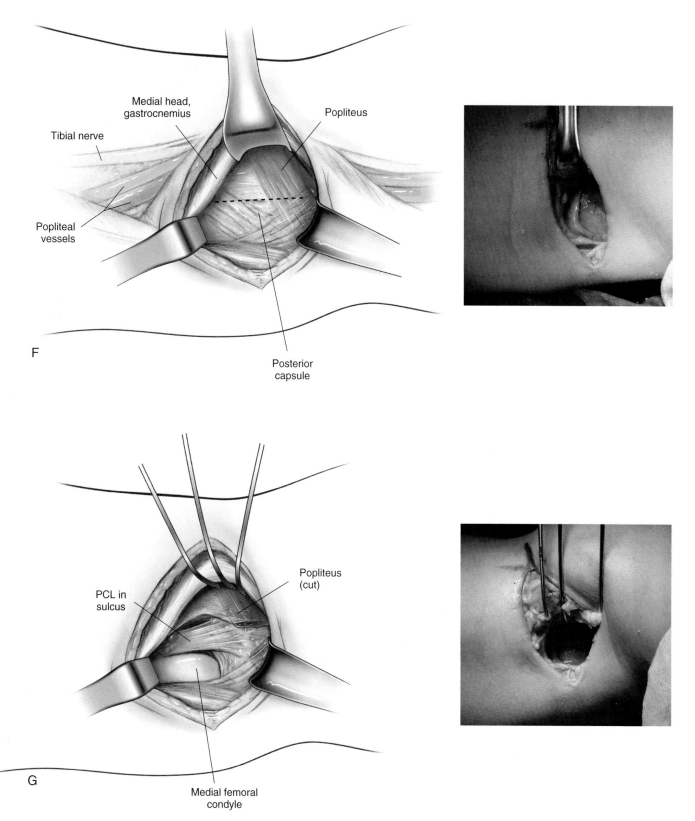

Medial head,
gastrocnemius

Popliteus

Tibial nerve

Popliteal
vessels

Posterior
capsule

F

PCL in
sulcus

Popliteus
(cut)

Medial femoral
condyle

G

FIGURE KL-21, cont'd   F, Vertical incision in the joint capsule. **G,** Steinmann pins retract the gastrocnemius for deep dissection.

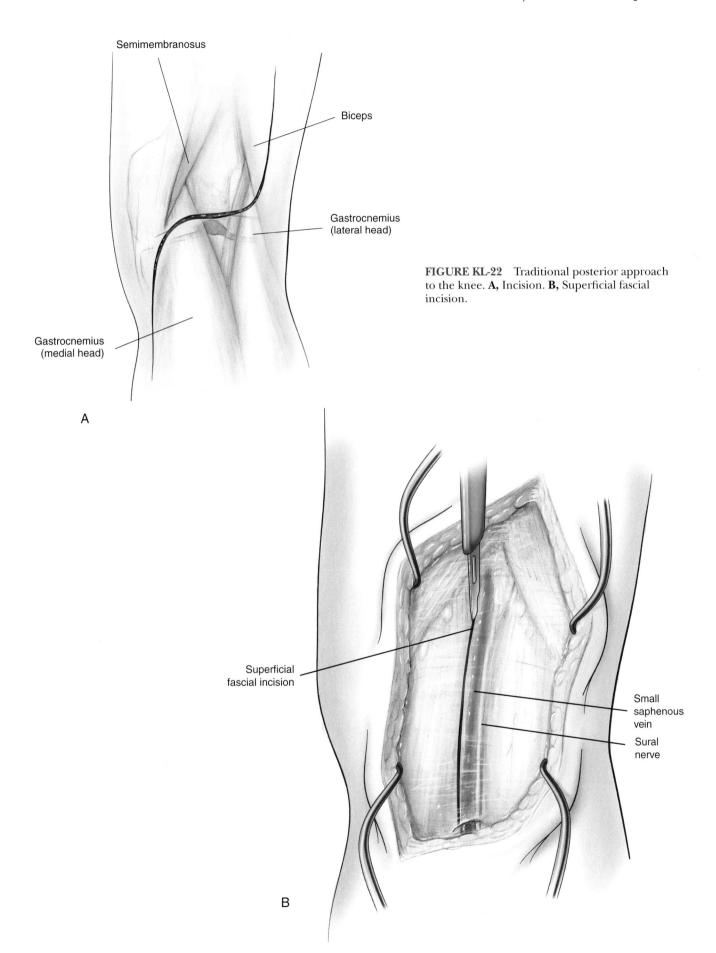

Semimembranosus

Biceps

Gastrocnemius
(lateral head)

Gastrocnemius
(medial head)

A

FIGURE KL-22 Traditional posterior approach to the knee. **A,** Incision. **B,** Superficial fascial incision.

Superficial
fascial incision

Small
saphenous
vein

Sural
nerve

B

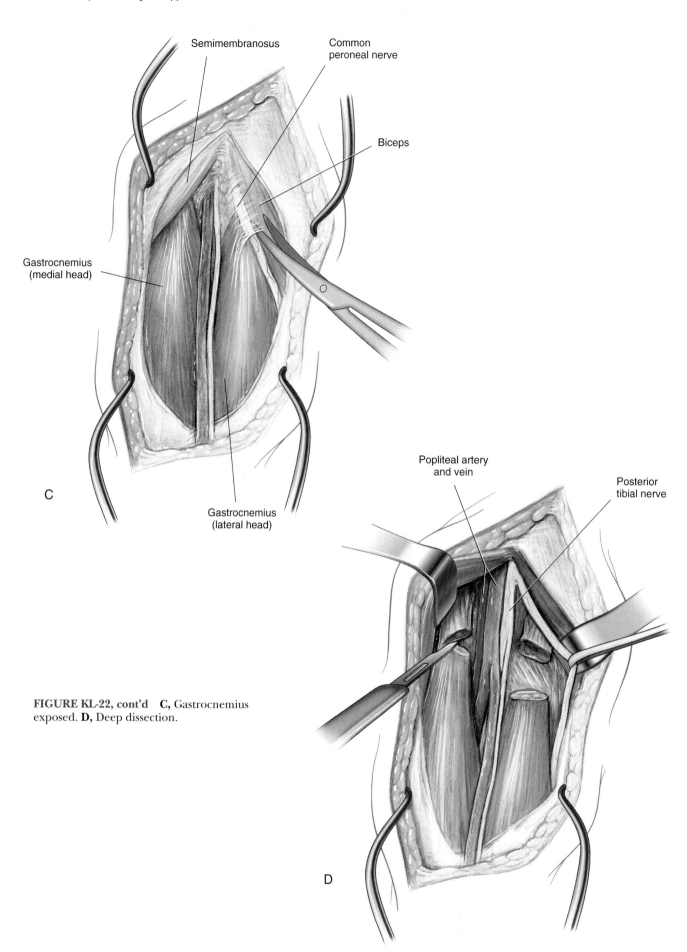

Semimembranosus

Common
peroneal nerve

Biceps

Gastrocnemius
(medial head)

Gastrocnemius
(lateral head)

C

Popliteal artery
and vein

Posterior
tibial nerve

D

FIGURE KL-22, cont'd   C, Gastrocnemius
exposed. **D,** Deep dissection.

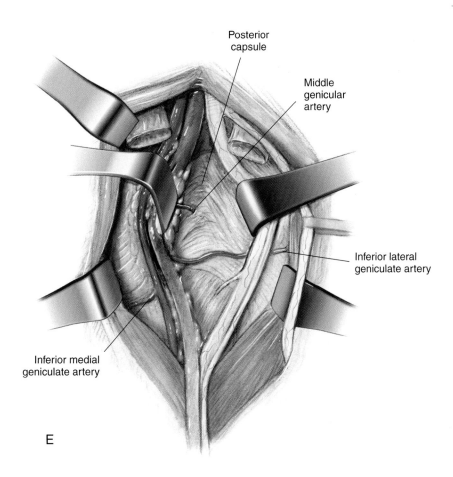

FIGURE KL-22, cont'd   E, Capsule is excised.

LATERAL APPROACH TO THE PROXIMAL TIBIA (Figure KL-23)

Indications: Lateral tibial plateau fracture

POSITIONING

- Patient is placed in a supine position on a radiolucent surgical table
- A bump or triangle is used to allow for knee flexion up to 90 degrees

INCISION

- 10 cm vertical lateral parapatellar skin incision

SUPERFICIAL DISSECTION

- The subcutaneous tissue is reflected laterally to expose the tibialis anterior fascia

DEEP DISSECTION

- A hockey-stick incision is made in the fascia, and the tibialis anterior is reflected laterally with an elevator to expose the proximal tibia
- The fascial incision should not be directly on bone to allow for primary closure
- An arthrotomy can be made through the proximal portion of the incision to inspect the joint
- When the level of the joint line is identified, the coronary ligaments are reflected perpendicular to the skin incision, and the meniscus is tagged with a nonabsorbable mattress stitch, which can be used to mobilize the meniscus and later to perform repair through the capsule
- The coronary ligaments and capsule can be sharply incised and the meniscus lifted up to allow better visualization

CLOSURE

- Additional nonabsorbable mattress sutures are placed into the meniscus with the ends of these sutures passed through the capsule with a free needle

- The capsule is closed and the meniscal sutures tied, completing the meniscal repair

- The tibialis anterior fascia should be closed primarily with a drain left deep to the muscle

- Subcutaneous and skin layers are closed in the usual fashion

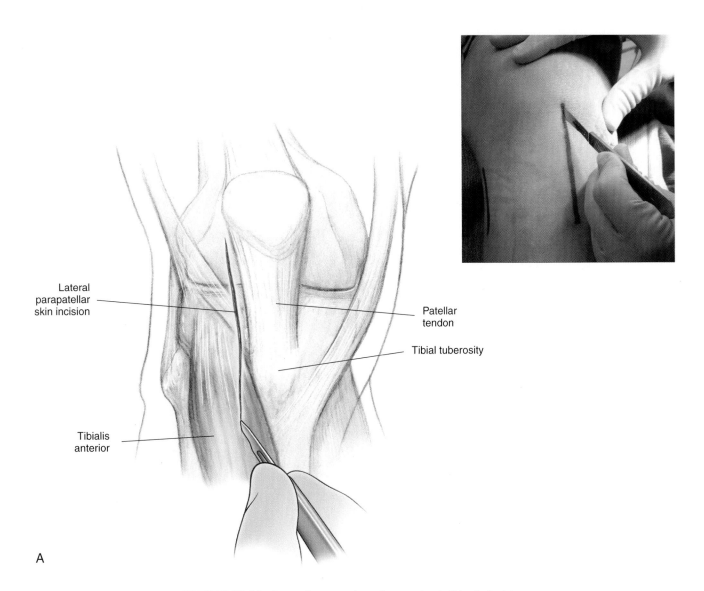

Lateral parapatellar skin incision

Patellar tendon

Tibial tuberosity

Tibialis anterior

A

FIGURE KL-23 Lateral approach to the proximal tibia. **A,** Incision.

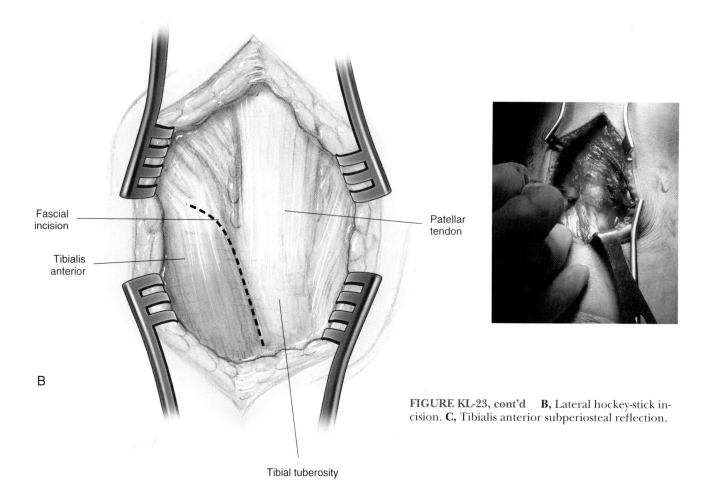

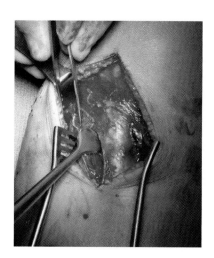

Fascial
incision

Tibialis
anterior

Patellar
tendon

B

Tibial tuberosity

FIGURE KL-23, cont'd **B,** Lateral hockey-stick incision. **C,** Tibialis anterior subperiosteal reflection.

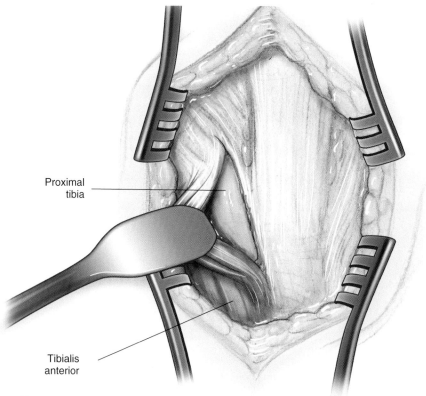

Proximal
tibia

Tibialis
anterior

C

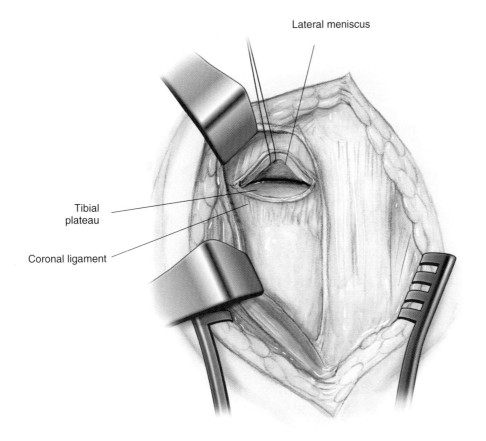

Lateral meniscus

Tibial
plateau

Coronal ligament

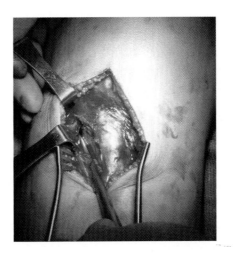

D

FIGURE KL-23, cont'd   D, Deep exposure.

MEDIAL APPROACH TO THE PROXIMAL TIBIA (Figure KL-24)

Indications: Medial tibial plateau fracture

POSITIONING

- Patient is placed in a supine position on a radiolucent surgical table
- A bump or triangle is used to allow for knee flexion up to 90 degrees

INCISION

- 10 cm medial parapatellar incision is made just behind the posteromedial border of the tibia

SUPERFICIAL DISSECTION

- Subcutaneous tissue and medial retinaculum is reflected to expose the medial head of the gastrocnemius and the semimembranosus

DEEP DISSECTION

- Develop the interval between the medial head of the gastrocnemius and the semimembranosus to expose the medial proximal tibia
- An arthrotomy can be made through the proximal portion of the incision to inspect the joint as described previously

CLOSURE

- Subcutaneous and skin layers are closed in the usual fashion

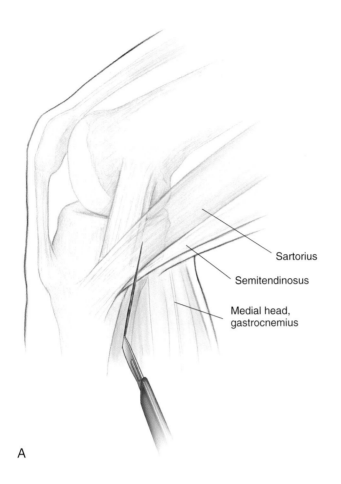

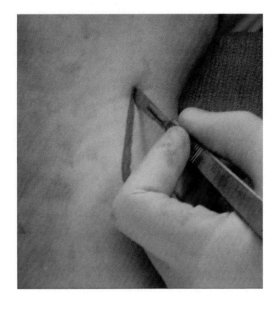

A

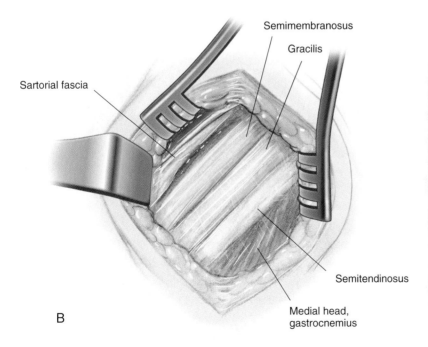

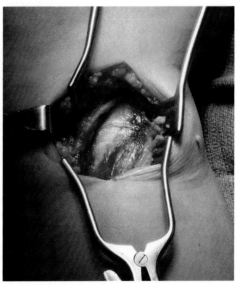

B

FIGURE KL-24   Medial approach to the proximal tibia. **A,** Incision. **B,** Interval between sartorius and semimembranosus.

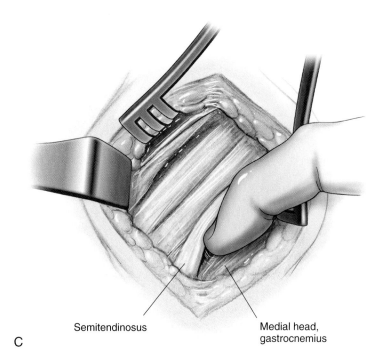

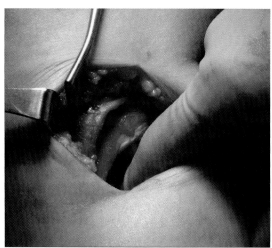

Semitendinosus

Medial head,
gastrocnemius

C

Semitendinosus

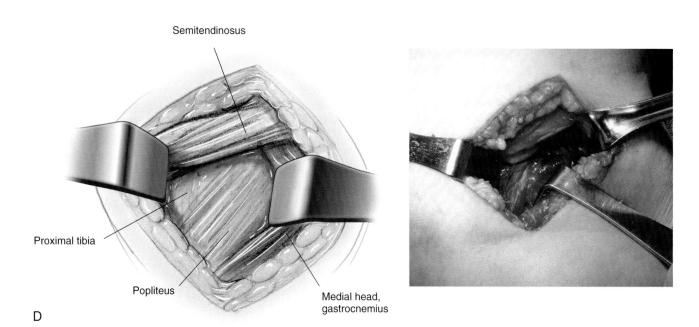

Proximal tibia

Popliteus

Medial head,
gastrocnemius

D

FIGURE KL-24, cont'd   **C** and **D,** Deep exposure.

LATERAL APPROACH TO THE LEG (Figure KL-25)

Indications: Compartment syndrome, fracture fixation

POSITIONING

- Supine with a bump
    - Padding of prominent structures is important

INCISION

- 10-15 cm longitudinal incision is made directly laterally
- For exertional compartment syndrome, 1-2 smaller incisions may be made

SUPERFICIAL DISSECTION

- Incise the fascia
- Protect the superficial peroneal nerve, which is located approximately 12 cm proximal to the distal tip of the lateral malleolus
- Identify the septum that divides the anterior and lateral compartments of the leg, and selectively release the fascia over the involved compartments, being careful not to go deep to the fascia

DEEP DISSECTION

- Exposure of the posterior tibia (e.g., for bone grafting) can be accomplished by dissecting posterior to the fibula and dissecting the deep posterior compartment (posterior tibialis) off the interosseous membrane to expose the tibia

CLOSURE

- Skin and subcutaneous tissues are closed in standard fashion

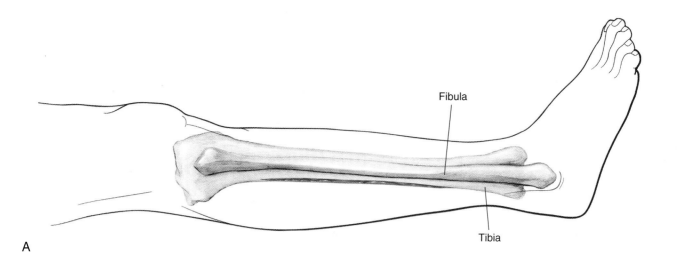

A

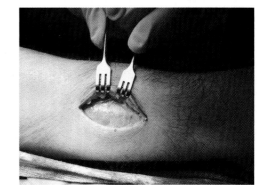

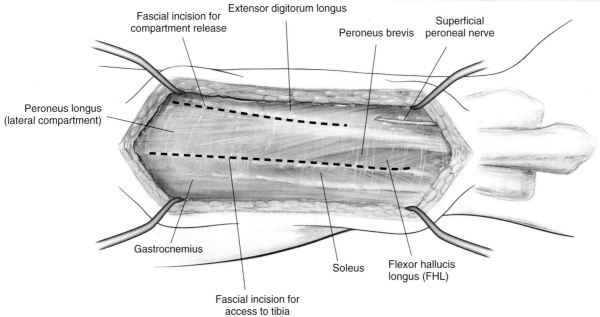

B

FIGURE KL-25   Lateral approach to the lower leg. **A,** Surface anatomy. **B,** Fascial incision.

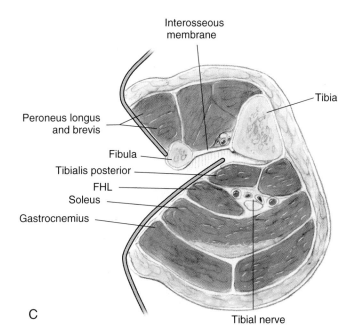

C

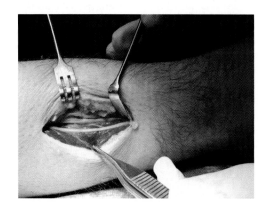

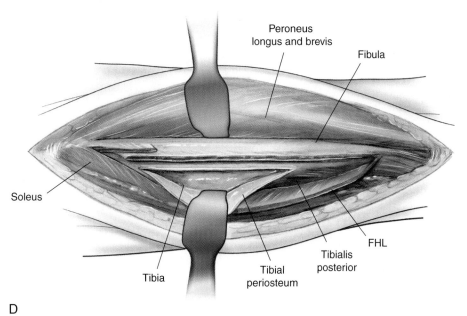

D

FIGURE KL-25, cont'd   **C,** Deep dissection **D,** Exposure of the compartments.

MEDIAL APPROACH TO THE LEG (Figure KL-26)

Indications: Compartment syndrome, fracture fixation

POSITIONING

- Supine with a bump
  - Padding of prominent structures is important

INCISION

- 10-15 cm longitudinal incision is made directly medially, just posterior to the tibia
- For exertional compartment syndrome, smaller incisions may be made

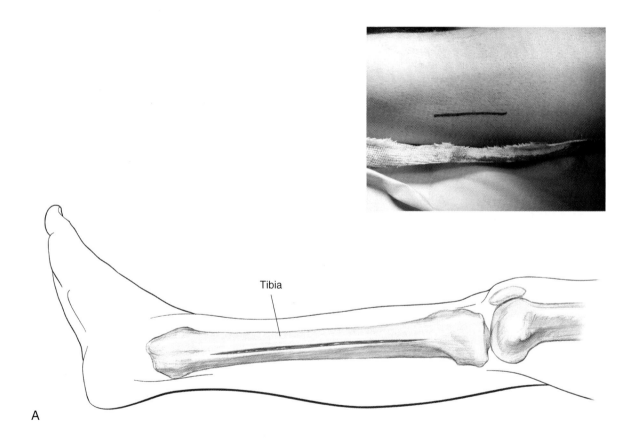

Tibia

A

FIGURE KL-26   Medial approach to the lower leg. **A,** Incision.

SUPERFICIAL DISSECTION

● Incise the fascia

DEEP DISSECTION

● Expose the posterior tibia

CLOSURE

● Skin and subcutaneous tissues are closed in standard fashion

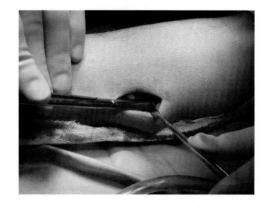

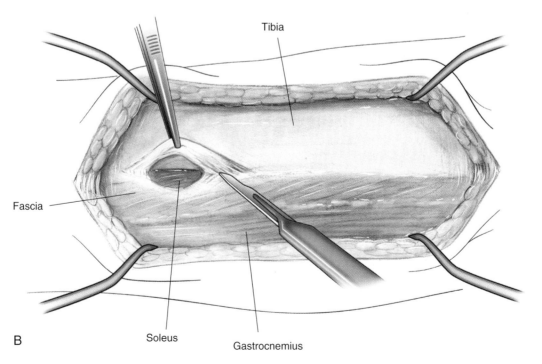

FIGURE KL-26, cont'd   B, Fascial incision.

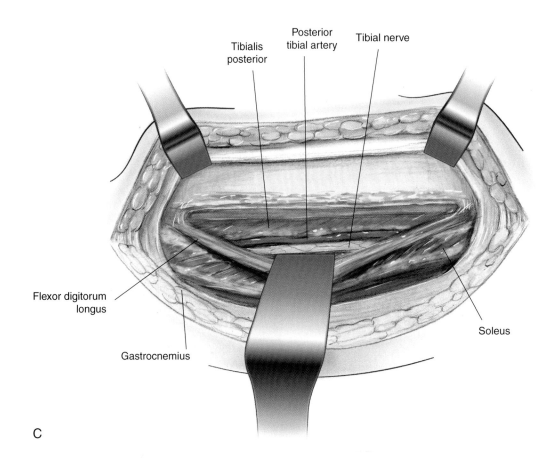

C

FIGURE KL-26, cont'd **C,** Deep dissection.

KNEE ARTHROSCOPY

Indications: Meniscal surgery, cruciate ligament repair or reconstruction, loose body removal, patellar procedures, articular cartilage procedures

POSITIONING (FIGURE KL-27)

- Supine with a leg holder or lateral post

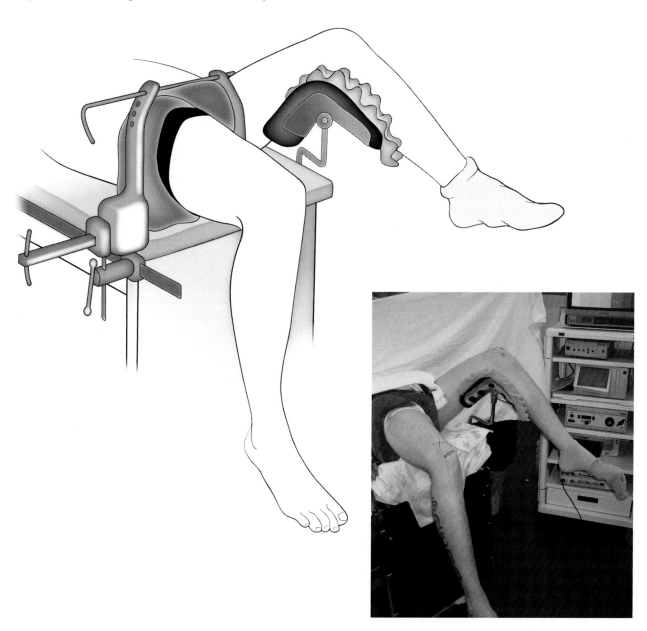

FIGURE KL-27   Positioning for knee arthroscopy.

PORTALS (FIGURES KL-28 THROUGH KL-31)

- **Inferolateral**
  - Location: just lateral to the patellar tendon and just above the joint line
  - Use: primary viewing portal

- **Inferomedial**
  - Location: just medial to the patellar tendon and just above the joint line
    - Some surgeons localize this portal from outside-in with a spinal needle before establishing the portal
  - Use: primary instrument portal
    - Also can be used for visualization based on access

- **Proximal portals**
  - Location: superior to the patella either lateral or medial
  - Use: optional use for inflow/outflow
    - Also can be used for visualization of patellar tracking

- **Posteromedial portal**
  - Location: just above the joint line, posterior to the joint
    - Typically located with a spinal needle while viewing the posteromedial aspect of the knee through a Gilquist or modified Gilquist portal (cannula is introduced into the back of the knee along the inferolateral aspect of the medial femoral condyle)
      - Care must be taken to avoid injuring the saphenous vein or nerve while establishing this portal
  - Use: posterior horn medial meniscus visualization, loose body removal, synovectomy

- **Posterolateral portal**
  - Location: just above the joint line, posterior to the joint
    - Typically located with a spinal needle while viewing the posterolateral aspect of the knee through the notch (cannula is introduced into the back of the knee along the inferomedial aspect of the lateral femoral condyle)
      - Care must be taken to avoid injuring the peroneal nerve while establishing this portal. *The portal must be anterior to the biceps tendon*
  - Use: posterior horn lateral meniscus visualization, loose body removal, synovectomy

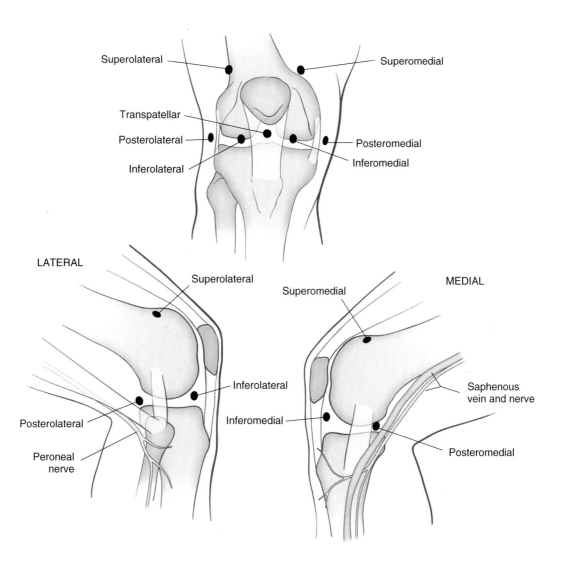

FIGURE KL-28   Portal for knee arthroscopy.

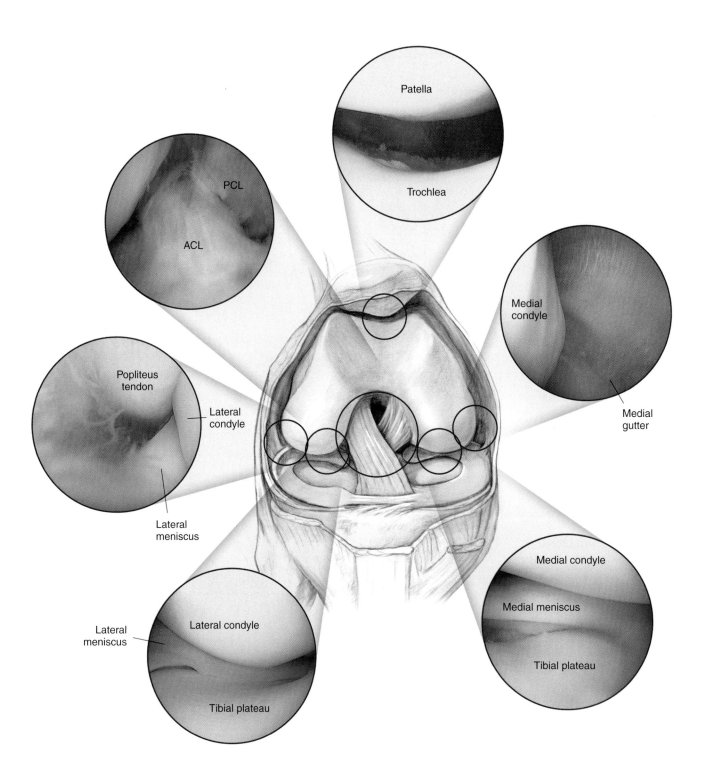

FIGURE KL-29   Arthroscopic visualization.

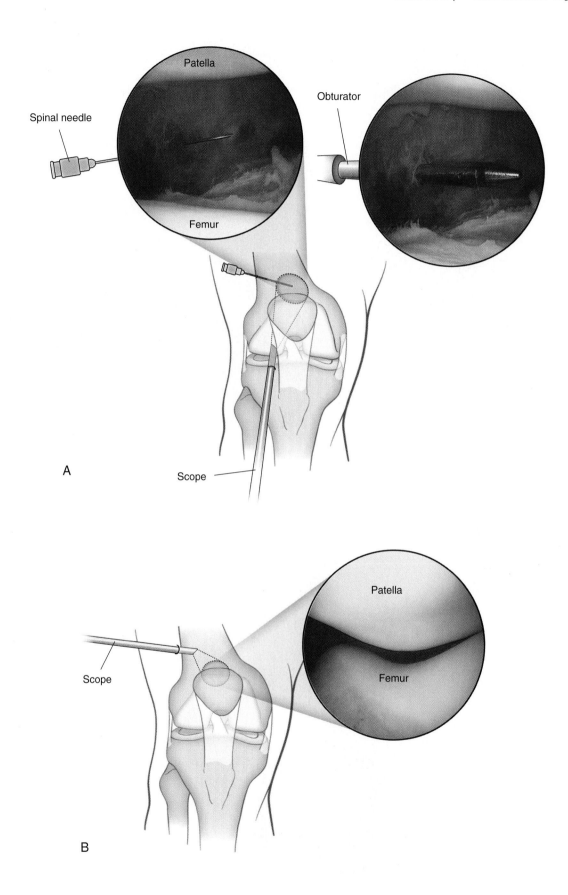

FIGURE KL-30 Proximal portal. **A,** Establishing the portal. **B,** View from the proximal portal.

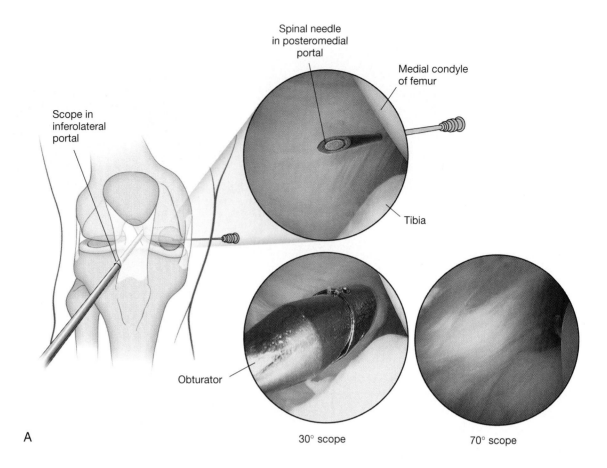

Spinal needle
in posteromedial
portal

Medial condyle
of femur

Scope in
inferolateral
portal

Tibia

Obturator

30° scope

70° scope

A

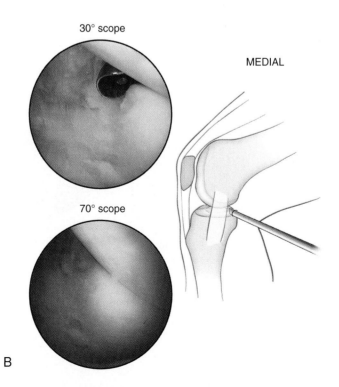

30° scope

MEDIAL

70° scope

B

FIGURE KL-31   Posterior portals. **A,** Posteromedial portal. **B,** View from the posteromedial portal.

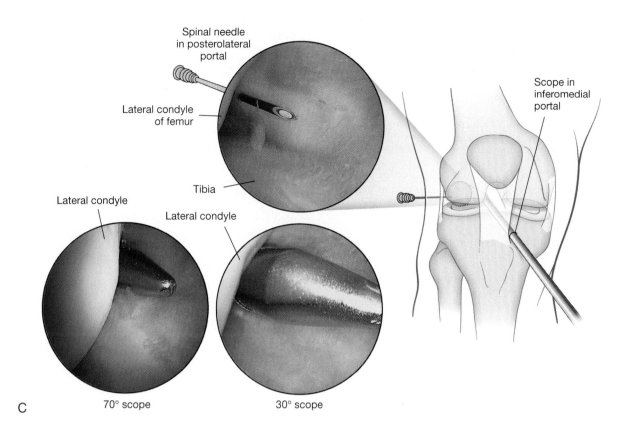

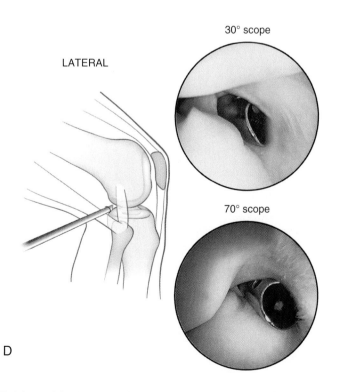

FIGURE KL-31, cont'd **C,** Posterolateral portal. **D,** View from the posterolateral portal.

REFERENCES

Arciero RA, Taylor DC: Inside-outside and all-inside meniscus repair: Indications, techniques, and results. Op Tech Orthop 5:58-69, 1995.

Berger RA, Deimengian CA, Della Valle CJ, et al: A technique for minimally invasive, quadriceps sparing total knee arthroplasty. J Knee Surg 19:63-70, 2006.

Burks RT, Schaffer JJ: A simplified approach to the tibial attachment of the posterior cruciate ligament. Clin Orthop 254:216-219, 1990.

Gold DL, Schaner PJ, Sapega AA: The posteromedial portal in knee arthroscopy: An analysis of diagnostic and surgical utility. Arthroscopy 11:139-145, 1995.

Miller MD, Osborne JR, Warner JJP, et al: Knee arthroscopy. In: MRI-Arthroscopy Correlative Atlas. Philadelphia, Saunders, 1997, pp 44-53.

Miller MD, Warner JJP, Harner CD: Meniscal repair. In Fu FH, Harner CD, Vince KG (eds): Knee Surgery. Baltimore, Williams & Wilkins, 1994, pp 615-630.

Mouhsine E, Garofalo R, Moretti B, et al: Two minimal incision fasciotomy for chronic exertional compartment syndrome of the lower leg. Knee Surg Sports Traumatol Arthrosc 14:193-197, 2006.

Noyes FR, Medvecky MJ, Bhargava M: Arthroscopically assisted quadriceps double-bundle tibial inlay posterior cruciate ligament reconstruction: An analysis of techniques and a safe operative approach to the popliteal fossa. Arthroscopy 19:894-905, 2003.

Palmeri M, Bartolozzi AR: Arthroscopic anterior cruciate ligament reconstruction with patellar tendon. Op Tech Orthop 6:126-134, 1996.

Scuderi GR, Tenholder M, Capeci C: Surgical approaches in mini-incision total knee arthroplasty. Clin Orthop 428:61-67, 2004.

Terry GC, LaPrade RF: The posterolateral aspect of the knee: Anatomy and surgical approach. Am J Sports Med 24:2-8, 1996.

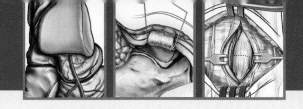

CHAPTER

8

FOOT AND ANKLE

——

SHEPARD R. HURWITZ

REGIONAL ANATOMY

Osteology

- **Talus (Figure FA-1)**

  - Three parts—body, neck, and head
  - No muscles or tendons attached
  - Superior surface is dome—large articular facet
  - Medial surface is rough inferiorly for attachment of the deltoid ligament and smooth superiorly with comma-shaped medial malleolar facet
  - Lateral surface has triangular lateral malleolar facet
  - These articulating surfaces—dome and medial and lateral malleolar facets—form the trochlea of the talus
  - Narrow posterior surface is directed medially ending as the posterior process of the talus and is grooved by the tendon of the flexor hallucis longus (FHL) into medial and lateral tubercles
  - Inferior surface has large concave posterior facet for calcaneus
  - Neck is directed forward and medially and bears the head, which articulates with navicular and plantar calcaneonavicular ligament and medially to deltoid ligament

- **Calcaneus (Figure FA-2)**

  - Thick, roughly rectangular bone that projects posteriorly, acting as a strong lever for the calf muscles
  - Posterior surface has an area for insertion of the Achilles tendon
  - Anterior surface is triangular, is concavoconvex, and articulates with the cuboid
  - Superior surface has 3 articular surfaces—posterior, middle, and anterior facets for the talus
  - The groove of the calcaneus is between the posterior and middle facets, and it opens laterally to a rough quadrangle
    - The groove with the talus above forms the sinus tarsi, where the interosseous talocalcaneal ligament attaches
    - The quadrangular ligament gives attachment to the inferior extensor retinaculum, the stem of the bifurcate ligament, and a part of the origin of the extensor digitorum brevis (EDB)
  - Inferior surface is marked by a groove and behind that by the anterior tubercle. Posteriorly are the lateral and the medial tubercles
  - Lateral surface has the peroneal tubercle or trochlea with the peroneus longus and brevis tendon grooving bone above and below
  - Medial surface is concave with an overhanging sustentaculum tali and projecting medial tubercle. The bridge of the flexor retinaculum between them converts the groove into a tunnel
  - The thick medial border of the sustentaculum, with the tendons of the tibialis posterior above and flexor digitorum longus (FDL) on its medial margin, is grooved inferiorly by the tendon of the FHL
    - The plantar calcaneonavicular (spring) ligament attaches to the medial margin of the sustentaculum anteriorly and the medial talocalcaneal ligament posteriorly

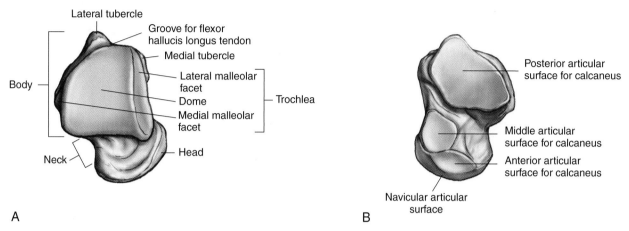

FIGURE FA-1 A, Talus—superior view. **B,** Talus—inferior view.

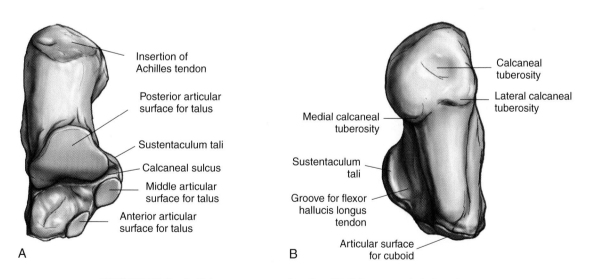

FIGURE FA-2   A, Calcaneus—superior view. **B,** Calcaneus—inferior view.

- Cuboid (Figure FA-3)

  - Pyramidal shaped
  - Anterior surface articulates with 4th-5th metatarsal base
  - Posterior surface articulates with calcaneus
  - Superior surface has ligamentous attachments
  - Inferior surface has tuberosity and groove for peroneus tendon
  - Lateral surface has groove for peroneus longus tendon and a small facet for the cartilage of the sesamoid bone
  - Medial surface articulates with the late cuneiform and with the navicular

- Navicular (see Figure FA-3)

  - Navicular means "boat-shaped" in Latin
  - Oval posterior facet for the talar head
  - Anterior surface is convex for the 3 cuneiforms
  - Spring ligament is attached to plantar surface, which also has the groove for tibialis posterior tendon
  - Lateral surface articulates with navicular
  - Superior surface merges with the medial and has the tuberosity to which the anterior fibers of the deltoid are attached along with the main insertion of the tibialis posterior tendon

- Cuneiforms (see Figure FA-3)

  - Means "wedge shaped"
  - There are 3 cuneiforms—medial, intermediate, and lateral
  - Medial cuneiform
    - Largest; articulates anteriorly with base of 1st metatarsal, posteriorly with navicular, laterally with intermediate cuneiform and medial side of base of 2nd metatarsal
  - Intermediate cuneiform
    - Smallest of 3 cuneiforms
  - Lateral cuneiform
    - Articulates with navicular, cuboid, intermediate cuneiform, and base of 3rd metatarsal; has medial and lateral facets for 2nd and 4th metatarsals

- Metatarsals (Figure FA-4)

  - Five metatarsals are located side by side in the forefoot and contribute to longitudinal and transverse arch
  - Each metatarsal consists of the base, shaft, and head
  - The heads touch the ground anteriorly and share the load of the body (1st metatarsal head bears double the weight compared with the rest)
  - 1st metatarsal is stout and strong, whereas the rest are long and slender

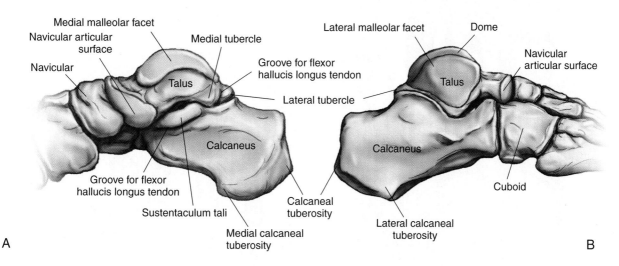

FIGURE FA-3　**A,** Hind foot—medial view. **B,** Hind foot—lateral view.

- ● Phalanges (see Figure FA-4)
  - ▤ There are 2 phalanges in the big toe and 3 in each of the others
  - ▤ Each phalanx possesses a shaft and a proximal base larger than its distal head
  - ▤ Both phalanges of the big toe are much heavier and stronger than the others
- ● Sesamoids
  - ▤ Bones that lie within tendons and have an articular surface covered with hyaline cartilage
  - ▤ Situated where tendons cross joints and change the direction of pull of tendons
  - ▤ Also improve mechanical advantage of tendon
  - ▤ Constant sesamoids are medial and lateral sesamoids
  - ▤ Inconstant sesamoids
    - ● Subhallux sesamoid
    - ● Sesamoid of tibialis posterior tendon
    - ● Sesamoid in the peroneus longus tendon
    - ● Sesamoids under metatarsal heads, commonly under 2nd and 5th heads

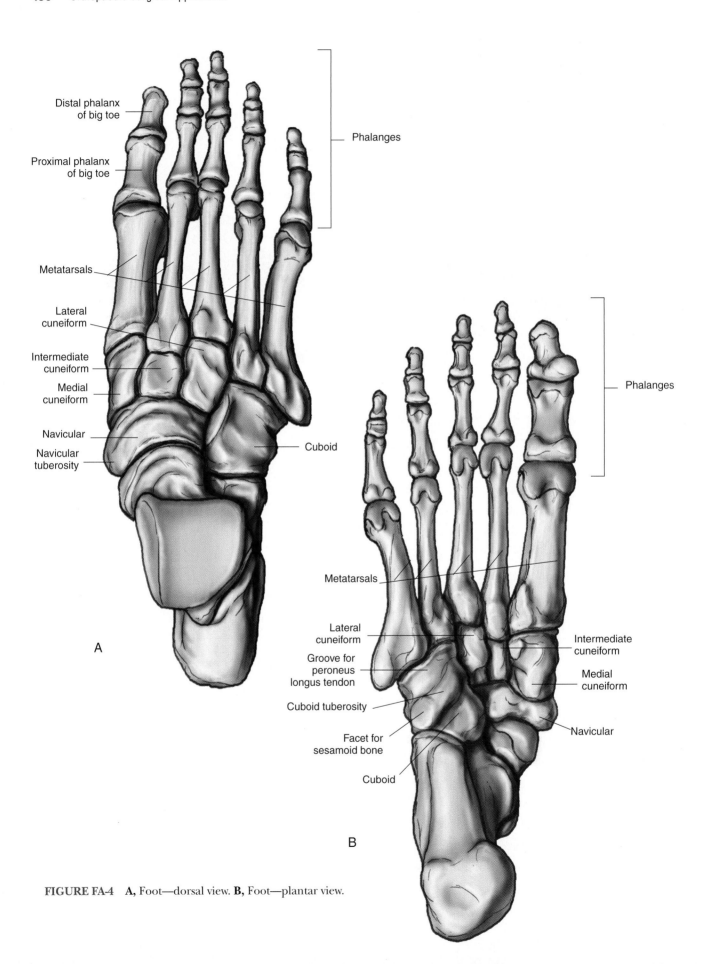

Distal phalanx
of big toe

Proximal phalanx
of big toe

Phalanges

Metatarsals

Lateral
cuneiform

Intermediate
cuneiform

Medial
cuneiform

Navicular

Navicular
tuberosity

Cuboid

A

Phalanges

Metatarsals

Lateral
cuneiform

Groove for
peroneus
longus tendon

Cuboid tuberosity

Facet for
sesamoid bone

Cuboid

Intermediate
cuneiform

Medial
cuneiform

Navicular

B

FIGURE FA-4   **A,** Foot—dorsal view. **B,** Foot—plantar view.

Arthrology

- Ankle joint (Figures FA-5, FA-6, and FA-7)

  - Strong and stable joint
  - Synovial hinge joint
  - Capsule encloses joint and is attached to bony articular margins
  - Ligaments
    - Medial/deltoid ligament
    - Lateral ligaments
    - Anterior talofibular ligament
    - Calcaneofibular ligament
    - Posterior talofibular ligament
  - Nerve supply
    - Deep peroneal and tibial nerve
  - Movements
    - Dorsiflexion
    - Plantar flexion

- Subtalar joint (see Figures FA-5, FA-6, and FA-7)

  - Plane synovial joint
  - Capsule attaches to articular margins of talus and calcaneus
  - Ligaments
    - Medial and lateral talocalcaneal ligaments
    - Interosseous talocalcaneal ligament (main support)
  - Movements
    - Inversion
    - Eversion

- Talocalcaneonavicular joint (see Figures FA-5, FA-6, and FA-7)

  - Synovial joint
  - Capsule incompletely encloses joint
  - Ligaments
    - Plantar calcaneonavicular ligament
  - Movements
    - Gliding and rotatory movements
    - Limited inversion and eversion

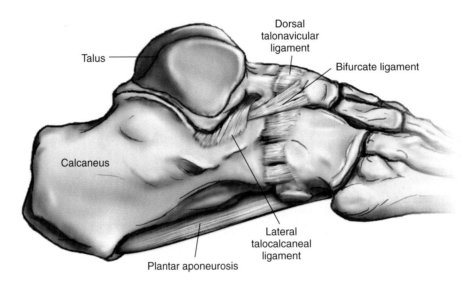

Talus

Dorsal
talonavicular
ligament

Bifurcate ligament

Calcaneus

Lateral
talocalcaneal
ligament

Plantar aponeurosis

FIGURE FA-5   Ligaments of the hind foot—lateral view.

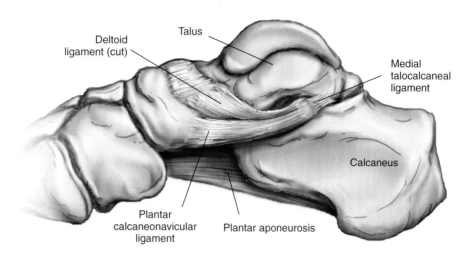

FIGURE FA-6   Ligaments of the hind foot—medial view.

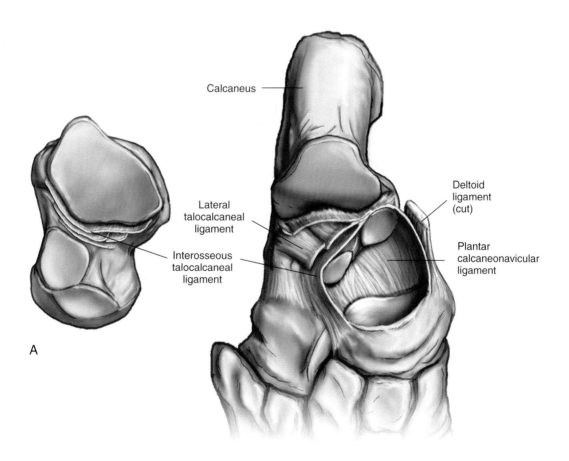

FIGURE FA-7   A, Inferior view of talus showing the interosseous ligament. **B,** Dorsal view of the hind foot (after removal of talus) showing the calcaneal facets with the spring ligaments.

- **Calcaneocuboid joint (Figure FA-8)**
  - Plane synovial
  - Capsule encloses the joint
  - Ligaments
    - Bifurcated "Y" ligaments
    - Long plantar ligament
    - Short plantar ligament
  - Movements
    - Limited inversion and eversion

- **Cuneonavicular (see Figure FA-8)**
  - Synovial joint of gliding variety between navicular and 3 cuneiforms
  - Capsule reinforced by dorsal and plantar ligaments
  - Joint cavity continuous with intercuneiform, cuneocuboid, cuneometatarsal, and intermetatarsal joints

- **Cuboideonavicular (see Figure FA-8)**
  - Fibrous joint
  - Dorsal, plantar, and interosseous ligaments reinforce joint stability

- **Intercuneiform and cuneocuboid (see Figure FA-8)**
  - Plane synovial joints
  - Stabilized by dorsal, plantar, and interosseous ligaments
  - Joint cavity communicates with cavity of cuneonavicular joint
  - Cuneocuboid joint is syndesmosis

- **Tarsometatarsal (Lisfranc joint) and intermetatarsal joints (see Figure FA-8)**
  - Plane synovial joints
  - Tarsometatarsal joint of great toe has separate joint cavity
  - Stabilized by dorsal, plantar, and interosseous ligaments
  - Movements
    - Plantar flexion–dorsiflexion—1st cuneometatarsal, 4th and 5th
    - Rotation

- **Metatarsophalangeal (MTP) and interphalangeal joints (see Figure FA-8)**
  - MTP joints are condyloid joints
  - Stabilized by plantar plates and oblique collateral ligaments
  - Deep transverse ligaments connect all 5 MTP joints
  - 2nd toe is long axis, and adduction-abduction is performed by interossei
  - Interphalangeal joints are hinge joints
    - Stabilized by collateral ligaments, capsular plantar ligament (fibrous plate)
    - Only plantar flexion movement

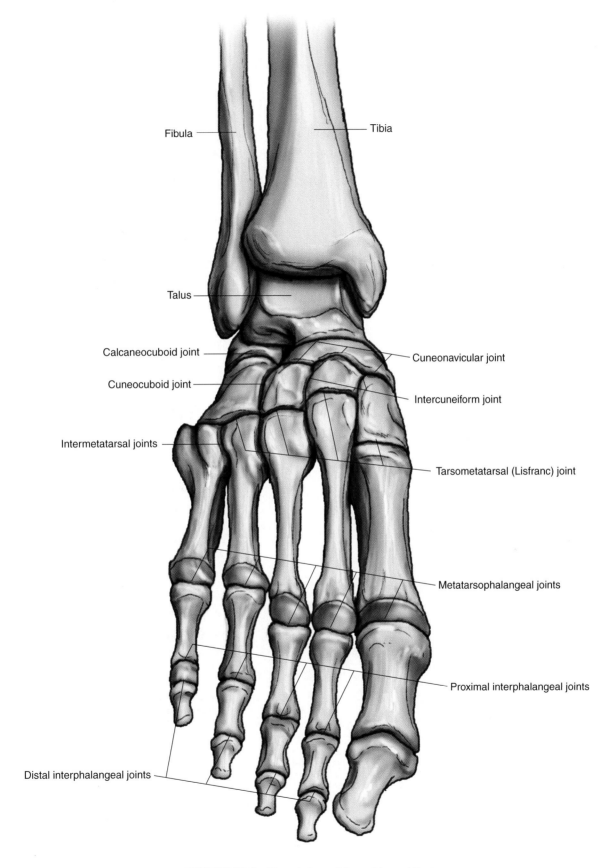

FIGURE FA-8 Dorsal view of the ankle and foot.

● Arches of the foot

  ■ Maintained by shape of bones, strong ligaments, tendons, and muscle tone
    ● Lateral longitudinal (Figure FA-9)
      ○ Lateral half of calcaneus, cuboid, 4th and 5th metatarsal bones
    ● Medial longitudinal (Figure FA-10)
      ○ Medial half of calcaneus, talus, navicular, 3 cuneiforms, and first 3 metatarsals
    ● Transverse arch (Figure FA-11)
      ○ Bases of metatarsal bones, cuboid, and 3 cuneiforms

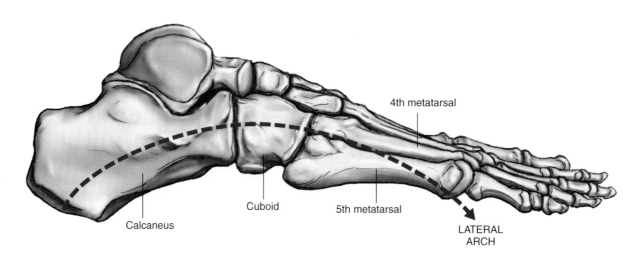

FIGURE FA-9 Lateral bony plantar arch.

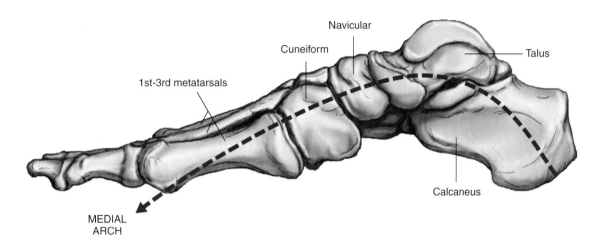

FIGURE FA-10   Medial bony plantar arch.

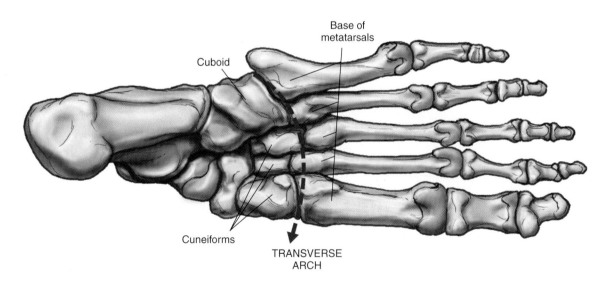

FIGURE FA-11   Transverse bony arch.

Muscles

- Extrinsic muscles
  - Muscles are in the leg, but their tendons function within the foot
    - Anterior compartment (innervated by deep peroneal/anterior tibial nerve) (Figure FA-12)
      - From medial to lateral—tibialis anterior, extensor hallucis longus (EHL), extensor digitorum longus (EDL), and peroneus tertius
    - Lateral compartment (innervated by superficial peroneal nerve) (Figure FA-13)
      - Peroneus longus and brevis muscle
      - Tendons descend together in a common tendon sheath underneath superior peroneal retinaculum
    - Posterior compartment (innervated by posterior tibial nerve) (Figures FA-14, FA-15, and FA-16)
      - Superficial layer
        - Triceps surae
      - Deep layer
        - FDL
        - Tibialis posterior
        - FHL
    - Functions
      - Plantar flexors
        - Triceps surae
        - Tibialis posterior
        - Assisted by peroneals, FHL, and FDL
      - Dorsiflexors
        - Tibialis anterior
        - Assisted by EHL, EDL, and peroneus tertius
      - Eversion
        - Peroneus longus, brevis, and tertius
      - Inversion
        - Tibialis anterior and posterior

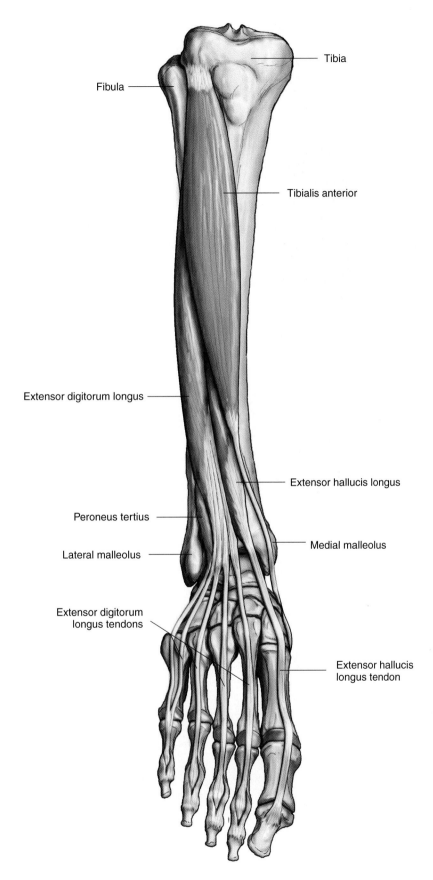

FIGURE FA-12 Muscles of the anterior compartment of the leg and dorsum of the foot.

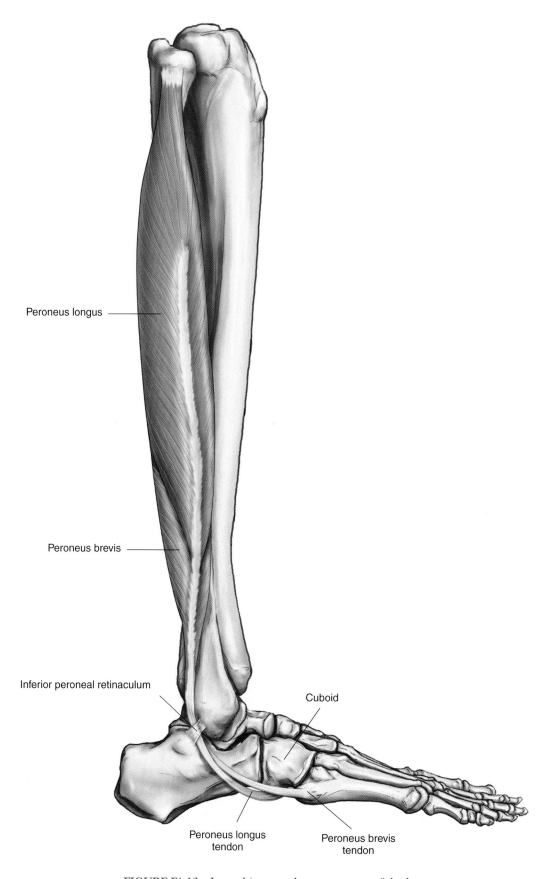

Peroneus longus

Peroneus brevis

Inferior peroneal retinaculum

Cuboid

Peroneus longus
tendon

Peroneus brevis
tendon

FIGURE FA-13 Lateral/peroneal compartment of the leg.

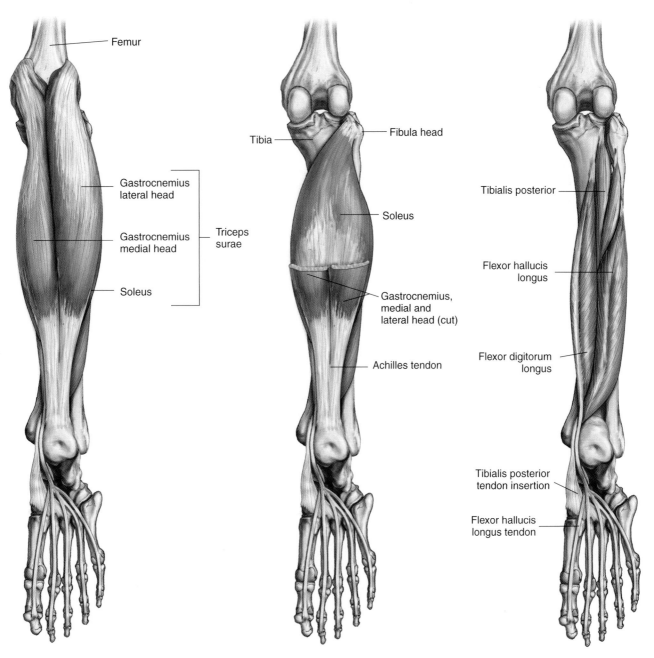

FIGURE FA-14 Posterior compartment of the leg (gastrocnemius).

FIGURE FA-15 Posterior compartment of the leg (soleus).

FIGURE FA-16 Posterior compartment of the leg (deep layers).

- Intrinsic muscles
  - Muscles that originate, insert, and function in the foot
    - EDB
      - Originates from lateral aspect of os calcis, the floor of tarsal sinus, and inserts into lateral aspect of extensor hood of the medial 4 toes; innervated by the deep peroneal nerve
  - Plantar intrinsic muscles lie in 4 layers
    - First layer (Figure FA-17)
      - Abductor hallucis
      - Flexor digitorum brevis
      - Abductor digiti minimi
    - Second layer (Figure FA-18)
      - FHL
      - FDL
      - Quadratus plantae
      - Lumbricals
    - Third layer (Figure FA-19)
      - Short intrinsic to great and small toes
      - Flexor hallucis brevis
      - Adductor hallucis
      - Flexor digiti minimi brevis
    - Fourth layer (Figure FA-20)
      - Interossei
      - Insertion of peroneus longus, tibialis anterior, and tibialis posterior

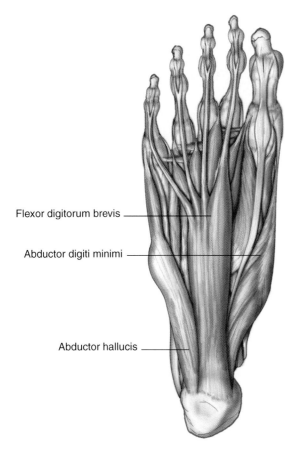

FIGURE FA-17   Muscles of the sole of the foot—1st layer.

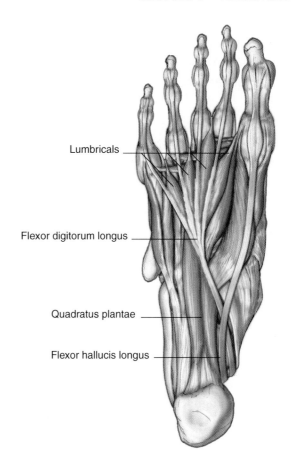

FIGURE FA-18   Muscles of the sole of the foot—2nd layer.

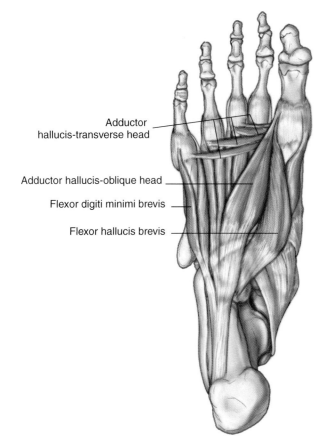

FIGURE FA-19   Muscles of the sole of the foot—3rd layer.

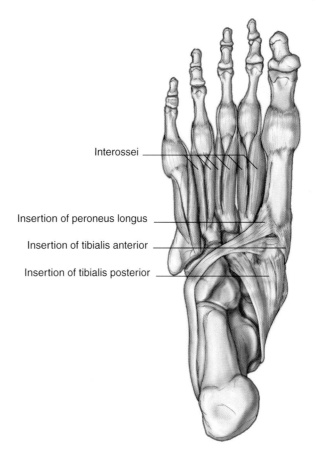

FIGURE FA-20 Muscles of the sole of the foot—4th layer.

Nerves (Figures FA-21 and FA-22)

- Most innervations are of sciatic origin (except for saphenous nerve)

- Sciatic nerve separates near the apex of the popliteal fossa to the medial popliteal (tibial nerve) and the lateral popliteal (common peroneal nerve)

  - Tibial nerve
    - Medial sural cutaneous
    - Medial plantar nerve
    - Lateral plantar nerve
  - Common peroneal nerve
    - Lateral sural cutaneous nerve
    - Superficial peroneal (musculocutaneous) nerve
    - Medial dorsal cutaneous nerve
    - Intermediate dorsal cutaneous nerve
    - Deep peroneal (anterior tibial) nerve
      - Dorsal digital nerves—adjacent sides of 1st and 2nd toes
  - Saphenous nerve
    - Largest cutaneous branch of femoral nerve
    - Follows saphenous vein, supplying medial side of leg, skin of the ankle, and further down along medial side of the foot up to base of great toe
  - Sural nerve
    - Formed by union of the medial sural cutaneous to the peroneal communicating branch of lateral sural cutaneous nerve
    - Supplies lower lateral side of leg and calcaneal branches to the heel; continues as lateral dorsal cutaneous nerve, supplying lateral side of foot and little toe

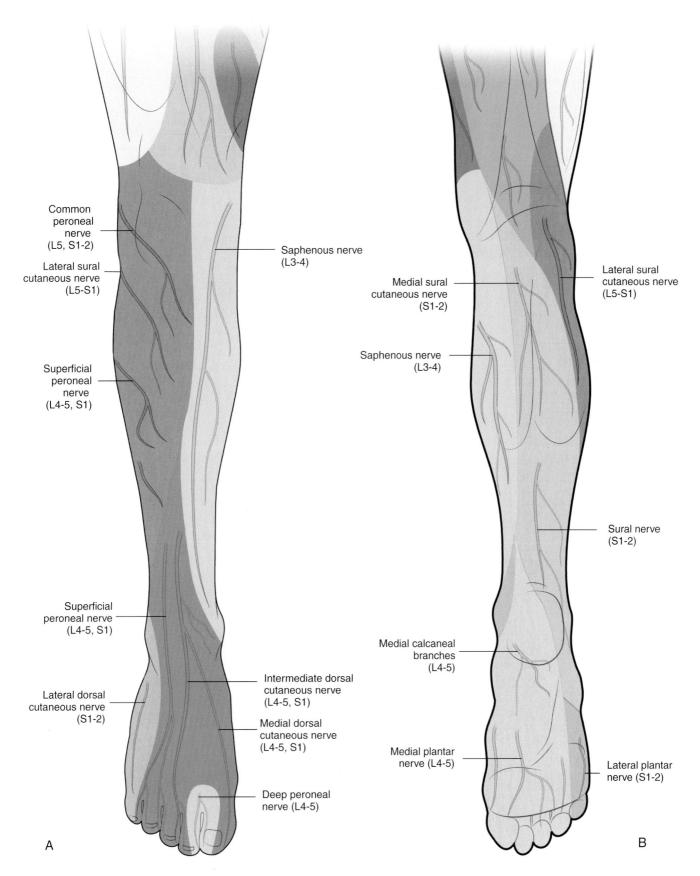

Common
peroneal
nerve
(L5, S1-2)

Lateral sural
cutaneous nerve
(L5-S1)

Saphenous nerve
(L3-4)

Superficial
peroneal
nerve
(L4-5, S1)

Medial sural
cutaneous nerve
(S1-2)

Lateral sural
cutaneous nerve
(L5-S1)

Saphenous nerve
(L3-4)

Sural nerve
(S1-2)

Superficial
peroneal nerve
(L4-5, S1)

Intermediate dorsal
cutaneous nerve
(L4-5, S1)

Medial calcaneal
branches
(L4-5)

Lateral dorsal
cutaneous nerve
(S1-2)

Medial dorsal
cutaneous nerve
(L4-5, S1)

Medial plantar
nerve (L4-5)

Lateral plantar
nerve (S1-2)

Deep peroneal
nerve (L4-5)

A

B

FIGURE FA-21   Cutaneous innervation of the leg and foot.

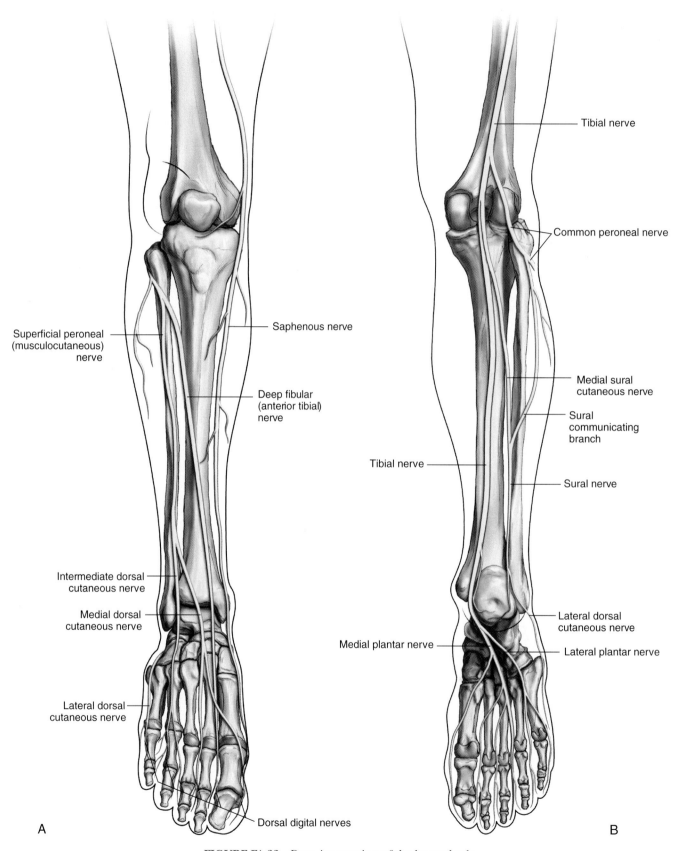

Superficial peroneal (musculocutaneous) nerve

Saphenous nerve

Deep fibular (anterior tibial) nerve

Intermediate dorsal cutaneous nerve

Medial dorsal cutaneous nerve

Lateral dorsal cutaneous nerve

Dorsal digital nerves

Tibial nerve

Common peroneal nerve

Medial sural cutaneous nerve

Sural communicating branch

Tibial nerve

Sural nerve

Lateral dorsal cutaneous nerve

Medial plantar nerve

Lateral plantar nerve

A

B

FIGURE FA-22   Deep innervation of the leg and sole.

Vascularity (Figures FA-23 and FA-24)

- Popliteal artery divides at lower border of the popliteus muscle into anterior and posterior tibial artery

  - Anterior tibial artery
    - Medial and lateral malleolar arteries
    - Dorsalis pedis artery
      - Lateral tarsal artery
      - Medial tarsal artery
        - Arcuate artery—forms arch at base of metatarsals
      - 1st dorsal metatarsal artery
      - Deep plantar artery
  - Posterior tibial artery
    - Peroneal artery arises 2-3 cm below popliteus muscle
      - Calcaneal
      - Posterior lateral malleolar branches
      - Perforating branch—to artery of tarsal sinus
    - Medial calcaneal branches
    - Medial plantar artery
    - Lateral plantar artery unites with deep plantar branch of dorsalis pedis to form plantar arch

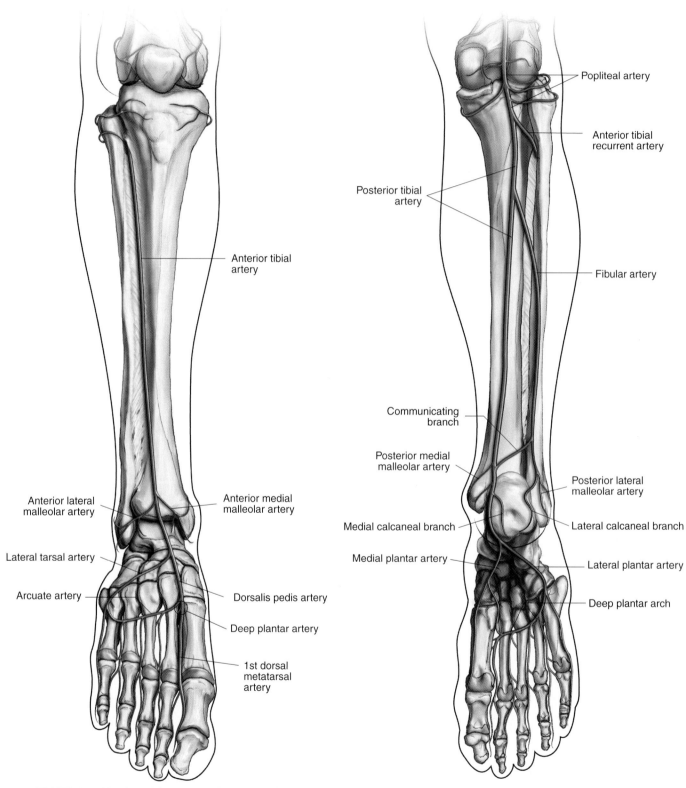

Anterior tibial
artery

Anterior lateral
malleolar artery

Anterior medial
malleolar artery

Lateral tarsal artery

Arcuate artery

Dorsalis pedis artery

Deep plantar artery

1st dorsal
metatarsal
artery

Popliteal artery

Anterior tibial
recurrent artery

Posterior tibial
artery

Fibular artery

Communicating
branch

Posterior medial
malleolar artery

Posterior lateral
malleolar artery

Medial calcaneal branch

Lateral calcaneal branch

Medial plantar artery

Lateral plantar artery

Deep plantar arch

FIGURE FA-23   Arterial system of the anterior leg and
dorsum of the foot.

FIGURE FA-24   Arterial system of the posterior leg and
sole of the foot.

● Blood supply of the talus (Figures FA-25 and FA-26)

- ▦ Neck of talus
  - ● Superior surface of neck
    - ○ Medial talar arteries—medial recurrent tarsal artery (branch of anterior tibial artery)
  - ● Inferior surface of the neck
    - ○ Artery of the tarsal canal (branch of posterior tibial artery)
  - ● Medial surface of body
    - ○ Deltoid branch (posterior tibial artery)
  - ● Posterior tubercle
    - ○ Direct branch from posterior tibial artery—infrequently from the peroneals
  - ● Lateral surface
    - ○ Artery of the tarsal sinus
- ▦ Head of talus
  - ● Superior neck vessels and branches of tarsal sinus artery
- ▦ Talar body
  - ● Tarsal canal artery supplies middle half to two thirds of the body
  - ● Internal anastomosis supplies the remainder
  - ● Deltoid branches combined with branches of the sinus tarsi artery provide significant source of vascularity

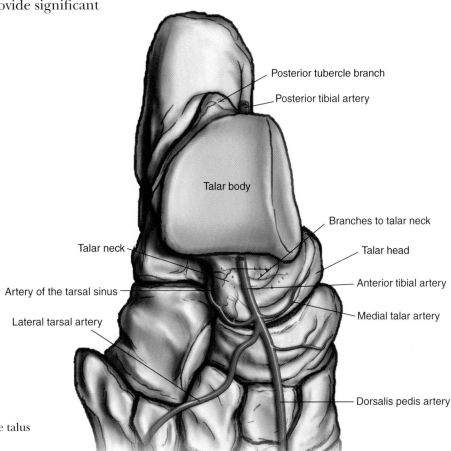

FIGURE FA-25 Arterial supply of the talus (distribution of blood supply).

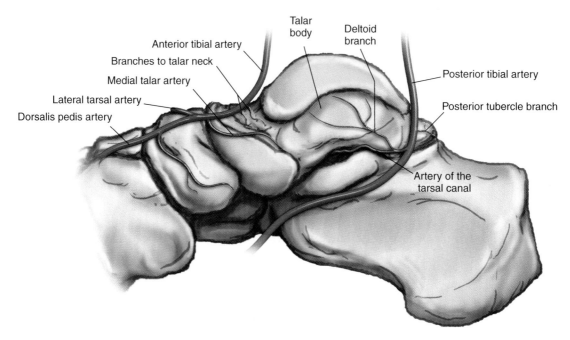

FIGURE FA-26 Arterial supply of the talus (main source of blood supply).

CROSS-SECTIONAL ANATOMY

- Lower tibia (Figure FA-27)
- Ankle (Figure FA-28)
- Foot (hind and mid parts) (Figures FA-29 and FA-30)

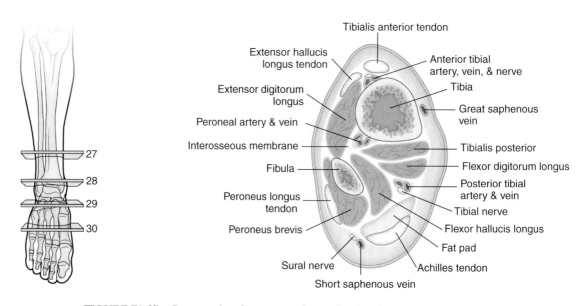

FIGURE FA-27 Cross-sectional anatomy—lower third of the leg.

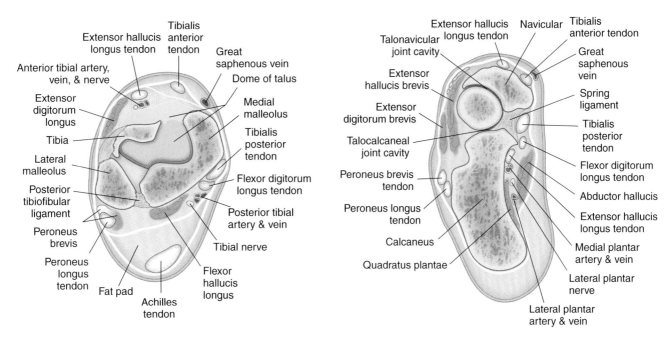

FIGURE FA-28 Cross-sectional anatomy—ankle joint.

FIGURE FA-29 Cross-sectional anatomy—hind foot.

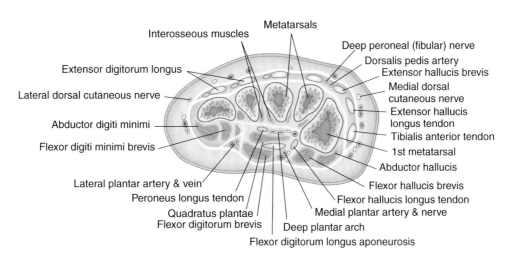

FIGURE FA-30 Cross-sectional anatomy—midfoot.

HAZARDS (Figures FA-31, FA-32, and FA-33)

- Medial neurovascular bundle, anterior neurovascular bundle, sural nerve, and dorsalis pedis artery

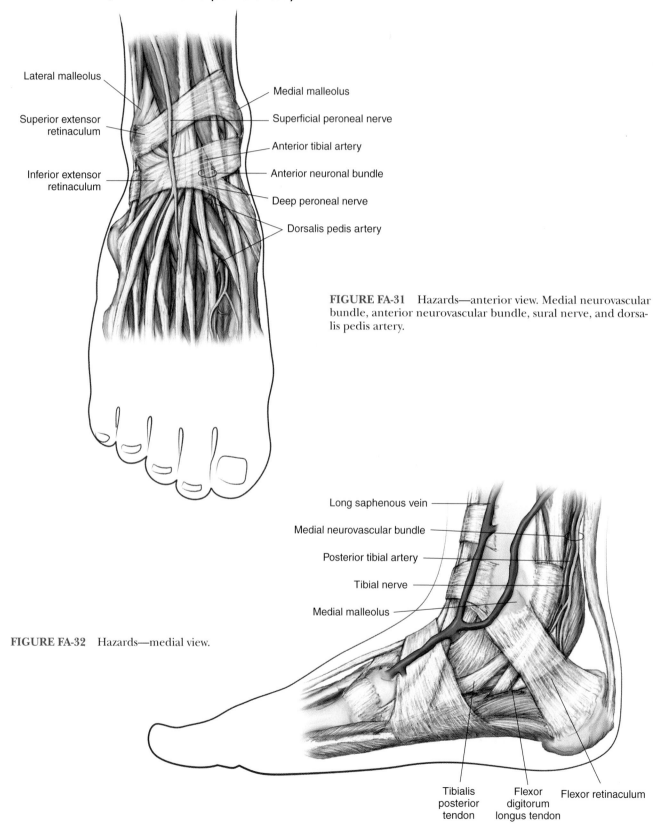

Lateral malleolus

Superior extensor retinaculum

Inferior extensor retinaculum

Medial malleolus

Superficial peroneal nerve

Anterior tibial artery

Anterior neuronal bundle

Deep peroneal nerve

Dorsalis pedis artery

FIGURE FA-31 Hazards—anterior view. Medial neurovascular bundle, anterior neurovascular bundle, sural nerve, and dorsalis pedis artery.

FIGURE FA-32 Hazards—medial view.

Long saphenous vein

Medial neurovascular bundle

Posterior tibial artery

Tibial nerve

Medial malleolus

Tibialis posterior tendon

Flexor digitorum longus tendon

Flexor retinaculum

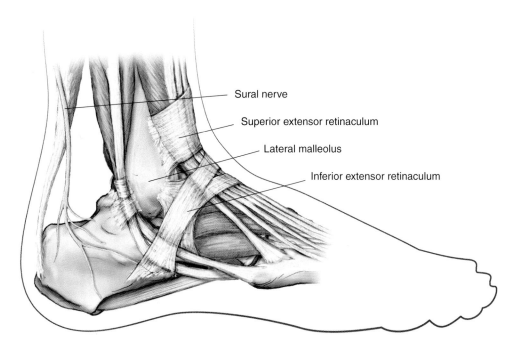

FIGURE FA-33   Hazards—lateral view.

Surface Landmarks (Figures FA-34 and FA-35)

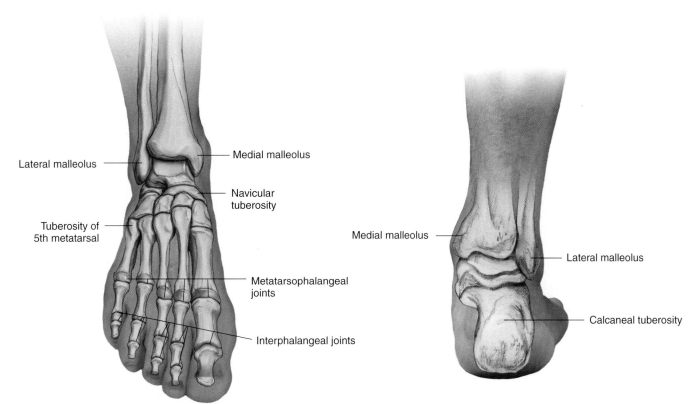

FIGURE FA-34   Superficial bony landmarks—dorsal view.

FIGURE FA-35   Superficial bony landmarks—posterior view.

ANTERIOR APPROACH TO THE ANKLE

Indications: Arthrotomy of ankle joint, loose body removal

POSITION (FIGURE FA-36)

- Supine
- Bump under ipsilateral buttock
- Calf tourniquet
- Exsanguinate by elevation for 3-5 minutes or Esmarch's bandage

INCISION

- Make 10-15 cm longitudinal incision crossing the ankle midway between the medial and lateral malleoli, then curving in a medial direction distal to the joint (Figure FA-37)

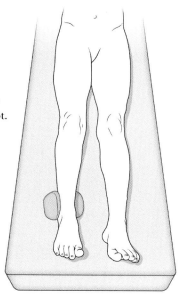

FIGURE FA-36 Position for surgery on dorsum of the foot.

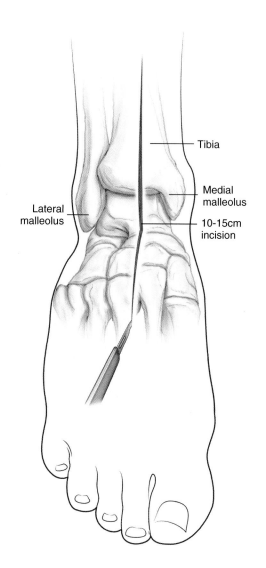

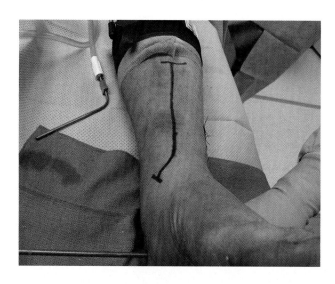

FIGURE FA-37 Skin marking. A 10-15 cm longitudinal incision crossing the ankle midway between the medial and lateral malleoli, then curving in a medial direction distal to the joint.

SUPERFICIAL DISSECTION

- Identify and protect superficial peroneal nerve (Figure FA-38)
- Deep fascia incised in line with skin incision
- Cut extensor retinaculum (Figure FA-39)
  - Medial to tibialis anterior tendon (desirable for exposure of proximal tibia)
  - Alternatively, identify plane between EHL tendon (medial) and EDL tendon (lateral) and the neurovascular bundle (deep peroneal nerve and anterior tibial artery) between them. Start a few centimeters above the ankle, and dissect the bundle carefully distally as the tendon of EHL crosses medially (this approach is desirable for distal extension to the dorsum of foot)

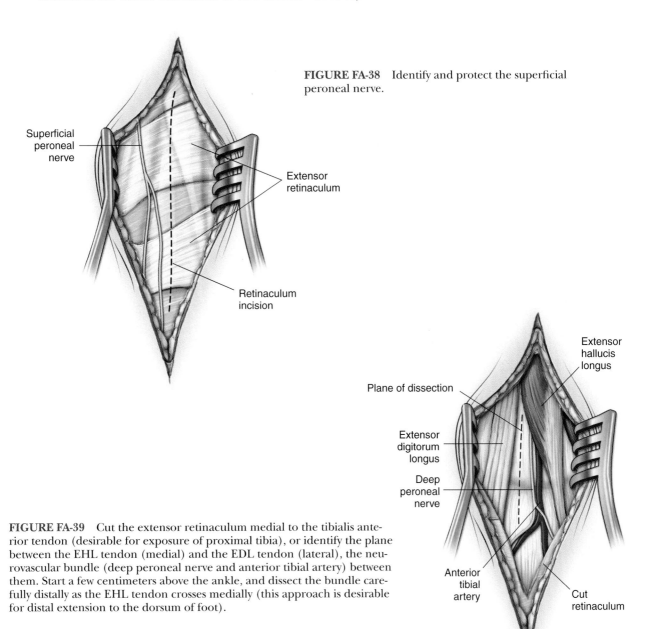

FIGURE FA-38   Identify and protect the superficial peroneal nerve.

FIGURE FA-39   Cut the extensor retinaculum medial to the tibialis anterior tendon (desirable for exposure of proximal tibia), or identify the plane between the EHL tendon (medial) and the EDL tendon (lateral), the neurovascular bundle (deep peroneal nerve and anterior tibial artery) between them. Start a few centimeters above the ankle, and dissect the bundle carefully distally as the EHL tendon crosses medially (this approach is desirable for distal extension to the dorsum of foot).

DEEP DISSECTION

- Retraction of tendons exposes the overlying fat above ankle joint capsule (Figure FA-40)
- Incise capsule longitudinally; expose the width of the ankle joint as required by sharp dissection and subperiosteal stripping

HAZARDS

- Superficial peroneal nerve—close to line of skin incision
- Deep peroneal nerve and anterior tibial artery (neurovascular bundle)

CLOSURE

- Depending on indication, a drain may be left
- Neurovascular bundle and tendons fall back into position
- Interrupted absorbable stitches for extensor retinaculum
- Standard 2-layer skin closure

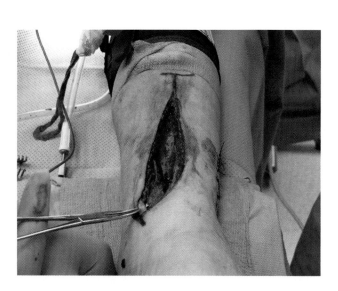

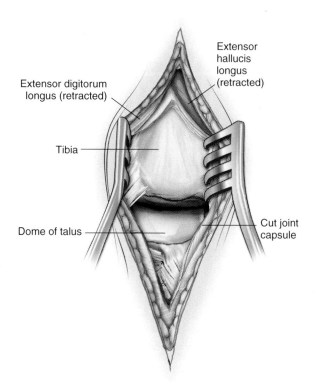

FIGURE FA-40 Retraction of the tendons exposes the overlying fat above the ankle joint capsule. Incise the capsule longitudinally to expose the width of the ankle joint.

APPROACH TO THE MEDIAL MALLEOLUS

Indications: Open reduction and internal fixation (ORIF) of the medial malleolar fractures

POSITION (FIGURE FA-41)

- Supine; sandbag/bump under opposite buttock

Anterior Incision

INCISION (FIGURE FA-42)

- Good view of medial malleolar fracture
- Visualization of anteromedial ankle joint
- Visualization of anteromedial dome of talus

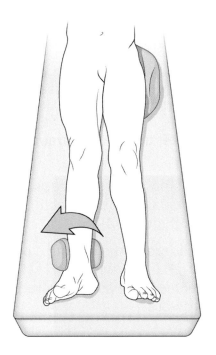

FIGURE FA-41   Position for surgery on medial aspect of the foot.

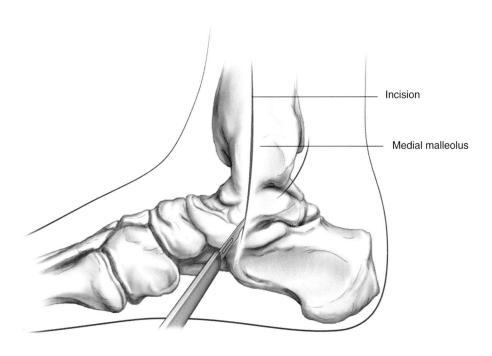

Incision

Medial malleolus

FIGURE FA-42   Skin incision with reference to the medial malleolus.

SUPERFICIAL DISSECTION

- 10-cm curved incision (longitudinal) centered over medial malleolus

- Dissect anterior and posterior flaps

- Identify and preserve great saphenous vein and saphenous nerve (best preserved together) (Figure FA-43)

DEEP DISSECTION (FIGURE FA-44)

- Preserve soft tissue attachments to bony fragment

- Small incision in anterior capsule aids in direct visualization of fracture reduction (Figure FA-45)

- Split the fibers of the deltoid—ensures better purchase of wires and screws and provides soft tissue coverage over hardware

HAZARDS

- Saphenous nerve

- Great saphenous vein

CLOSURE

- Standard 2-layer skin closure (interrupted/continuous)

- Posterior incision

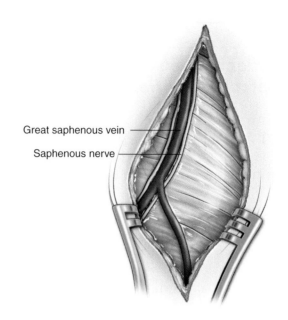

Great saphenous vein

Saphenous nerve

FIGURE FA-43 Raise medial and lateral flaps with identification of the saphenous vein and nerve.

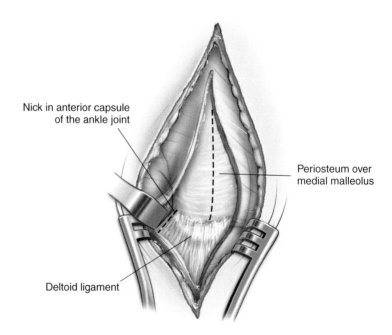

Nick in anterior capsule of the ankle joint

Periosteum over medial malleolus

Deltoid ligament

FIGURE FA-44 Deep dissection. Small incision in the anterior ankle joint capsule with partial detachment of the deltoid ligament.

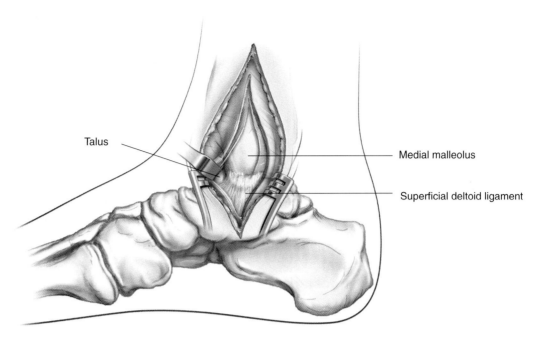

FIGURE FA-45 Bony exposure. Small incision in the anterior ankle joint capsule aids in assessing reduction of the medial malleolus.

INCISION (FIGURE FA-46)

- Open reduction and fixation of medial malleolar fractures
- Visualization of posterior margin of tibia (aids in reduction of fractured posterior malleolus)

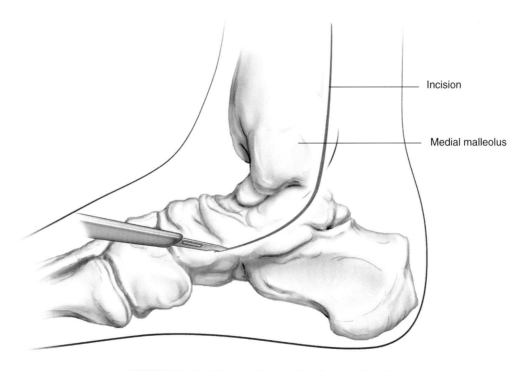

FIGURE FA-46 Skin incision and surface landmarks.

SUPERFICIAL DISSECTION (FIGURE FA-47)

- 10-cm curved incision centered on medial side of ankle

- Raise anterior and posterior flaps

DEEP DISSECTION (FIGURE FA-48)

- Protect soft tissue attachments to fracture piece

- Incise retinaculum behind posterior border of medial malleolus (watch and protect tendon of tibialis posterior)

  - External rotation of leg aids in better exposure of the posterior malleolus

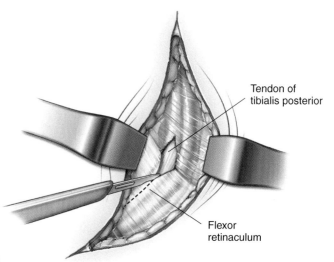

FIGURE FA-47 Superficial dissection with identification of the tibialis posterior tendon.

HAZARDS

- Careful deep dissection needed to identify and protect structures passing behind medial malleolus

  - From front to back—tibialis posterior tendon, FDL, posterior tibial artery, posterior tibial nerve

CLOSURE

- Reattach flexor retinaculum

- Standard 2-layer skin closure (interrupted/continuous)

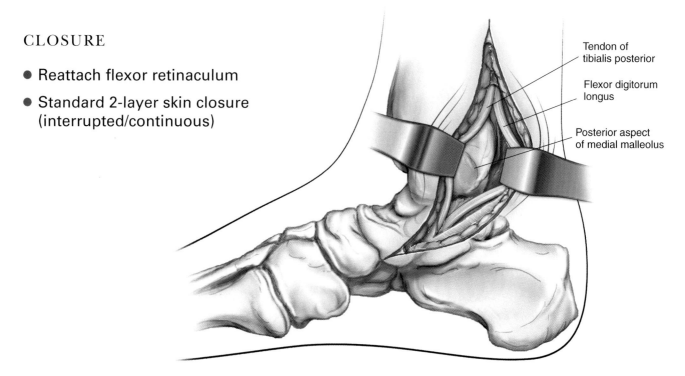

FIGURE FA-48 Deep dissection through the flexor retinaculum and capsule to expose the ankle joint and the posterior malleolus.

Straight Midline

INCISION

- Direct straight incision centered over medial malleolus (Figure FA-49)

- Allows anterior access to ankle joint for visualization of fracture reduction

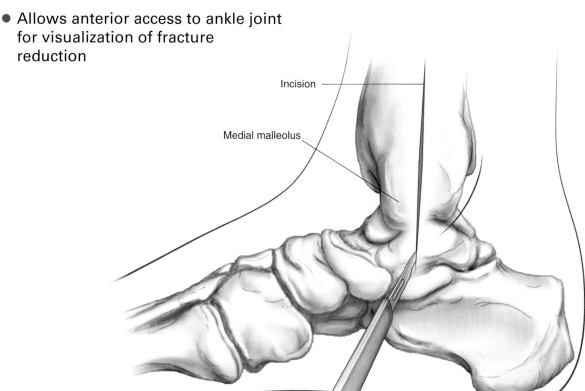

Incision

Medial malleolus

FIGURE FA-49   Direct straight incision centered over the medial malleolus.

Approach to the Medial Side of Ankle

Indications: Ankle arthrodesis, loose body and osteochondral fragment removal, ORIF for displaced talar neck fractures, ORIF for fractures of the dome or body of talus

POSITION

- Supine

- Bump under opposite buttock

- Calf tourniquet

- Exsanguinate by elevation for 3-5 minutes or Esmarch's bandage

INCISION

- 10-12 cm longitudinal incision centered over tip of the medial malleolus (curve lower half of the incision forward toward mid part of the foot) (Figure FA-50)

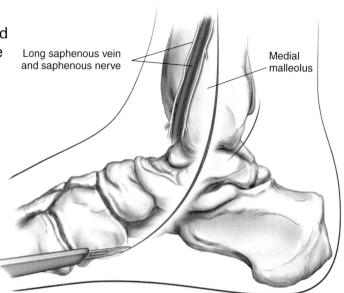

FIGURE FA-50 Skin incision. A 10-12 cm longitudinal incision centered over the tip of the medial malleolus (curve the lower half of the incision forward toward the mid part of the foot).

SUPERFICIAL DISSECTION

- Raise anterior and posterior flaps by blunt dissection, carefully protecting great saphenous vein and saphenous nerve under anterior flap (Figure FA-51)

DEEP DISSECTION

- Expose borders of the medial malleolus (Figure FA-52)

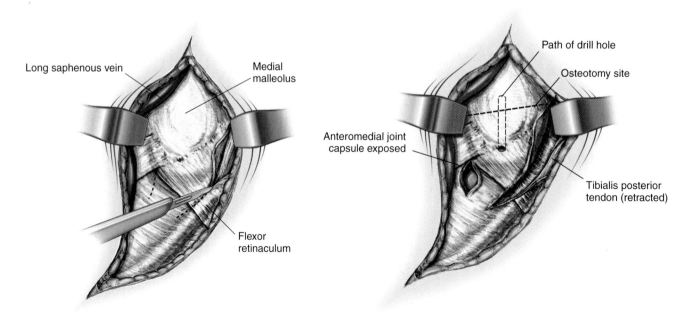

FIGURE FA-51 Raise the anterior and posterior flaps by blunt dissection, carefully protecting the great saphenous vein and the saphenous nerve under the anterior flap.

FIGURE FA-52 Expose the borders of the medial malleolus—incise the ankle joint capsule anterior to the medial malleolus, and carefully divide the flexor retinaculum from the posterior border of the malleolus after identifying the tibialis posterior tendon.

> ▣ Incise ankle joint capsule anterior to the medial malleolus, and carefully divide flexor retinaculum from posterior border of the malleolus after identifying tibialis posterior tendon

- Leave attachment of deltoid ligaments intact
- Osteotomize medial malleolus (Figure FA-53)

  - ▣ First drill and tap medial malleolus, then make an oblique cut from top to bottom—reflect medial malleolus downward
  - ▣ This exposes the dome of the talus and the articulating surface of the tibia into view (eversion of the foot improves the exposure further) (Figure FA-54)

HAZARDS

- Saphenous nerve and great saphenous vein
- Tibialis posterior tendon

CLOSURE

- Secure medial malleolus osteotomy with screws and modified tension band wiring
- Reattach flexor retinaculum to posterior border of medial malleolus
- Standard 2-layer closure of subcutaneous tissue and skin

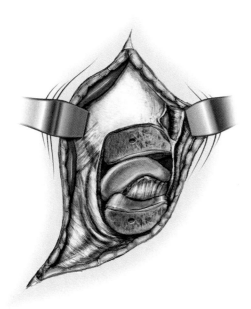

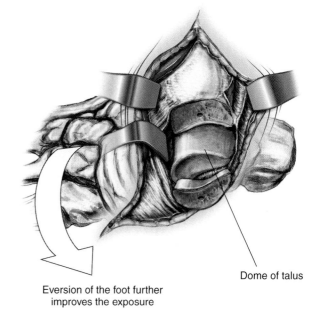

Eversion of the foot further improves the exposure

Dome of talus

FIGURE FA-53   Osteotomize the medial malleolus—first drill and tap the medial malleolus, then make an oblique cut from top to bottom; reflect the medial malleolus downward.

FIGURE FA-54   Eversion of the foot improves the exposure further.

APPROACH TO THE TARSAL TUNNEL

Indications: Tarsal tunnel syndrome

POSITION

- Supine with sand bag under opposite hip
- Calf tourniquet
- Exsanguinate by elevation for 3-5 minutes or Esmarch's bandage

INCISION

- Incision begins between the medial malleolus and medial aspect of the tuberosity of the calcaneus extending down to about 1 cm below the navicular tuberosity (Figure FA-55)

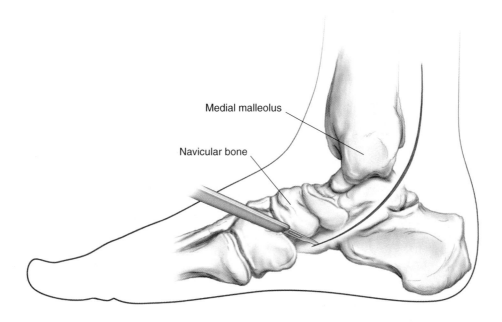

Medial malleolus

Navicular bone

FIGURE FA-55   Skin incision begins between the medial malleolus and the medial aspect of the tuberosity of the calcaneus extending down to about 1 cm below the navicular tuberosity.

SUPERFICIAL DISSECTION

- Cauterize and ligate veins connecting the plantar and saphenous systems (Figure FA-56)

- Divide investing fascia of the calf proximally and medial side of the foot distally

DEEP DISSECTION (FIGURE FA-57)

- Identify proximal and distal borders of flexor retinaculum and neurovascular bundles before the bundle disappears underneath the flexor retinaculum

- Release the retinaculum from proximal to distal direction until you reach the muscle fibers of abductor hallucis

HAZARDS

- Sometimes medial calcaneal branch penetrates flexor retinaculum and becomes damaged resulting in painful neuroma

- Neurovascular bundles that pass behind medial malleolus

CLOSURE

- Standard closure of subcutaneous tissue and skin only

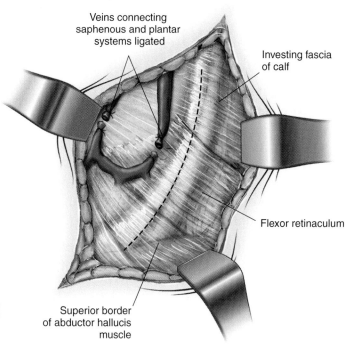

FIGURE FA-56 Cauterize and ligate the veins connecting the plantar and the saphenous systems. Divide the investing fascia of the calf proximally and the medial side of the foot distally.

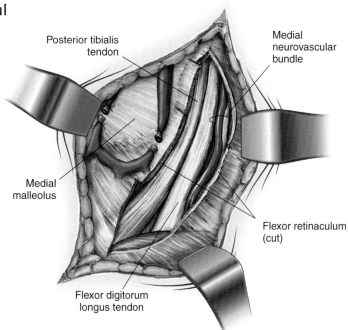

FIGURE FA-57 Identify the proximal and distal borders of the flexor retinaculum and the neurovascular bundles before the bundle disappears underneath the flexor retinaculum, and release the retinaculum from proximal to distal up to the muscle fibers of the abductor hallucis.

POSTEROMEDIAL APPROACH TO THE ANKLE

Indications: Exposure of posterior malleolus, clubfoot correction in pediatric patients

POSITION

- Supine with flexion of hip and knee; place lateral side of affected ankle on opposite knee

- Lateral position with affected leg nearest table; flexion of opposite knee moves its ankle out of the way

INCISION (FIGURE FA-58)

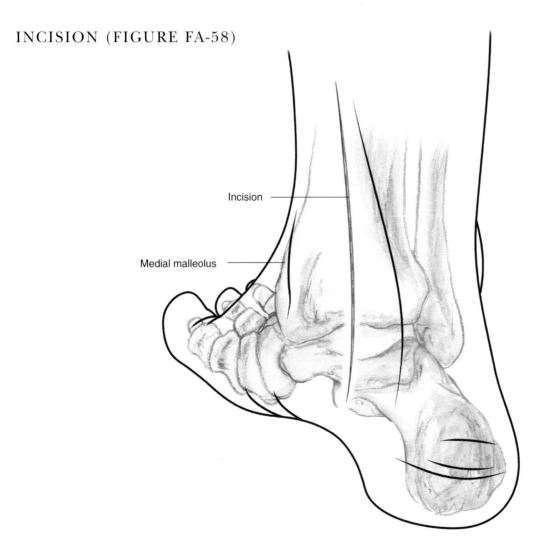

Incision

Medial malleolus

FIGURE FA-58 Surface landmark and skin incision.

SUPERFICIAL DISSECTION (FIGURES FA-59 AND FA-60)

- 8-10 cm incision midway between medial malleolus and Achilles tendon

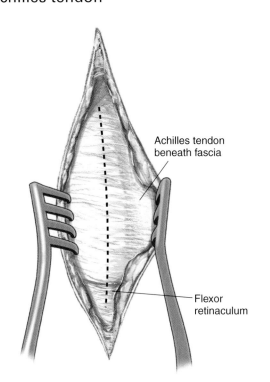

Achilles tendon beneath fascia

Flexor retinaculum

FIGURE FA-59   Superficial dissection.

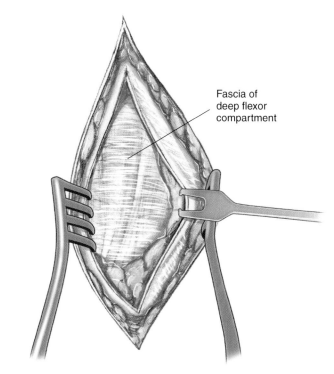

Fascia of deep flexor compartment

FIGURE FA-60   Superficial dissection. Exposure of the flexor retinaculum.

DEEP DISSECTION

- Using blunt dissection, identify fat plane between the Achilles tendon and the structures that pass behind the medial malleolus (Figure FA-61)

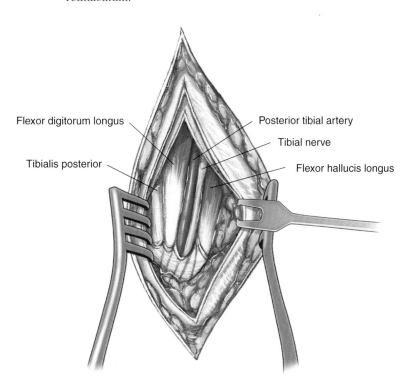

Flexor digitorum longus

Tibialis posterior

Posterior tibial artery

Tibial nerve

Flexor hallucis longus

FIGURE FA-61   Exposure of the contents of the flexor retinaculum.

- Retract Achilles tendon and retrotendinous fat laterally—exposes the fascia of deeper flexor compartment (Figure FA-62)

- Identify fascial plane in anterior flap that covers tendons of flexor retinaculum

   - Incise this deep fascia along the length of the incision, and one by one expose and identify the contents of the flexor retinaculum
   - This facilitates medial retraction of the structures, aiding exposure of the posterior malleolus and the posterior part of the ankle joint

HAZARDS

- Tendons and neurovascular contents of flexor retinaculum

CLOSURE

- Do not attempt to close flexor retinaculum

- Standard 2-layered closure of subcutaneous tissue and skin

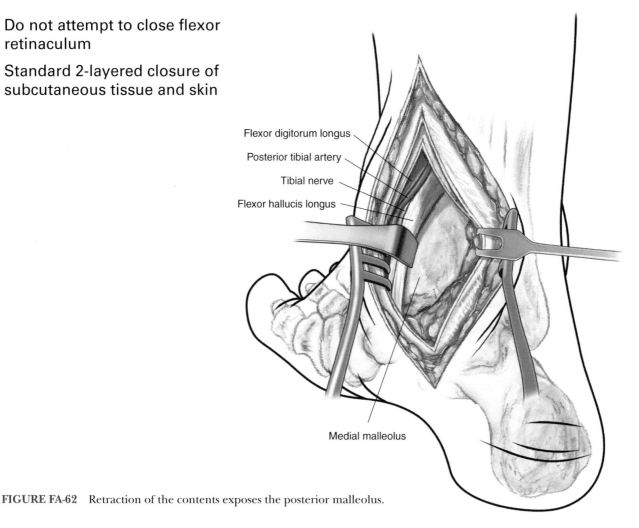

Flexor digitorum longus

Posterior tibial artery

Tibial nerve

Flexor hallucis longus

Medial malleolus

FIGURE FA-62   Retraction of the contents exposes the posterior malleolus.

APPROACH TO THE ACHILLES TENDON

Indications: Acute or chronic rupture of Achilles tendon, insertional tendinitis

POSITION (FIGURE FA-63)

- Prone position
- Calf tourniquet
- Exsanguinate by elevation for 3-5 minutes or Esmarch's bandage

INCISION (FIGURE FA-64)

- Make 10-15 cm long posteromedial/ posterolateral incision about 1 cm from tendon, and extend it just proximal to where the shoe counter strikes the heel

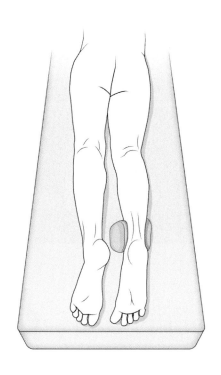

FIGURE FA-63   Prone position for surgery on the posterior part of the foot.

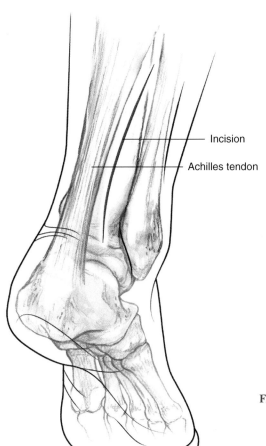

Incision

Achilles tendon

A

FIGURE FA-64   **A** to **C,** Surface landmarks and skin incision
Continued

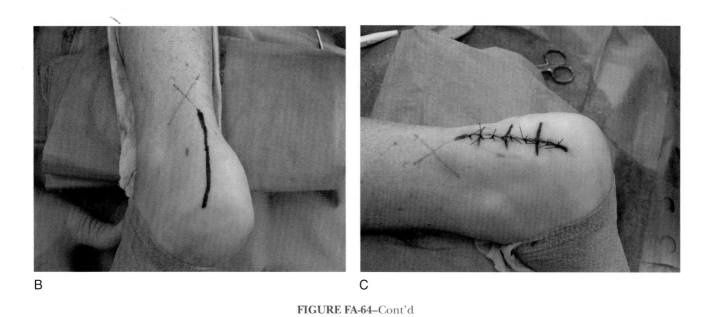

B   C

FIGURE FA-64–Cont'd

SUPERFICIAL DISSECTION (FIGURE FA-65)

- Watch for cutaneous divisions of sural nerve lateral to the tendon

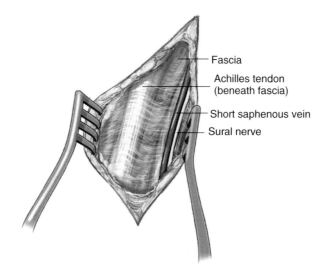

Fascia

Achilles tendon
(beneath fascia)

Short saphenous vein

Sural nerve

FIGURE FA-65   Superficial dissection.

DEEP DISSECTION (FIGURE FA-66)

● Carry sharp dissection through subcutaneous tissue and tendon sheath—reflect as 1 layer to minimize subcutaneous tissue dissection

HAZARDS

● Cutaneous branches of sural nerve and short saphenous vein on lateral border of Achilles tendon

CLOSURE

● Close tendon sheath with interrupted nonabsorbable suture

● Standard subcutaneous tissue and skin closure

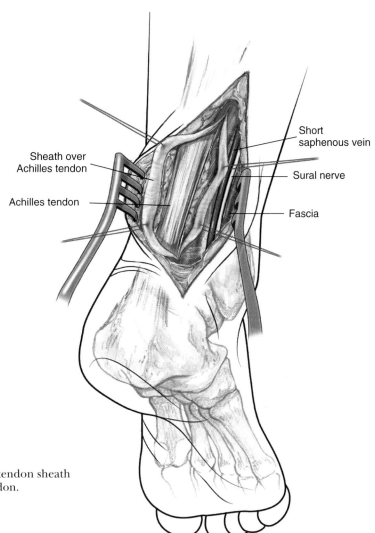

Short saphenous vein

Sheath over Achilles tendon

Sural nerve

Achilles tendon

Fascia

FIGURE FA-66 Deep dissection to expose the tendon sheath and incise the sheath to expose the Achilles tendon.

POSTEROLATERAL APPROACH TO THE ANKLE

Indications: ORIF of posterior malleolar fractures, reconstruction and lengthening of peroneal tendons and Achilles tendon, arthrodesis of posterior facet of subtalar joint, access to ankle joint for débridement and excision of sequestra, benign tumor or mass in distal tibia and ankle joint

POSITION

- Prone position

- Place sandbag or bump under the ankle, leaving foot free for manipulation

- Calf tourniquet

- Exsanguinate by elevation for 3-5 minutes or Esmarch's bandage

INCISION (FIGURE FA-67)

- Define borders of lateral malleolus and Achilles tendon, and make 10-12 cm longitudinal incision between them

   - Note the internervous plane between the peroneus brevis (superficial peroneal nerve) and FHL (tibial nerve)

SUPERFICIAL DISSECTION (FIGURE FA-68)

- Raise the skin flaps carefully—watch for short saphenous vein and sural nerve behind lateral malleolus

- Incise deep fascia in line of the skin incision

- Identify the 2 peroneal tendons (brevis is more muscular and is anterior behind the fibula at this level)

- Incise peroneal retinaculum to mobilize the tendons laterally, which exposes the FHL (this too is muscular at this level)

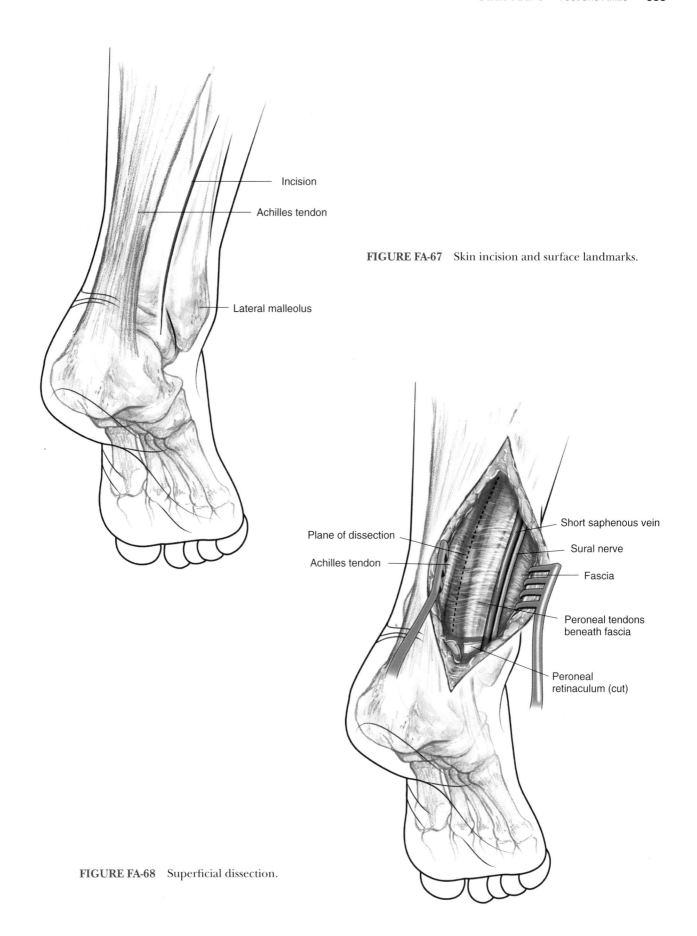

Incision

Achilles tendon

Lateral malleolus

FIGURE FA-67   Skin incision and surface landmarks.

Plane of dissection

Achilles tendon

Short saphenous vein

Sural nerve

Fascia

Peroneal tendons beneath fascia

Peroneal retinaculum (cut)

FIGURE FA-68   Superficial dissection.

DEEP DISSECTION

- Incise fascia over FHL to expose muscle fibers (Figure FA-69)
- Using sharp dissection, lift off the fibers of FHL from fibula (Figure FA-70)
- Retract FHL medially to expose periosteum; further subperiosteal reflection exposes posterior surface of the tibia and ankle joint
- For proximal extension, develop muscular plane between the peroneals and the lateral head of gastrocnemius soleus

  - The FHL is reflected from the fibula and retracted medially; further exposure can be achieved medially across the interosseous membrane and posterior surface of tibia

HAZARDS

- Short saphenous vein and sural nerve

CLOSURE

- FHL muscle falls back into place
- Repair peroneal retinaculum
- Standard 2-layer closure of skin

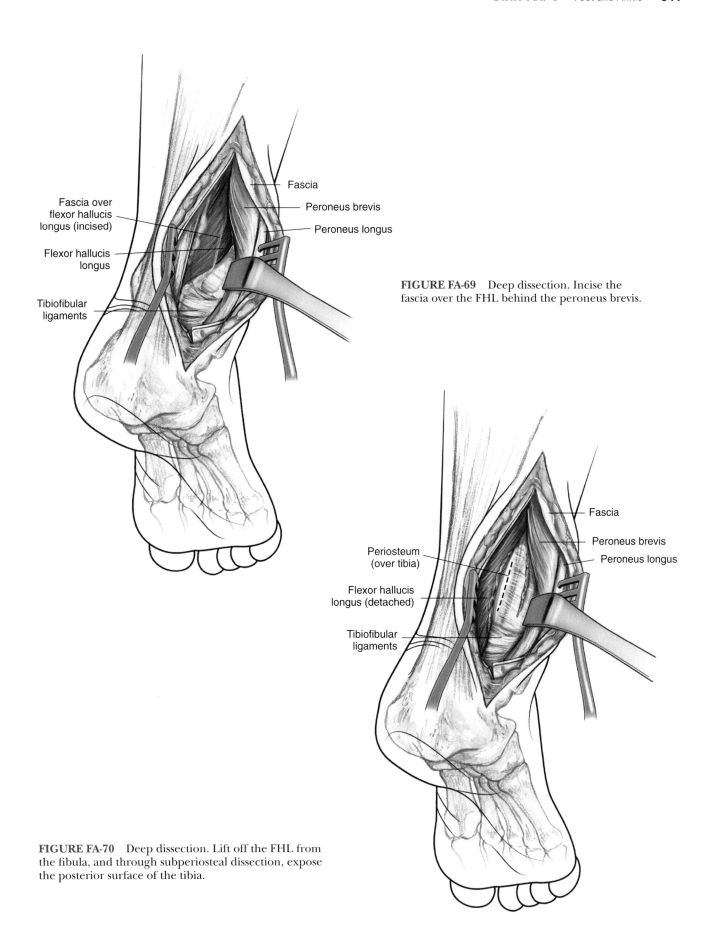

Fascia

Peroneus brevis

Peroneus longus

Fascia over
flexor hallucis
longus (incised)

Flexor hallucis
longus

Tibiofibular
ligaments

FIGURE FA-69   Deep dissection. Incise the
fascia over the FHL behind the peroneus brevis.

Periosteum
(over tibia)

Flexor hallucis
longus (detached)

Tibiofibular
ligaments

Fascia

Peroneus brevis

Peroneus longus

FIGURE FA-70   Deep dissection. Lift off the FHL from
the fibula, and through subperiosteal dissection, expose
the posterior surface of the tibia.

APPROACH TO THE LATERAL MALLEOLUS

Indications: ORIF of lateral malleolar fractures

- Can be exploited to expose posterolateral aspect of tibia

POSITION (FIGURE FA-71)

- Supine with sandbag or bump underneath ipsilateral hip
- Calf tourniquet
- Exsanguinate by elevation for 3-5 minutes or Esmarch's bandage

INCISION

SUPERFICIAL DISSECTION

- Make 12-15 cm incision along posterior border of the fibula up to its distal end; the distal end can be either straight or be curved forward (Figure FA-72)

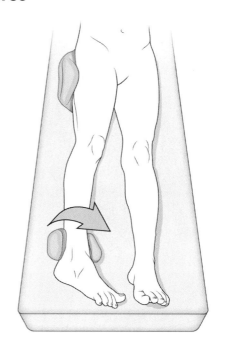

FIGURE FA-71   Position for surgery on lateral aspect of foot.

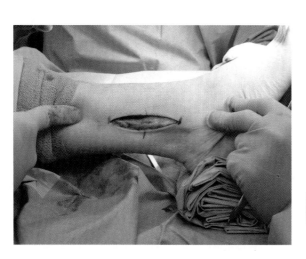

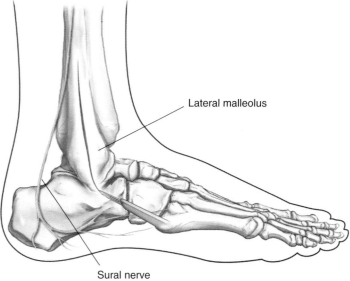

Lateral malleolus

Sural nerve

FIGURE FA-72   Skin incision. A 12-15 cm incision along the posterior border of the fibula up to its distal end. The distal end can be either straight or curved forward.

- Elevate anterior and posterior skin flaps, taking care to protect short saphenous vein posterior to lateral malleolus (Figure FA-73)

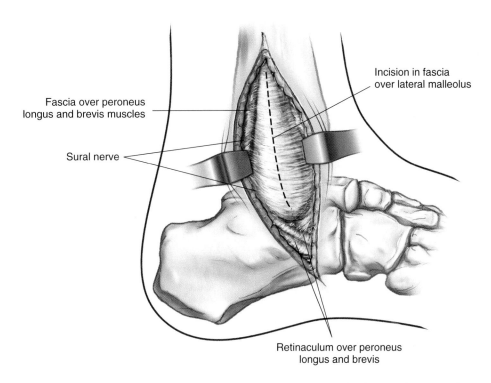

Fascia over peroneus longus and brevis muscles

Incision in fascia over lateral malleolus

Sural nerve

Retinaculum over peroneus longus and brevis

FIGURE FA-73 Elevate anterior and posterior skin flaps, taking care to protect the short saphenous vein posterior to the lateral malleolus.

DEEP DISSECTION

- Limit subperiosteal dissection of subcutaneous surface of fibula to a minimum, limiting stripping to fractured ends of bone (Figure FA-74)

- Proximal extension is possible by extending incision along posterior border of fibula and developing a plane between the peroneal and the flexor group

- Distal extension is possible by curving incision forward and along lateral side of foot, dividing peroneal retinaculum and excising fat pad from sinus tarsi and lifting off origin of EDB, exposing calcaneocuboid joint

HAZARDS

- Sural nerve
- Terminal branches of peroneal artery (deep to medial surface of distal fibula)

CLOSURE

- Meticulous closure of subcutaneous tissue to cover plate over lateral malleolus
- Standard skin closure

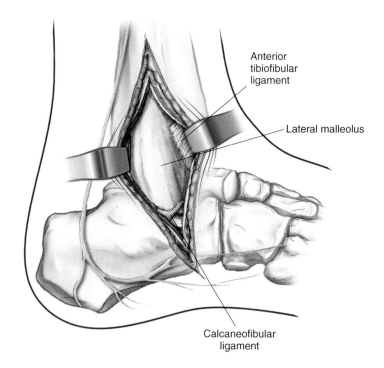

Anterior tibiofibular ligament

Lateral malleolus

Calcaneofibular ligament

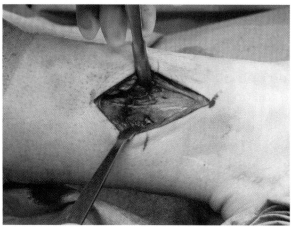

FIGURE FA-74 Limit the subperiosteal dissection of the subcutaneous surface of the fibula to a minimum.

ANTEROLATERAL APPROACH TO THE ANKLE

Indications: Ankle arthrodesis, ORIF of pilon fracture

POSITION

- Supine with sandbag underneath ipsilateral bump
- Calf tourniquet
- Exsanguinate by elevation for 3-5 minutes or Esmarch's bandage

INCISION (FIGURE FA-75)

- A 12-15 cm incision is made along anterolateral aspect of ankle, slightly anterior to anterior border of fibula; curve the incision down, crossing the ankle joint 2 cm medial to tip of lateral malleolus

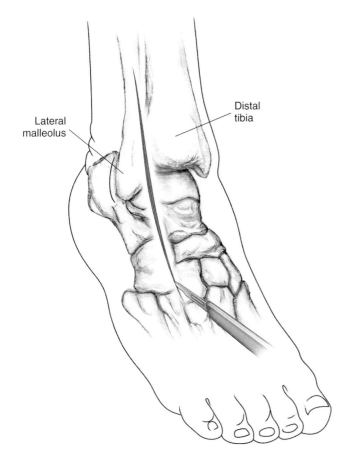

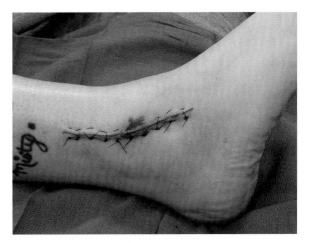

FIGURE FA-75   Surface marking of the skin incision for anterolateral approach to the ankle.

SUPERFICIAL DISSECTION (FIGURE FA-76)

- Incise fascia in line with skin incision

- Divide superior and inferior extensor retinaculum (Figure FA-77)

- Carefully dissect off dorsal cutaneous branches of superficial peroneal nerve as it crosses the field

- Identify peroneus tertius and EDL, and go down to tibia just lateral to these muscles

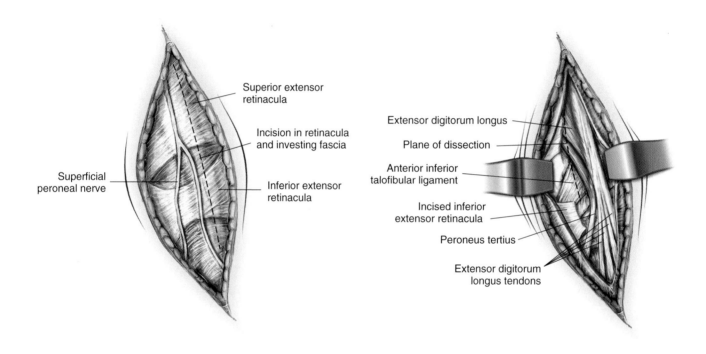

FIGURE FA-76 Superficial dissection. Watch for the branch of the superficial peroneal nerve.

FIGURE FA-77 Divide the extensor retinaculum, and identify the plane lateral to the EDL and the peroneus tertius.

DEEP DISSECTION (FIGURES FA-78 AND FA-79)

- Medial retraction of extensor muscle group exposes anterior aspect of distal tibia and anterior ankle joint capsule

- Proximal extension to explore anterior compartment

- Distal extension to expose sinus tarsi, calcaneocuboid joint, and tarsometatarsal joint on lateral half of foot

HAZARDS

- Dorsal cutaneous branch of superficial peroneal nerve
- Deep peroneal nerve
- Anterior tibial artery

CLOSURE

- Extensor muscles fall back into place
- Standard 2-layer closure of skin

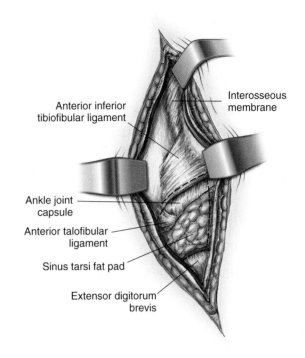

Anterior inferior tibiofibular ligament

Interosseous membrane

Ankle joint capsule

Anterior talofibular ligament

Sinus tarsi fat pad

Extensor digitorum brevis

FIGURE FA-78   Deep dissection to expose the ankle joint and dome of the talus.

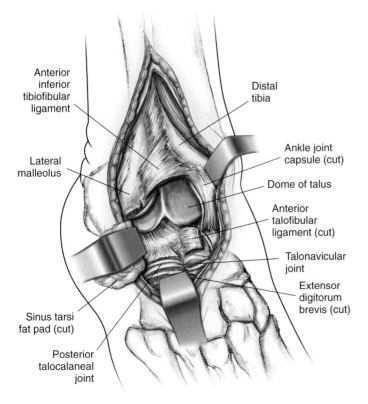

Anterior inferior tibiofibular ligament

Lateral malleolus

Sinus tarsi fat pad (cut)

Posterior talocalaneal joint

Distal tibia

Ankle joint capsule (cut)

Dome of talus

Anterior talofibular ligament (cut)

Talonavicular joint

Extensor digitorum brevis (cut)

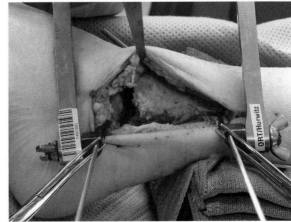

FIGURE FA-79   Deep dissection to expose the ankle joint and dome of the talus.

ANTEROLATERAL APPROACH TO THE HIND FOOT

Indications: Approach to subtalar joint, calcaneocuboid joint, talonavicular joint, sinus tarsi

POSITION

- Supine with sandbag underneath ipsilateral bump
- Calf tourniquet
- Exsanguinate by elevation for 3-5 minutes or Esmarch's bandage

INCISION (FIGURE FA-80)

- Straight incision from anterior border of tip of fibula to base of 4th-5th metatarsal

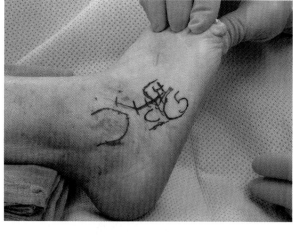

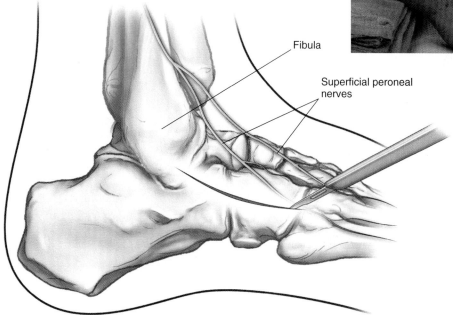

FIGURE FA-80   Surface marking and skin incision for anterolateral approach to the hind foot.

SUPERFICIAL DISSECTION

- Incise deep fascia in line with length of incision

- Carefully preserve dorsal cutaneous branches of superficial peroneal nerve (Figure FA-81)

- Identify origin of EDB from calcaneus (Figure FA-82)

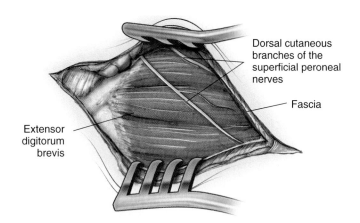

FIGURE FA-81   Tendinous origin of the fibers of the EDB and the dorsal cutaneous branches of the superficial peroneal nerves.

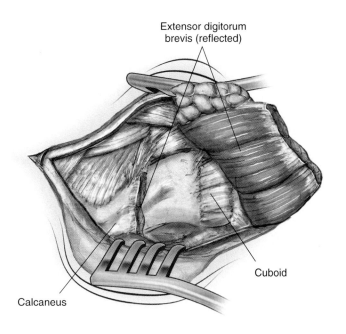

FIGURE FA-82   Reflection of the origin of the EDB muscle from the calcaneus.

DEEP DISSECTION

- Detach origin of EDB from calcaneus, and reflect it distally
- Identify capsule of calcaneocuboid joint and talonavicular joint
- In proximal part of incision, reflect and remove fat pad over sinus tarsi—this exposes talocalcaneal joint (subtalar) (Figure FA-83)
- Incise capsule as desired for joint to be exposed
- Plantar flexion and inversion aids further exposure

HAZARDS

- Cutaneous branches of superficial peroneal nerve

CLOSURE

- Reattach extensor digitorum muscle to periosteum of calcaneus
- Standard subcutaneous tissue and skin closure

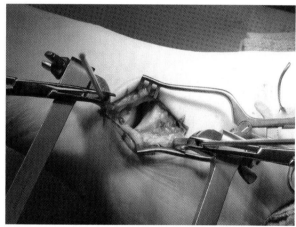

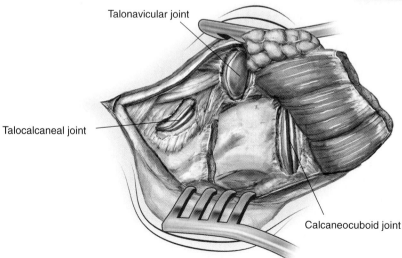

FIGURE FA-83 Reflect and remove the fat pad over the sinus tarsi—exposes the talocalcaneal joint (subtalar). Incise the capsule as desired for the joint to be exposed.

APPROACH TO THE TIBIALIS POSTERIOR TENDON

Indications: Débridement, repair of incomplete tears, reconstruction and tendon transfer for complete tears and insufficiency

POSITION

- Supine with sandbag or bump under opposite hip
- Calf tourniquet
- Exsanguinate by elevation for 3-5 minutes or Esmarch's bandage
- Rest foot in gravity equinus

INCISION (FIGURE FA-84)

- Start at inferior edge of navicular tuberosity, and carry incision proximally about 1 cm posterior to medial malleolus, and extend it 3-4 cm above flexor retinaculum

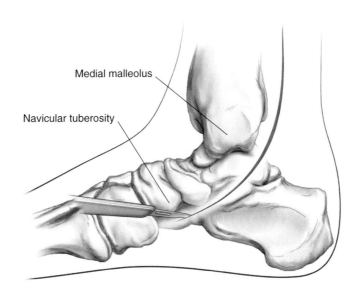

FIGURE FA-84   Surface landmark for the approach to the tibialis posterior tendon.

SUPERFICIAL DISSECTION

- Identify tendon at inferior margin, and trace it up proximally until muscle belly is seen (Figure FA-85)

FIGURE FA-85 Identify the tendon at the inferior margin, and trace it up proximally until the muscle belly is seen.

DEEP DISSECTION (FIGURE FA-86)

- Release pulley behind medial malleolus and deep investing fascia of distal leg
- Trace distal plantar slip of tendon around 1 cm distal to the tuberosity

HAZARDS

- Tibialis posterior tendon
- Neurovascular structures that run behind tendon (posterior tibial vessels and nerve)

CLOSURE

- Leave flexor retinaculum open
- Standard closure of subcutaneous tissue and skin

FIGURE FA-86 Release the pulley behind the medial malleolus and the deep investing fascia of the distal leg, and trace the distal plantar slip of the tendon around 1 cm distal to the tuberosity.

EXTENSILE LATERAL APPROACH TO THE CALCANEUS

Indications: ORIF of calcaneal fracture

POSITION (FIGURE FA-87)

- Lateral position
- Calf tourniquet
- Exsanguinate by elevation for 3-5 minutes or Esmarch's bandage

INCISION

- Make L-shaped incision—start midway between posterior border of fibula and Achilles tendon, and curve the incision forward about 1 cm from calcaneal tuberosity toward calcaneocuboid joint (Figure FA-88)

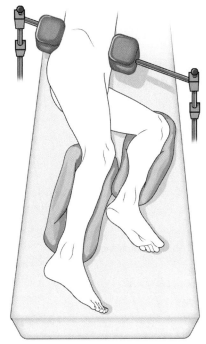

FIGURE FA-87 Lateral decubitus position for surgery on lateral border/calcaneus.

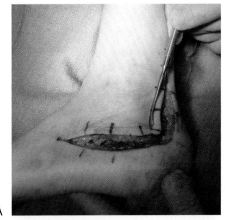

A

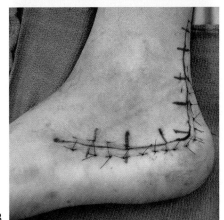

B

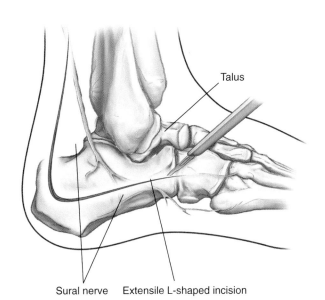

Talus

Sural nerve   Extensile L-shaped incision

FIGURE FA-88 Extensile L-shaped incision.

SUPERFICIAL DISSECTION

- Incise soft tissues sharply, and carry incision down to periosteum of lateral wall

- Watch for branches of sural nerve at both ends of limb of incision (Figure FA-89)

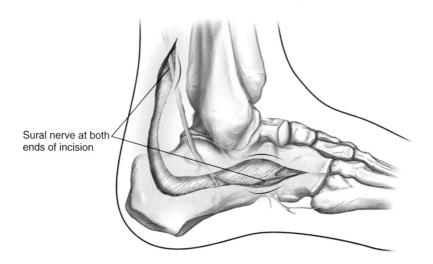

Sural nerve at both ends of incision

FIGURE FA-89   Branches of the sural nerve at both ends of the limb of the incision.

DEEP DISSECTION

- With strict subperiosteal dissection along lateral wall, elevate flap in 1 layer, and retract it with 2 Kirschner wires placed into talus (Figure FA-90)

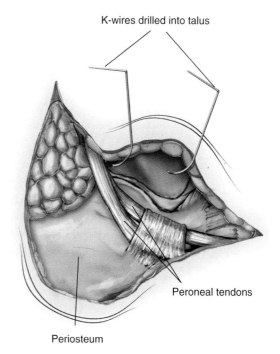

K-wires drilled into talus

Peroneal tendons

Periosteum

FIGURE FA-90   Elevate the flap in 1 layer, and drill 2 Kirschner wires into the talus (aids exposure and retraction). Proximal dissection exposes the posterior facet of the calcaneus, and distal dissection reflects the peroneal tendon with its pulley.

- Expose entire lateral wall of calcaneus distally to calcaneocuboid joint (Figure FA-91)

- Dissect above and below peroneal tendons—it may be reflected with its pulley if coming in way of fixation

- Dissect proximally to expose posterior facet of calcaneus

HAZARDS

- Sural nerve at proximal and distal ends of exposure

CLOSURE

- Reattach peroneal retinaculum to periosteum (if elevated)

- Meticulous closure of the flap after securing hemostasis

- Desirable to use horizontal mattress sutures for skin

- Fluffs and wool dressing with limb elevation also play a part in reducing incidence of flap necrosis

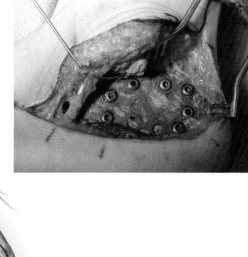

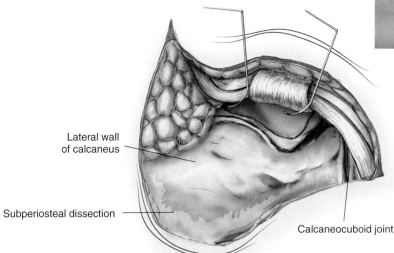

FIGURE FA-91   Subperiosteal dissection exposes the lateral surface of the calcaneus and calcaneocuboid joint.

ANTEROLATERAL APPROACH TO TALUS NECK

Indications: ORIF of head and neck of talus

POSITION

- Supine with sandbag or bump underneath ipsilateral hip
- Calf tourniquet
- Exsanguinate by elevation for 3-5 minutes or Esmarch's bandage

INCISION

- A 5 cm incision over sinus tarsi extending toward base of 4th metatarsal (Figure FA-92)

SUPERFICIAL DISSECTION

- Dissect carefully to protect dorsal intermediate cutaneous nerve (Figure FA-93)

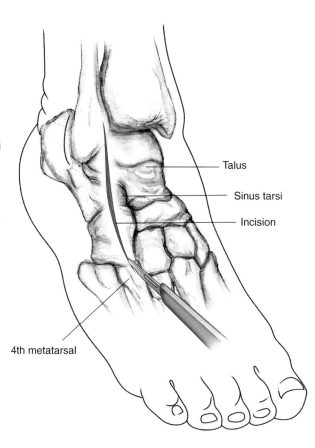

FIGURE FA-92 Skin marking. A 5 cm incision over the sinus tarsi extending toward the base of the 4th metatarsal.

DEEP DISSECTION

- Incise inferior extensor retinaculum, and retract peroneus tertius medially to expose sinus tarsi and EDB (Figure FA-94)
- Reflect EDB plantarward to expose fracture (Figure FA-95)

HAZARDS

- Dorsal intermediate cutaneous nerve of foot

CLOSURE

- EDB falls into place
- Standard subcutaneous tissue and skin closure

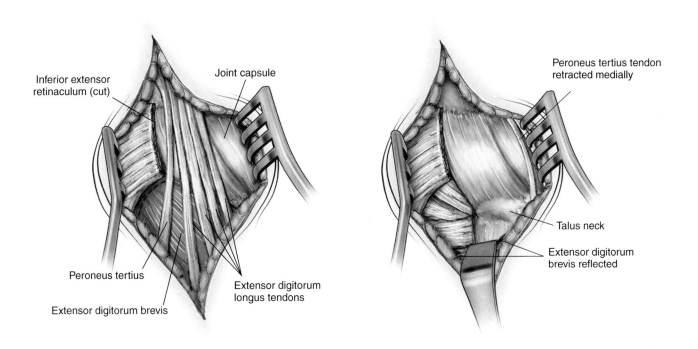

FIGURE FA-93   Protect the dorsal intermediate cutaneous nerve.

FIGURE FA-94   Incise the inferior extensor retinaculum, and retract the peroneus tertius tendon medially.

FIGURE FA-95   Reflect the EDB plantarward to expose the fracture.

DORSOMEDIAL APPROACH TO TALUS NECK

Indications: ORIF of fractures of head and neck of talus

POSITION

- Supine with sandbag or bump underneath ipsilateral hip
- Calf tourniquet
- Exsanguinate by elevation for 3-5 minutes or Esmarch's bandage

INCISION

- Take 7-10 cm long incision, starting proximally, just anterior to medial malleolus, curving distally and toward sole of foot, ending on medial side of body of navicular (Figure FA-96)

SUPERFICIAL DISSECTION (FIGURE FA-97)

- Avoid incising tibialis posterior tendon and neurovascular structures, which pass behind medial malleolus

DEEP DISSECTION (FIGURE FA-98)

- Preserve as many soft tissue attachments as possible around head and neck of talus

HAZARDS

- Tibialis posterior tendon
- Neurovascular structures that pass behind medial malleolus (posterior tibial vessels and nerve)

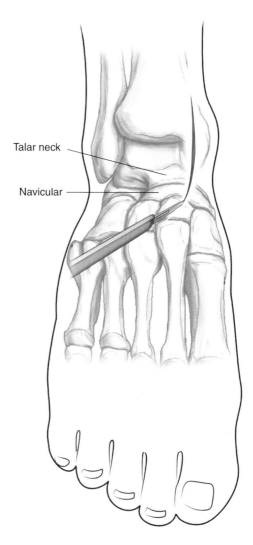

Talar neck

Navicular

FIGURE FA-96   Skin incision. A 7-10 cm long incision, starting proximally, just anterior to the medial malleolus, curving distally and toward the sole of the foot, ending on the medial side of the body of the navicular.

CLOSURE

- ## Standard closure of subcutaneous tissue and skin

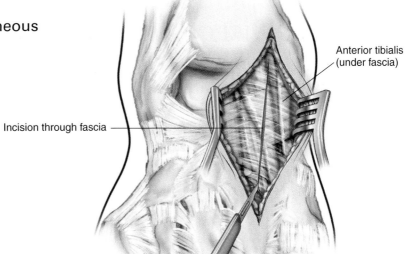

Anterior tibialis (under fascia)

Incision through fascia

FIGURE FA-97   Incise the capsule and the periosteum to expose the talar neck.

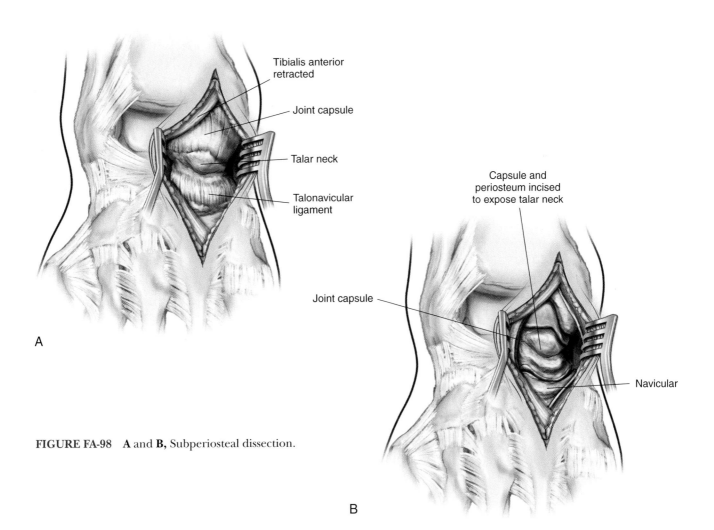

Tibialis anterior retracted

Joint capsule

Talar neck

Talonavicular ligament

A

Capsule and periosteum incised to expose talar neck

Joint capsule

Navicular

FIGURE FA-98   A and **B,** Subperiosteal dissection.

B

ANTEROLATERAL APPROACH FOR SUBTALAR DISLOCATION

Indications: Irreducible lateral subtalar dislocation

POSITION

- Supine with sandbag or bump underneath ipsilateral hip
- Calf tourniquet
- Exsanguinate by elevation for 3-5 minutes or Esmarch's bandage

INCISION

- A 7-10 cm longitudinal anterolateral incision from just proximal to ankle to cuboid (Figure FA-99)

SUPERFICIAL DISSECTION

- Protect medial and lateral dorsal cutaneous branches of superficial peroneal nerve

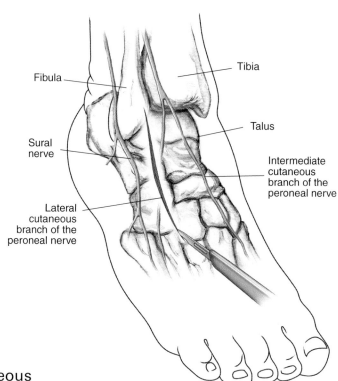

FIGURE FA-99 Skin marking. A 7-10 cm longitudinal anterolateral incision from just proximal to the ankle joint to the cuboid—watch for medial and lateral dorsal cutaneous branches of the superficial peroneal nerve.

DEEP DISSECTION

- Divide extensor retinaculum (Figure FA-100)
- Retract EDL and EHL medially and peroneus tertius tendon laterally to expose talus and midtarsal joints (Figure FA-101)
- Incise capsule over head and neck of talus, and extend incision into midtarsus (Figure FA-102)
- Leverage and traction aids in further exposure and aids in reduction of dislocated subtalar and talonavicular joints

HAZARDS

- Medial and lateral dorsal cutaneous branches of superficial peroneal nerve

CLOSURE

● Allow retracted tendons to fall into place

● Standard subcutaneous tissue and skin closure

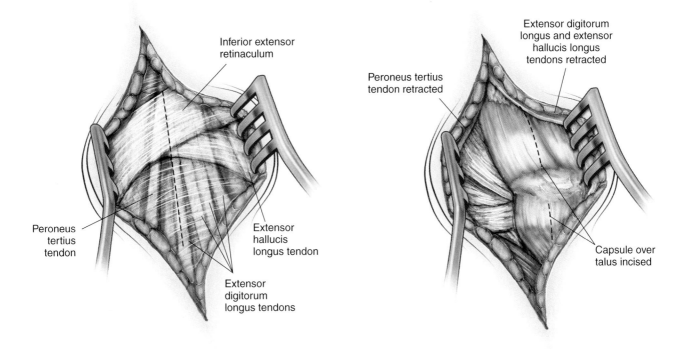

FIGURE FA-100 Divide the extensor retinaculum as shown.

FIGURE FA-101 Retract the EDL and EHL medially and the peroneus tertius tendon laterally to expose the talus and the midtarsal joints.

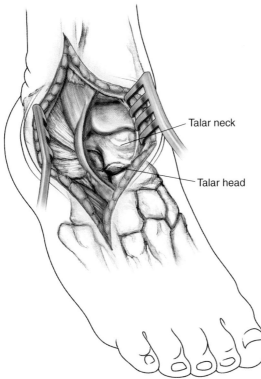
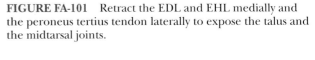

FIGURE FA-102 Incise the capsule over the head and neck of the talus, and extend the incision into the midtarsus.

EXTENSILE DORSOMEDIAL EXPOSURE TO THE MIDFOOT

Indications: ORIF of Lisfranc's fracture dislocation, tarsometatarsal arthrodesis, intermetatarsal arthrodesis

POSITION

- Supine with sandbag or bump underneath ipsilateral hip
- Calf tourniquet
- Exsanguinate by elevation for 3-5 minutes or Esmarch's bandage

INCISION

- Make 5-8 cm dorsal incision, lateral to EHL tendon over interval between base of 1st-2nd metatarsal (Figure FA-103)

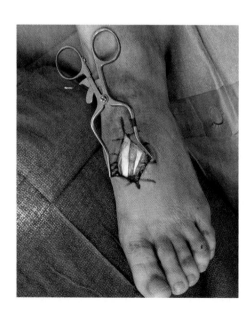

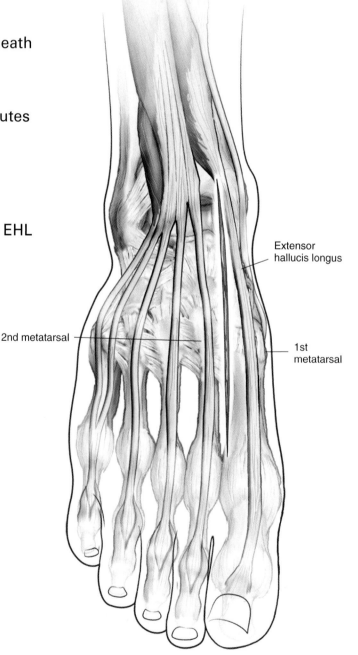

Extensor hallucis longus

2nd metatarsal

1st metatarsal

FIGURE FA-103 Skin marking. A 5-8 cm dorsal incision, lateral to the EHL tendon over the interval between the base of the 1st and 2nd metatarsals.

SUPERFICIAL DISSECTION (FIGURES FA-104 AND FA-105)

- Preserve dorsal medial cutaneous branch of peroneal nerve
- Incise inferior extensor retinaculum

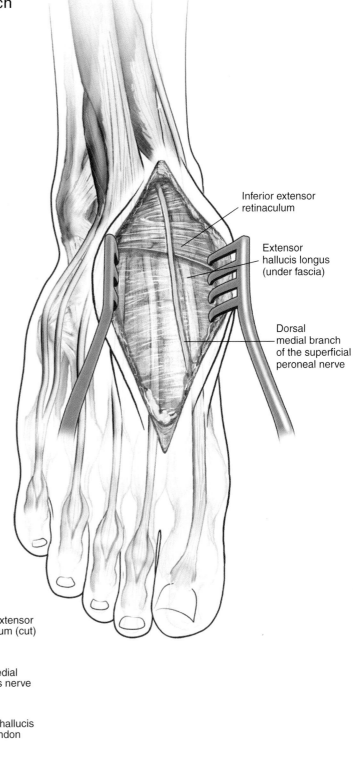

FIGURE FA-104   Preserve the dorsal medial branch of the superficial peroneal nerve. Incise the inferior extensor retinaculum.

Inferior extensor retinaculum

Extensor hallucis longus (under fascia)

Dorsal medial branch of the superficial peroneal nerve

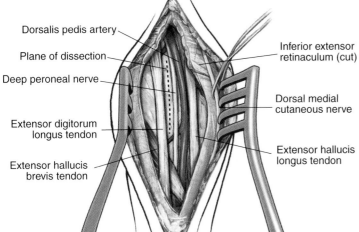

Dorsalis pedis artery

Plane of dissection

Deep peroneal nerve

Extensor digitorum longus tendon

Extensor hallucis brevis tendon

Inferior extensor retinaculum (cut)

Dorsal medial cutaneous nerve

Extensor hallucis longus tendon

FIGURE FA-105   Incision of inferior extensor retinaculum exposes its contents.

DEEP DISSECTION

- Isolate dorsalis pedis and deep peroneal nerve with loop for medial or lateral retraction as needed (Figure FA-106)

HAZARDS

- Dorsal medial cutaneous branches
- Dorsalis pedis artery
- Deep peroneal nerve

CLOSURE

- Retracted neurovascular structures and extensor hallucis tendon fall into place
- Standard subcutaneous tissue and skin closure

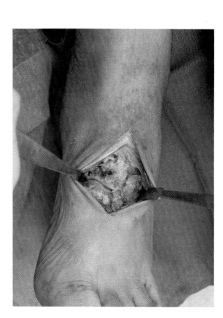

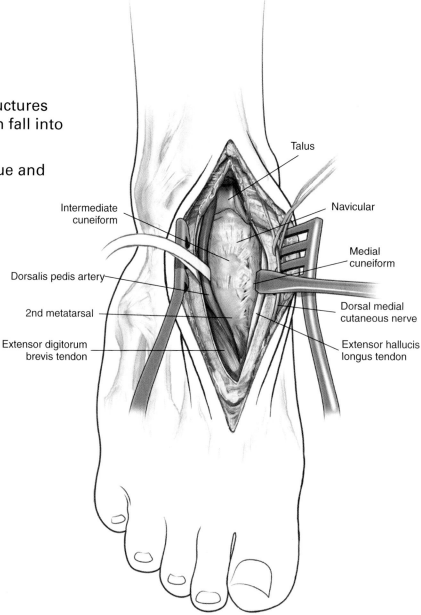

FIGURE FA-106   Isolate the dorsalis pedis and the deep peroneal nerve with a loop for medial or lateral retraction as needed.

DORSAL APPROACH TO THE IST AND 2ND METATARSAL

Indications: Corrective proximal metatarsal osteotomies for hallux valgus

POSITION

- Supine with sandbag or bump underneath ipsilateral hip

- Calf tourniquet

- Exsanguinate by elevation for 3-5 minutes or Esmarch's bandage

INCISION

- Make 5-6 cm longitudinal incision, lateral to long extensor tendon to big toe (Figure FA-107)

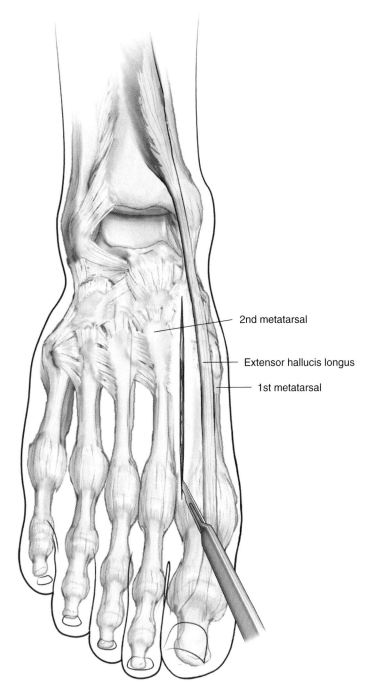

2nd metatarsal

Extensor hallucis longus

1st metatarsal

FIGURE FA-107   A 5-6 cm longitudinal incision, lateral to the long extensor tendon to the big toe.

SUPERFICIAL DISSECTION

- Protect dorsal cutaneous branches of superficial peroneal nerve (Figure FA-108)

- Identify plane between long and short extensor (Figure FA-109)

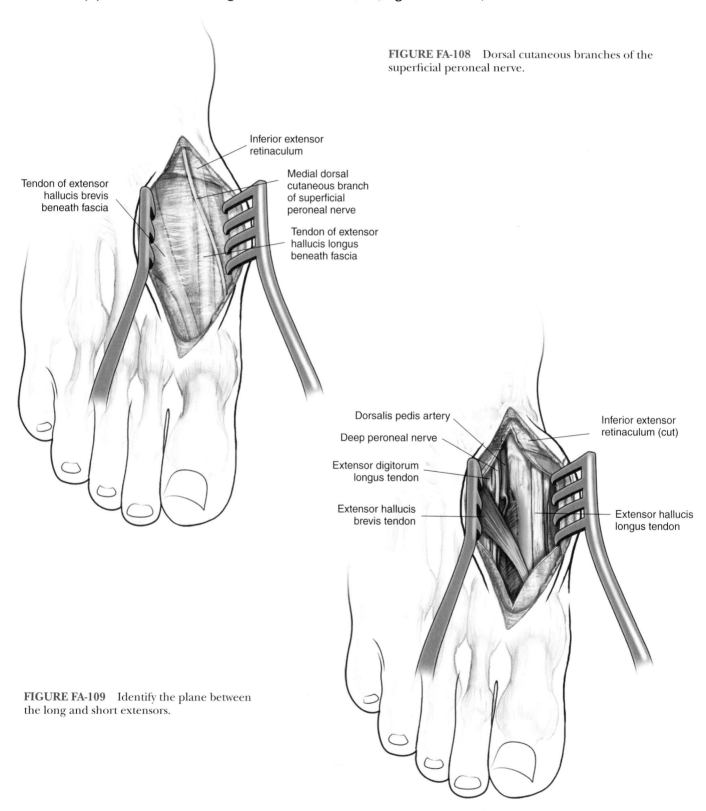

FIGURE FA-108 Dorsal cutaneous branches of the superficial peroneal nerve.

Inferior extensor retinaculum

Tendon of extensor hallucis brevis beneath fascia

Medial dorsal cutaneous branch of superficial peroneal nerve

Tendon of extensor hallucis longus beneath fascia

Dorsalis pedis artery

Deep peroneal nerve

Extensor digitorum longus tendon

Extensor hallucis brevis tendon

Inferior extensor retinaculum (cut)

Extensor hallucis longus tendon

FIGURE FA-109 Identify the plane between the long and short extensors.

DEEP DISSECTION

- Incise periosteum over 1st metatarsal shaft
- Subperiosteally elevate periosteum to expose base and proximal part of 1st metatarsal (Figure FA-110)

HAZARDS

- Cutaneous branch of superficial sural nerve

CLOSURE

- Standard subcutaneous tissue and skin closure

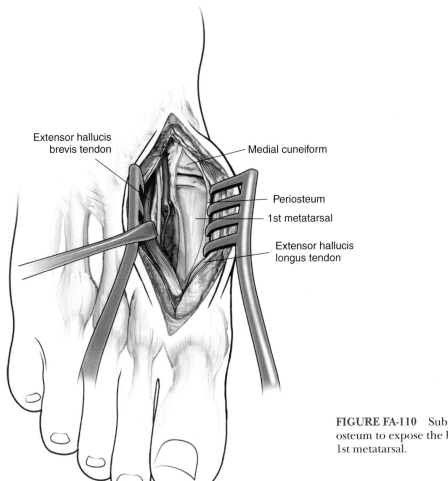

Extensor hallucis brevis tendon

Medial cuneiform

Periosteum

1st metatarsal

Extensor hallucis longus tendon

FIGURE FA-110 Subperiosteally elevate the periosteum to expose the base and proximal part of the 1st metatarsal.

APPROACH FOR PHALANGEAL DISLOCATION

Indications: Irreducible dislocations of interphalangeal joints

POSITION

- Supine with sandbag or bump underneath ipsilateral hip
- Calf tourniquet
- Exsanguinate by elevation for 3-5 minutes or Esmarch's bandage

INCISION

- Dorsal inverted L–shaped incision with transverse limb at joint and longitudinal limb dorsolateral (Figure FA-111)

SUPERFICIAL DISSECTION

- Preserve EHL insertion to distal phalanx (Figure FA-112)

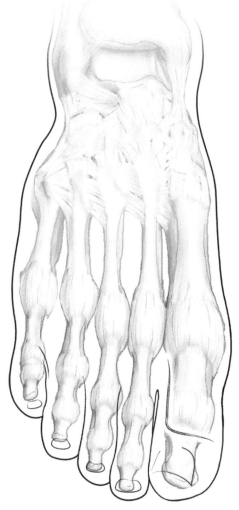

FIGURE FA-111 Dorsal inverted L–shaped incision with the transverse limb at the joint and the longitudinal limb dorsolateral.

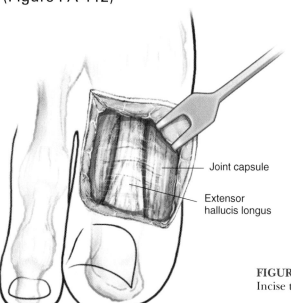

Joint capsule

Extensor hallucis longus

FIGURE FA-112 Preserve the EHL insertion to the distal phalanx. Incise the dorsal capsule.

DEEP DISSECTION

- Identify plantar plate on any one side of EHL (Figure FA-113)

- Divide plantar plate by making 3-4 mm incision into it

- Traction and manipulation with Freer elevator aids in further exposure and reduction (Figure FA-114)

HAZARDS

- EHL tendon

- Digital nerves and vessels

CLOSURE

- Standard skin closure

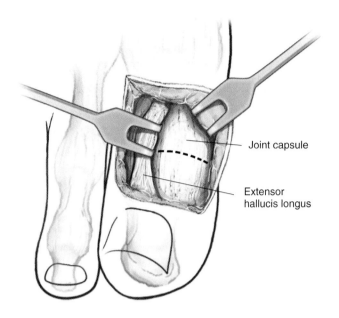

FIGURE FA-113   Identify the plantar plate on any one side of the EHL. Divide the plantar plate by making a 3-4 mm incision into it.

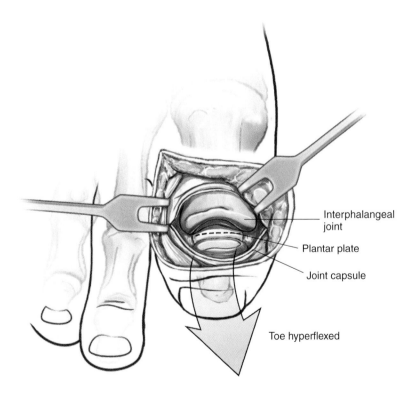

FIGURE FA-114   Traction and manipulation with a Freer elevator aids in further exposure and reduction.

Dorsal and Dorsomedial Approach to the 1st MTP Joint

Indications: Corrective surgeries for hallux valgus (distal metatarsal osteotomies, soft tissue corrections, tenotomies, proximal phalanx corrective osteotomies), excision of bunions, excision of metatarsal head, arthrodesis of MTP joint, replacement of MTP (arthroplasty)

POSITION

- Supine with sandbag or bump underneath ipsilateral hip
- Calf tourniquet
- Exsanguinate by elevation for 3-5 minutes or Esmarch's bandage

Dorsal

INCISION

- Place incision medial and parallel to tendon of EHL, starting 2-3 cm proximal to MTP joint, and extend it distally just proximal to interphalangeal joint (Figure FA-115)

SUPERFICIAL DISSECTION (FIGURE FA-116)

- Incise deep fascia in line with skin incision
- Retract tendon of EHL laterally

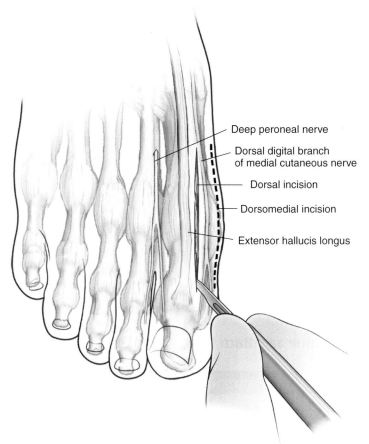

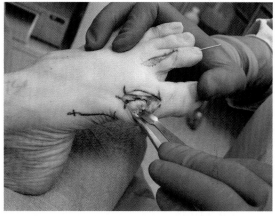

FIGURE FA-115 Place the incision medial and parallel to the tendon of EHL, starting 2-3 cm proximal to the MTP joint, and extend it distally just proximal to the interphalangeal joint.

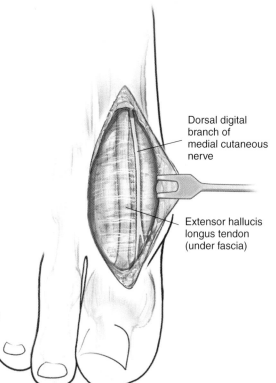

FIGURE FA-116 Incise the deep fascia in line with the skin incision, and dissect out the dorsal digital branch of the medial cutaneous nerve. Retract the tendon of EHL laterally.

DEEP DISSECTION

- Incise capsule—either straight or U-shaped incision (Figure FA-117)

- Make longitudinal incision in periosteum of proximal phalanx and 1st metatarsal longitudinally (Figure FA-118)

- Extent of subperiosteal stripping is dictated by type of procedure to be done

Dorsomedial

INCISION

- Incision starts at medial aspect of shaft of metatarsal about 2-3 cm proximal to MTP joint, curves over dorsal aspect of MTP joint, medial to the tendon of EHL, continuing dorsomedially over great toe ending just proximally to interphalangeal joint

SUPERFICIAL DISSECTION

- Incise deep fascia in line with skin incision

- Dissect out dorsal digital branch of medial cutaneous nerve, and retract it with lateral skin flap

DEEP DISSECTION

- Make either straight or U-shaped incision in capsule

- Make longitudinal incision in periosteum of proximal phalanx and 1st metatarsal longitudinally

- Extent of subperiosteal stripping is dictated by type of procedure to be done

HAZARDS

- Tendon of EHL

- Tendon of FHL can be displaced from its groove during subperiosteal stripping on undersurface of proximal phalanx

- Dorsal digital branch of medial cutaneous nerve (saphenous nerve)

CLOSURE

- Repair capsule/reefing dictated by surgical indication
- Standard closure of subcutaneous tissue and skin

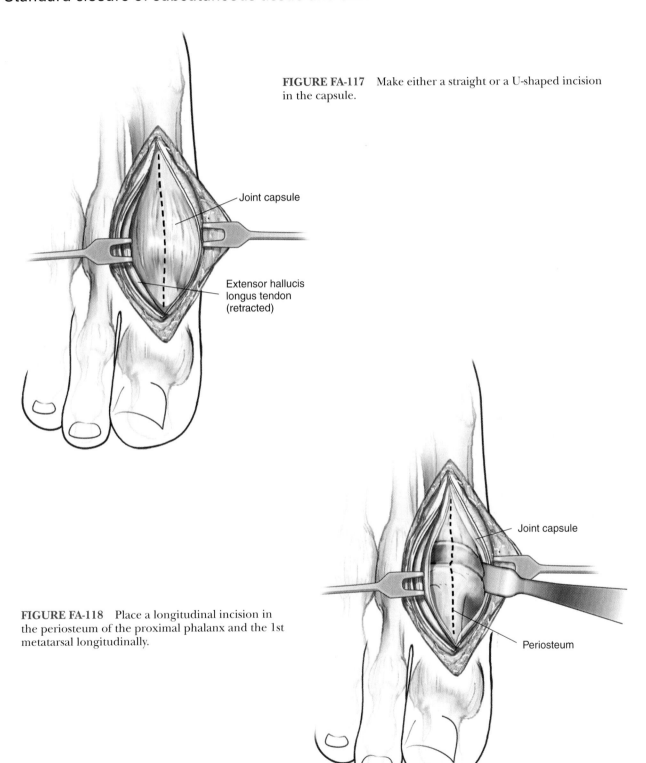

FIGURE FA-117 Make either a straight or a U-shaped incision in the capsule.

Joint capsule

Extensor hallucis longus tendon (retracted)

FIGURE FA-118 Place a longitudinal incision in the periosteum of the proximal phalanx and the 1st metatarsal longitudinally.

Joint capsule

Periosteum

MEDIAL APPROACH TO 1ST MTP JOINT

Indications: Excision of bunion, distal metatarsal osteotomy, proximal phalangeal osteotomy

POSITION

- Supine with sandbag or bump underneath ipsilateral hip
- Calf tourniquet
- Exsanguinate by elevation for 3-5 minutes or Esmarch's bandage

INCISION

- Make longitudinal medial incision along proximal two thirds of proximal phalanx, and extend it over medial eminence to distal third of metatarsal shaft (Figure FA-119)

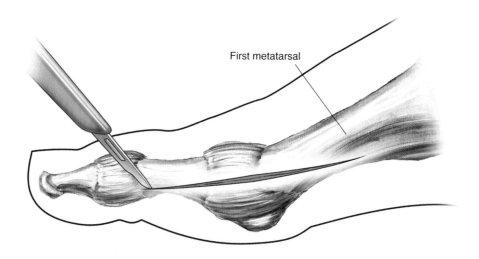

First metatarsal

FIGURE FA-119   Marking of skin incision—longitudinal medial incision—along the proximal two thirds of the proximal phalanx, and extend it over the medial eminence to the distal third of the metatarsal shaft.

SUPERFICIAL DISSECTION (FIGURE FA-120)

- Raise dorsal and ventral flaps
- Watch for dorsal cutaneous branch of saphenous nerve as dorsal flap is raised

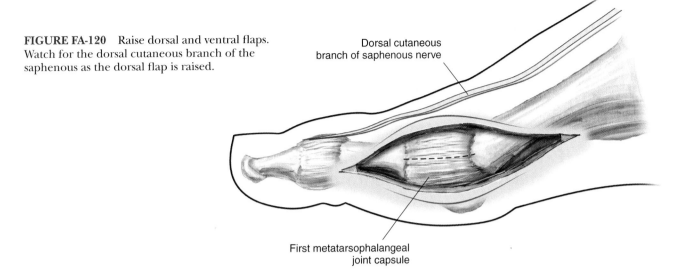

FIGURE FA-120   Raise dorsal and ventral flaps. Watch for the dorsal cutaneous branch of the saphenous as the dorsal flap is raised.

Dorsal cutaneous branch of saphenous nerve

First metatarsophalangeal joint capsule

DEEP DISSECTION

- Using sharp dissection, incise capsule along length of incision, and reflect capsule surrounding exostosis to expose medial eminence (Figure FA-121)

- Preserve as much of proximal capsular attachment to metatarsal neck as possible

HAZARDS

- Dorsal cutaneous branch of saphenous nerve

CLOSURE

- Repair/reefing capsule is dictated by surgical indication

- Standard closure of subcutaneous tissue and skin

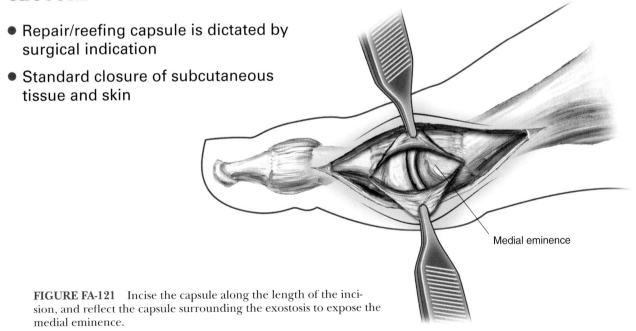

Medial eminence

FIGURE FA-121   Incise the capsule along the length of the incision, and reflect the capsule surrounding the exostosis to expose the medial eminence.

Dorsal Approach to the MTP Joints of the 2nd-5th Toes with Proximal Interphalangeal Joint Exposure

Indications: Excision of metatarsal heads, capsulotomies, tenotomies, distal metatarsal osteotomy, claw and hammer toe corrective surgeries

POSITION

- Supine with sandbag or bump underneath ipsilateral hip
- Calf tourniquet
- Exsanguinate by elevation for 3-5 minutes or Esmarch's bandage

INCISION (FIGURE FA-122)

- Make 3-4 cm incision over dorsolateral aspect of involved MTP joint (incision is longitudinal, but lateral and parallel to extensor tendon)
- Alternatively, exposure to 2 adjacent joints can be made through a single incision placed between 2 MTP joints

SUPERFICIAL DISSECTION

- Deep fascia is incised medial to long extensor tendon in line with length of incision (Figure FA-123)

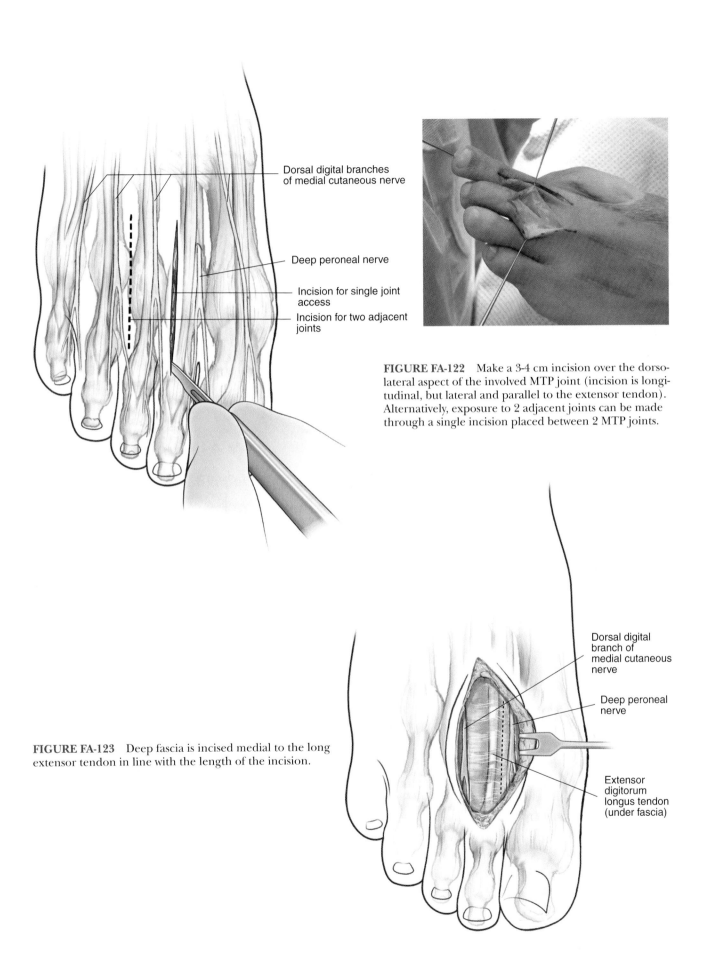

Dorsal digital branches
of medial cutaneous nerve

Deep peroneal nerve

Incision for single joint
access

Incision for two adjacent
joints

FIGURE FA-122 Make a 3-4 cm incision over the dorso-lateral aspect of the involved MTP joint (incision is longi-tudinal, but lateral and parallel to the extensor tendon). Alternatively, exposure to 2 adjacent joints can be made through a single incision placed between 2 MTP joints.

FIGURE FA-123 Deep fascia is incised medial to the long extensor tendon in line with the length of the incision.

Dorsal digital
branch of
medial cutaneous
nerve

Deep peroneal
nerve

Extensor
digitorum
longus tendon
(under fascia)

DEEP DISSECTION

- Retract tendon laterally to expose capsule over MTP joint (Figure FA-124)
- Make longitudinal incision over capsule (Figure FA-125)
- Retract capsule to expose joint

HAZARDS

- Long extensor tendon
- Plantar nerves and vessels deep to transverse metatarsal ligaments

CLOSURE

- Standard subcutaneous tissue and skin closure

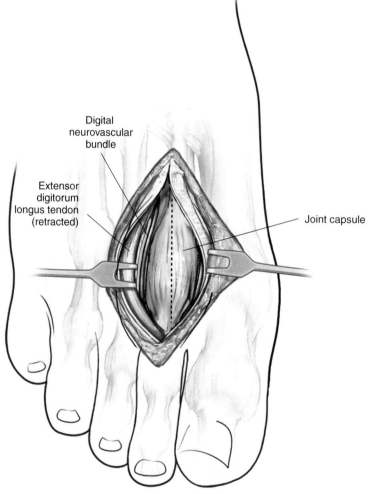

FIGURE FA-124   Retract the tendon laterally to expose the capsule over the MTP joint.

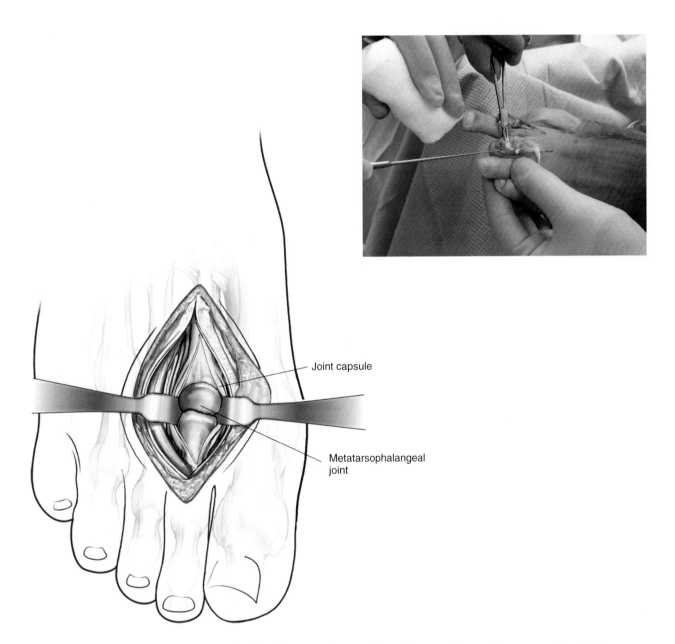

Joint capsule

Metatarsophalangeal joint

FIGURE FA-125   Make a longitudinal incision over the capsule, and retract the capsule to expose the joint.

LATERAL APPROACH TO THE 5TH MTP JOINT

Indications: Excision of metatarsal head, bunionette excision

POSITION

- Supine with sandbag or bump underneath ipsilateral hip
- Calf tourniquet
- Exsanguinate by elevation for 3-5 minutes or Esmarch's bandage

INCISION

- Make straight lateral incision from distal third of 5th metatarsal shaft to midshaft of proximal phalanx (Figure FA-126)

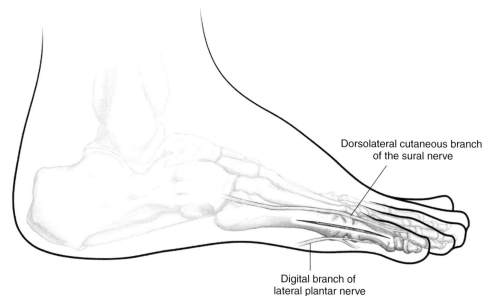

Dorsolateral cutaneous branch of the sural nerve

Digital branch of lateral plantar nerve

FIGURE FA-126   Skin incision. Straight lateral incision from the distal third of the 5th metatarsal shaft to the midshaft of the proximal phalanx.

SUPERFICIAL DISSECTION

- Straight incision passes between dorsolateral cutaneous branch of sural nerve and digital branch of lateral plantar nerve to the 5th toe (Figure FA-127)
- Tendon of insertion of abductor digiti minimi passes plantar to midline

DEEP DISSECTION

● Incise capsule and periosteum in straight line 2-3 mm dorsal to midline (Figure FA-128)

● With sharp dissection, elevate capsule dorsally and plantarward to expose metatarsal head (Figure FA-129)

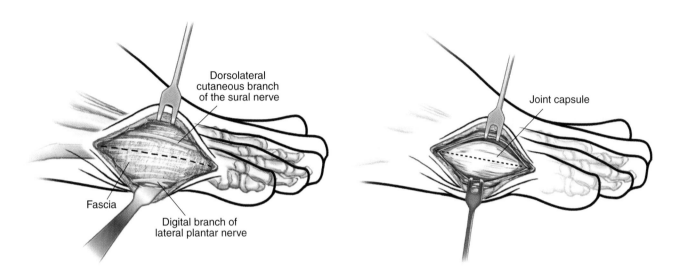

FIGURE FA-127 Dorsolateral cutaneous branch of the sural nerve and digital branch of the lateral plantar nerve to the 5th toe.

FIGURE FA-128 Capsule and the periosteum exposed.

HAZARDS

● Dorsolateral cutaneous branch of sural nerve

● Digital branch of lateral plantar nerve to 5th nerve

● Tendon of insertion of abductor digiti minimi

CLOSURE

● Imbricate capsule repair

● Standard subcutaneous tissue and skin closure

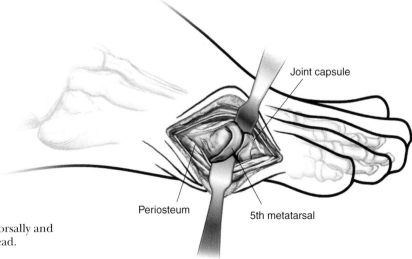

FIGURE FA-129 Elevate the capsule dorsally and plantarward to expose the metatarsal head.

APPROACH TO THE DORSAL WEB SPACE

Indications: Excision of interdigital neuroma, drainage of web space infections, exploration of cleft toes

POSITION

- Supine with sandbag or bump underneath ipsilateral hip
- Calf tourniquet
- Exsanguinate by elevation for 3-5 minutes or Esmarch's bandage

INCISION

- Spread 2 toes of affected web space, and make 3-4 cm longitudinal incision centered over web space (Figure FA-130)

SUPERFICIAL DISSECTION

- Carefully dissect off dorsal cutaneous nerves and vessels by blunt dissection (Figure FA-131)

DEEP DISSECTION

- Identify deep transverse metatarsal ligament, and incise it with a pair of scissors (Figure FA-132)

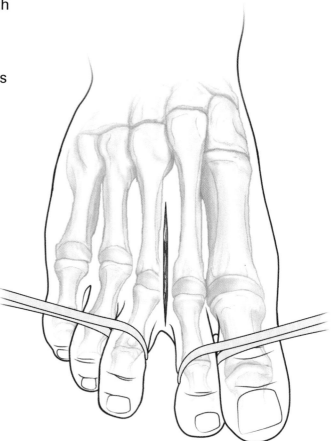

FIGURE FA-130   Skin marking. Spread the 2 toes of the affected web space, and make a 3-4 cm longitudinal incision centered over the web space.

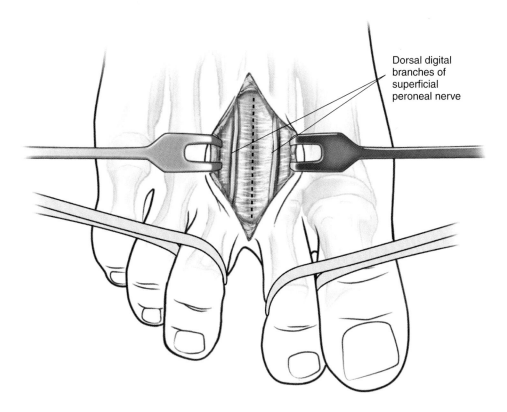

FIGURE FA-131 Carefully dissect off the dorsal cutaneous nerves and vessels by blunt dissection.

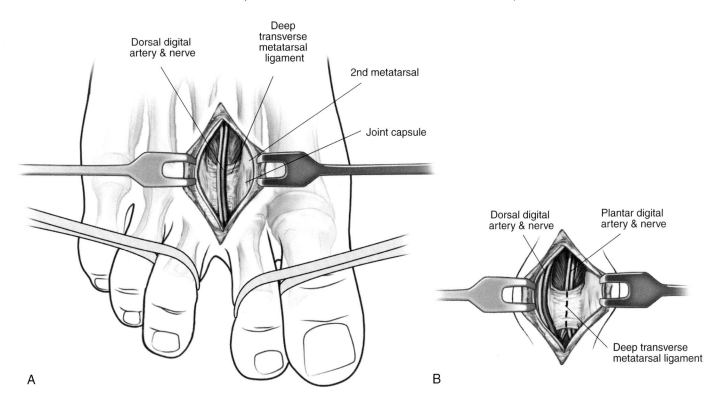

A

B

FIGURE FA-132 **A,** Identify the deep transverse metatarsal ligament. **B,** Incise deep transverse metatarsal ligament with a pair of scissors.

- Neurovascular bundle with the neuroma, which, if present, bulges out (Figure FA-133)

HAZARDS

- Dorsal digital nerves and vessels
- Plantar digital nerves and vessels

CLOSURE

- Standard subcutaneous tissue and skin closure

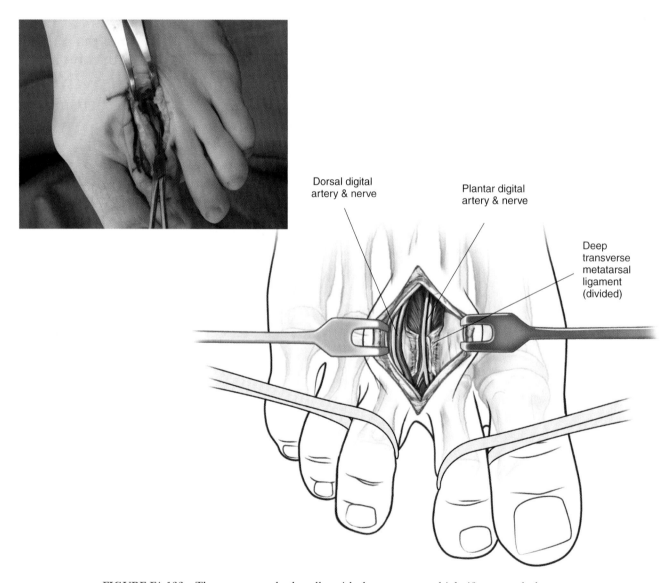

Dorsal digital artery & nerve

Plantar digital artery & nerve

Deep transverse metatarsal ligament (divided)

FIGURE FA-133 The neurovascular bundles with the neuroma, which, if present, bulges out.

Dorsal Approach to the Metatarsal Heads

Indications: excision of metatarsal heads, Clayton's forefoot arthroplasty, ORIF of multiple metatarsal fractures

POSITION

- Supine with sandbag or bump underneath ipsilateral hip
- Calf tourniquet
- Exsanguinate by elevation for 3-5 minutes or Esmarch's bandage

INCISION

- Make transverse curved incision over metatarsal heads from 1st-5th metatarsal heads (Figure FA-134)

  - Note that the incision is convex-shaped.

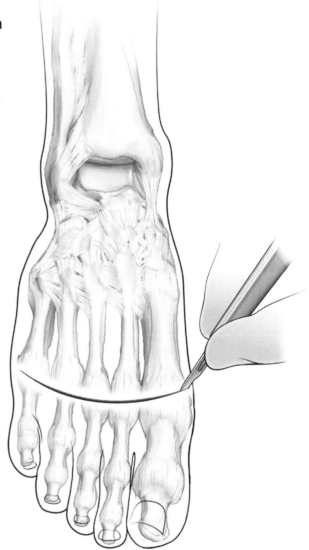

FIGURE FA-134 Skin incision. Transverse curved incision over the metatarsal heads from the 1st through the 5th metatarsal heads.

SUPERFICIAL DISSECTION

● Incise deep fascia medial to extensor tendon (Figure FA-135)

● Protect dorsal cutaneous branches as far as possible

● Protect dorsal veins as far as possible

DEEP DISSECTION

● Retract extensor tendon laterally and carefully with blunt dissection to protect digital neurovascular bundles in intermetatarsal spaces (Figure FA-136)

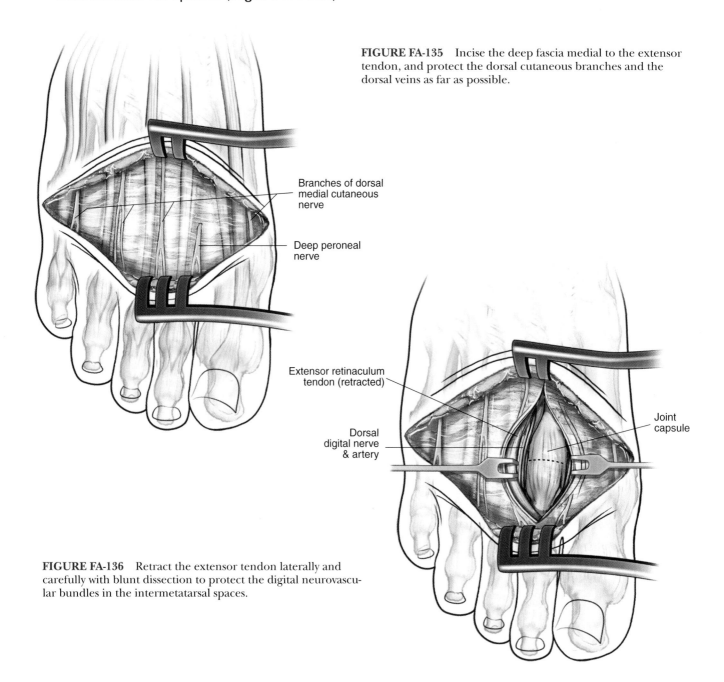

FIGURE FA-135 Incise the deep fascia medial to the extensor tendon, and protect the dorsal cutaneous branches and the dorsal veins as far as possible.

Branches of dorsal medial cutaneous nerve

Deep peroneal nerve

Extensor retinaculum tendon (retracted)

Dorsal digital nerve & artery

Joint capsule

FIGURE FA-136 Retract the extensor tendon laterally and carefully with blunt dissection to protect the digital neurovascular bundles in the intermetatarsal spaces.

- Incise capsule along length of incision (Figure FA-137)
- Strip soft tissue circumferentially around distal portion of metatarsal head and neck using Freer or periosteal elevator

HAZARDS

- Dorsal cutaneous branches of saphenous and sural nerves
- Digital neurovascular bundles in intermetatarsal space

CLOSURE

- Standard subcutaneous tissue and skin closure

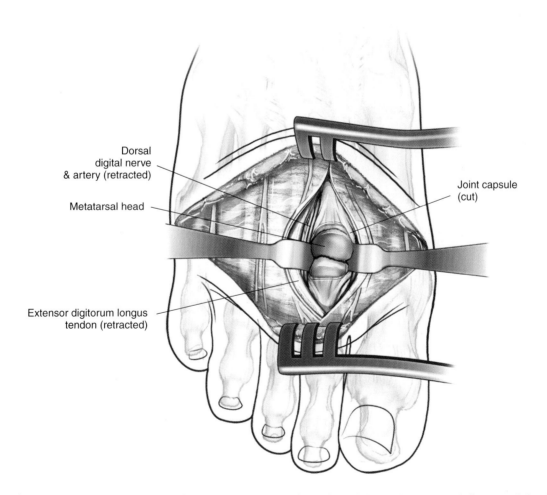

Dorsal
digital nerve
& artery (retracted)

Metatarsal head

Joint capsule
(cut)

Extensor digitorum longus
tendon (retracted)

FIGURE FA-137   Incise the capsule along the length of the incision. Strip the soft tissue circumferentially around the distal portion of the metatarsal head and neck using Freer or periosteal elevator.

APPROACH FOR SESAMOID FRACTURE

Indications: Painful sesamoids, fracture

POSITION

- Supine with sandbag or bump underneath ipsilateral hip
- Calf tourniquet
- Exsanguinate by elevation for 3-5 minutes or Esmarch's bandage

INCISION

- A 5 cm longitudinal skin incision on medial plantar part of 1st ray, centered over MTP joint (Figure FA-138)

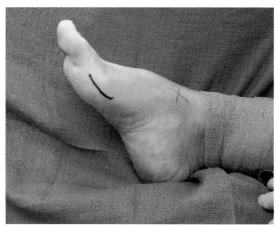

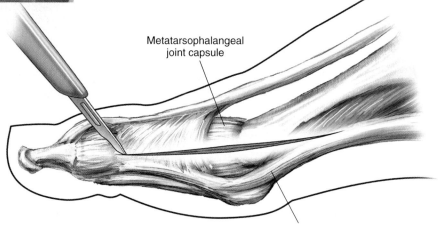

Metatarsophalangeal joint capsule

Abductor hallucis tendon

FIGURE FA-138 Surface marking. Longitudinal skin incision on the medial plantar part of the 1st ray, centered over the MTP joint.

SUPERFICIAL DISSECTION

● Identify capsule and abductor hallucis tendon, and divide
   along length of incision (Figure FA-139)

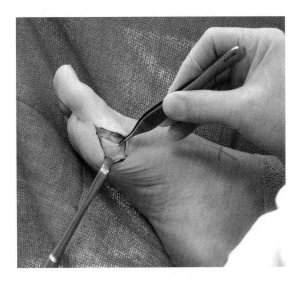

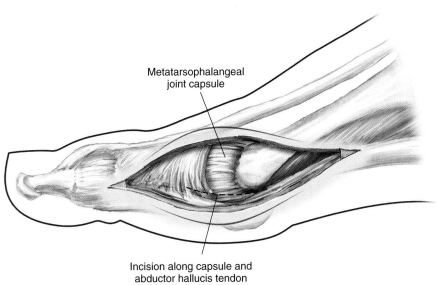

Metatarsophalangeal
joint capsule

Incision along capsule and
abductor hallucis tendon

FIGURE FA-139   Identify the capsule and the abductor hallucis tendon, and divide along the length of the incision.

DEEP DISSECTION

● Joint is entered dorsal to tibial sesamoid (Figure FA-140)

● Retraction exposes articular surface of each sesamoid further

HAZARDS

● Medial digital nerve and plantar digital nerve in deep exposure

CLOSURE

● Standard closure of subcutaneous tissue and skin

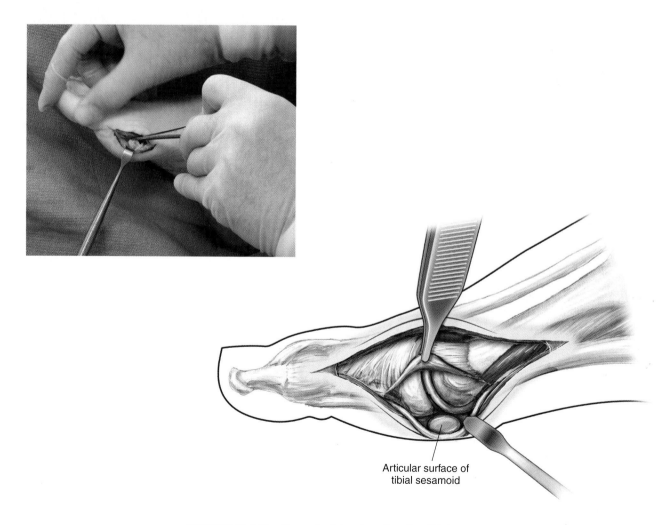

Articular surface of
tibial sesamoid

FIGURE FA-140   Enter the joint dorsal to the tibial sesamoid.

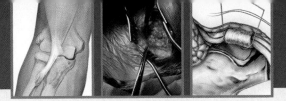

Index

A

Abductor digiti minimi muscle, in myology of hand and wrist, 153*t*, 156*f*

Abductor digiti minimi tendon, in cross-section of hand and wrist, 162*f*

Abductor pollicis brevis muscle
  in cross-section of hand and wrist, 162*f*
  in myology of hand and wrist, 153*t*, 156*f*
  scaphoid bone and, 146

Abductor pollicis longus muscle
  in cross-sectional anatomy of elbow, 82*f*
  in myology of elbow, 69*f*, 70*t*
  in myology of hand and wrist, 157*f*
  in Thompson approach to forearm, 131, 132*f*, 134, 134*f*–135*f*

Abductor pollicis longus tendon, in cross-section of hand and wrist, 162*f*

AC joint. *See* Acromioclavicular joint

Acromial artery, as hazard, 22*f*

Acromial extremity, of clavicle, 9*f*

Acromioclavicular joint
  approach to, 41–43
  in shoulder arthrology, 12, 13*f*

Acromion
  angle of, 8*f*
  as landmark, 19*f*
  fractures of, 34
  in acromioclavicular joint approach, 41*f*–43*f*
  in lateral approach to shoulder, 38*f*
  in shoulder arthrology, 13*f*
  in shoulder osteology, 8, 8*f*
  in superior approach to supraspinatus fossa, 44*f*
  in superolateral approach to shoulder, 34, 35*f*, 37, 37*f*

Adductor pollicis muscle
  in compartment release in hand approach, 208
  in cross-section of hand and wrist, 162*f*
  in myology of hand and wrist, 153*t*, 156*f*

Adhesive capsulitis, 54

Alar ligament
  in spinal arthrology, 217*f*

Amphiarthrodial joints, 4

Anconeus muscle
  in Bryan-Morrey approach to elbow, 104*f*, 105, 105*f*–106*f*
  in Kocher approach to elbow, 98, 98*f*, 99, 99*f*–101*f*
  in myology of elbow, 69*f*, 70*t*
  in ulnar shaft approach, 137*f*

Annular ligament
  in elbow arthrology, 67*f*
  in elbow arthroscopy, 119*f*
  in Kocher approach to elbow, 99, 99*f*, 100, 100*f*

Antebrachial cutaneous nerve
  as hazard, 84
  in anterior approach to elbow, 87, 87*f*–88*f*, 90
  in arm and shoulder neurology, 16*f*–17*f*
  in cross-sectional anatomy, 19*f*
  in dorsal forearm compartment release, 143*f*
  in elbow arthroscopy, 116, 117*f*, 120
  in elbow neurology, 72

Antebrachial cutaneous nerve *(Continued)*
  in Henry approach to arm, 129
  in Henry approach to forearm, 125
  in medial approach to elbow and humerus, 93, 93*f*, 96
  in volar forearm compartment release, 140, 140*f*, 141

Anterior approach
  to elbow, 85–90
  to humerus, 49–50
  to shoulder, 23–29

Anterior interosseous artery, in elbow and arm vasculature, 81*f*

Anterior interosseous nerve, in elbow neurology, 73, 74*f*

Anterior longitudinal ligament, in anterior approach to cervical spine, 240, 241*f*

Anterior longitudinal ligament, in spinal arthrology, 216*f*–218*f*

Anterior occipito-atlantal ligament
  in spinal arthrology, 216*f*

Anterior scalene muscle
  in spinal myology, 219*f*

Anterior transthoracic approach, to thoracic spine, 242–252

Anterior tubercle
  in spinal osteology, 213*f*
  of atlas
    in spinal arthrology, 216*f*

Anterolateral approach, to elbow, 77*f*

Apical ligament
  in spinal arthrology, 216*f*

APL. *See* Abductor pollicis longus muscle

Appendicular skeleton, 3*f*

Approaches
  anterior, to cervical spine, 232–241
  for compartment release of hand, 208–209
  for external wrist fixator, 185–187
  for median nerve exposure, 176–180
  for olecranon osteotomy, 112–114
  to acromioclavicular joint, 41–43
  to cervical spine, anterior, 232–241
  to clavicle, 46–48
  to elbow
    anterior, 85–90
    anterolateral, 77*f*
    Bryan-Morrey, 102–107
    distal volar, 78*f*
    Henry, 78*f*
    Kocher, 77*f*, 97–101
    medial, 76*f*, 91–96
    middle volar, 78*f*
    proximal volar, 78*f*
    Thompson, 79*f*
    triceps sparing, 102–107
    triceps splitting, 108–111
  to fingers
    dorsal, 197–199
    for infections, 205–207
    midlateral, 203–204
    volar, 200–201
  to forearm
    Henry, 124–129, 169
    Thompson, 130–135

Approaches *(Continued)*
  to forearm compartment release, volar, 139–141
  to humerus
    anterior, 49–50
    medial, 91–96
    posterior, 51–53
  to metacarpals, dorsal, 194–196
  to shoulder
    anterior, 23–29
    lateral, 38–40
    posterior, 30–33
    superior, 44–45
    superolateral, 34–37, 35*f*–37*f*
  to supraspinatus fossa, superior, 44–45
  to ulnar artery, 181–184
  to ulnar nerve, 181–184
  to ulnar shaft, 136–139
  to wrist
    dorsal, 164–168
    Henry, 169–175
    volar, 169–175
  ulnar shaft, 79*f*

Arcade of Struthers, in medial approach to elbow and humerus, 93*f*

Arcuate artery, as hazard, 22, 22*f*

Arm, positioning of, in anterior approach to cervical spine, 233

Arteries. *See* Vasculature; *individual arteries*

Arthrodesis
  metacarpophalangeal joints, 197
  proximal interphalangeal joint, 197
  wrist, 164

Arthrology
  of elbow, 65–66, 67*f*
  of hand and wrist, 149, 150*f*, 151, 152*f*
  of shoulder, 12, 13*f*
  of spine, 216–218, 216*f*–218*f*
  overview of, 4

Arthroplasty
  metacarpophalangeal joint, 197
  proximal interphalangeal joint, 197, 200
  radial head, 97
  shoulder, 23, 38
  total elbow, 102, 108
  ulnohumeral, 108
  volar plate, 200

Arthroscopy
  elbow, 115–123
  shoulder, 54–59
  wrist, 188–193

Articular facet
  in spinal osteology, 213*f*, 215*f*

Articular process
  inferior
    in spinal arthrology, 218*f*
  superior
    in spinal arthrology, 218*f*

Articular tubercle
  in spinal osteology, 213*f*

Atlantoaxial articulation
  in spinal arthrology, 217, 217*f*

Atlas. *See* C1 vertebra

Axial skeleton, 3*f*

Note: Information presented in tables and figures is represented by *t* and *f*, respectively.